Demystifying Research for Medical & Healthcare Students

To my wife, Clair.

Thank you for all your love and support – and for making it fun!

Demystifying Research for Medical & Healthcare Students

An Essential Guide

JOHN L. ANDERSON
Brighton & Sussex Medical School, Brighton, UK

WILEY Blackwell

Registered Offices
John Wiley & Sons, Inc., 111 River Street, Hoboken, NJ 07030, USA
John Wiley & Sons Ltd, The Atrium, Southern Gate, Chichester, West Sussex, PO19 8SQ, UK

Editorial Office
9600 Garsington Road, Oxford, OX4 2DQ, UK

For details of our global editorial offices, customer services, and more information about Wiley products visit us at **www.wiley.com**.

Wiley also publishes its books in a variety of electronic formats and by print-on-demand. Some content that appears in standard print versions of this book may not be available in other formats.

Library of Congress Cataloging-in-Publication Data

Names: Anderson, John L. (Medical sociologist) author.
Title: Demystifying research for medical & healthcare students :
    an essential guide / John L. Anderson.
Other titles: Demystifying research for medical and healthcare students
Description: Hoboken, NJ : Wiley-Blackwell, 2022. | Includes
    bibliographical references and index.
Identifiers: LCCN 2021028312 (print) | LCCN 2021028313 (ebook) |
    ISBN 9781119701378 (hardback) | ISBN 9781119701361 (Adobe PDF) |
    ISBN 9781119701385 (epub)
Subjects: MESH: Biomedical Research–methods | Research Design | Students, Medical
Classification: LCC R853.C55 (print) | LCC R853.C55 (ebook) | NLM W 20.5
    | DDC 610.72/4–dc23
LC record available at https://lccn.loc.gov/2021028312
LC ebook record available at https://lccn.loc.gov/2021028313

Cover Design: Wiley
Cover Image: © DeMango/iStock/Getty Images

Set in 10/12pt STIX Two Text by Straive, Pondicherry, India
Printed and bound by CPI Group (UK) Ltd, Croydon, CR0 4YY

C9781119701378_170522

Contents

Preface

When I signed the contract for this book in December 2019, I was overjoyed and eager to get started in the New Year. However, 2020 was been a funny sort of year! On the second of January I had a stroke – I couldn't move my right arm or leg! Fortunately, thanks to my wife Clair's quick thinking, I was bundled into the car and driven to Musgrove Park Hospital in Taunton. Within an hour of my first symptoms, I had been assessed in A&E by the stroke team, had had my CT and MMR scans and been given my first dose of Aspirin. I was kept in, but to my shame, I am afraid that I kept trying to do things on my own, only to be told off by the ward staff and by Clair and my lovely granddaughter Anna. So, I was off work for three months, and to tell the truth, I was glad of the break from work. I had been overdoing it and my stroke was probably the result. And then came 'Lockdown'! I must say that I enjoyed this period of time, because, as a family, we were suddenly released from the very many sets of demands on our time. Working from home was fine for me – all of what I had to do, including my teaching, could be done online. And I could get on with writing this book!

It was more difficult not having access to the usual library facilities and so on. But I was able to locate most of the research papers I needed to cite, from home. I had to rest a lot more – one of the legacies of my stroke has been the fatigues and I have to lie down for a rest every couple of hours. But I got there. So, I guess I lost about four months' time from my writing and have had to hurry more that I would have liked to complete this project. Now let me say a bit more about what has driven me to teach as I have and to write this book.

I have felt proud to be a sociologist. My tuition at Aberdeen provided me with a particular world view which has allowed me to question orthodoxy, and inequalities. My only disappointment in Sociology and in my chosen branch of sociology – medical sociology – has been my peers who have tended to make so many of their activities pretty much obscure to non-sociologists and therefore, with the jargon of the subject, this puts people off. I believe that every scientific discipline is guilty of that failing. In fact they tend to pride themselves in the elegance of their academic snobbery. The very fact that they engage in a language which the non-expert audience can not access is partly what makes a profession different from all the others.

In my career – which began in survey research, then very quickly moved into teaching in medicine – I very soon learned that it was a fruitless endeavour to try to teach sociology to medical students in the same way as it is taught to sociologists. So, from the beginning, in 1973, when sociology was first introduced into the medical school as a formally-taught, and examinable subject, I realised from the response of my students to the subject, that a large part of the challenge for me was to make my subject accessible to my students. It is a very lonely place, being a sole sociologist in a medical school. Not only were my students antagonistic about having to learn this subject, but the other staff in the medical school were mostly the same, and I believe, their antagonism fired the students' resentment. So reaching out to them was an essential process. I tried to make sociology both relevant and understandable for them.

When I joined the Brighton & Sussex Medical School Institute of Postgraduate Medicine (as it was then) in 2009, I was given the responsibility for teaching research methods and co-ordinating the Dissertation Panel. All our Master's students had to complete the research methods module and every student had to complete a research dissertation. My goal was to make research methods as accessible to them as possible. I remember one of the first students I taught saying that the research methods module was known as 'the killer' because students had such difficulty with it. His class gave me one of the most positive reviews (feedback) that I have had. Over the last 11 years I have become better at it. I have supervised over 70 student's dissertations and I seem to have a knack of connecting with their uncertainties, identifying what they are trying to get at in their projects and putting them at their ease. I have learned something from all of them and have appreciated the enrichment they have brought into my life.

So, this book is mostly based upon my lectures and the research skills workshops I have taught. I thought it would be an easy job to translate my lecture-notes into chapters, but it has been more work (interesting work) than I imagined. I still feel enthusiastic about research and slightly evangelical about promoting it. But I like to ensure that it makes sense and is not too over-complicated. I hope my positive attitude (can do!) comes over in this book, and I hope that it will give heart to those of you who are anxious about doing research.

I apologise in advance for my little Anecdotes, most of which were edited out! I can't resist telling a story. I like to breath some life and humanity into the subject. I hope it helps break up the material and gives you something to smile about at times!

Many people have provided me with inspiration over the years, from my first boss Ann Cartwright (who I didn't get on with very much, but who I respected for her knowledge) right up to Seb, one of my students and now a colleague and a friend, who has impressed me with his appreciation of the subject, his insights and his energy! (You will meet him in several chapters.) Mick Bloor, a great friend and researcher of over 50 years (!) and whose work I cite constantly throughout this book is, to my mind, one of the world's best qualitative researchers. He has been a source of friendship, advice and support over the years. Too many others to mention have influenced me in so very many ways. I thank you all.

My wife Clair and our granddaughter Anna are my beloved angels. It is like having a constant source of love, respect and common-sense surround me at all times. Clair has been so understanding and supportive throughout the process of writing this book. She keeps coming up with useful sources and new bits of information. Both she and Anna have read most of the chapters of the book and laughed at the right places. I am so proud of you both and love you so much.

Thank you.

John L. Anderson
January 2022

About the Companion Website

This book is accompanied by a companion website.

www.wiley.com/go/Anderson/DemystifyingResearch

This website includes:

- Lecture slides available to download in PowerPoint

CHAPTER 1

Introduction

What is 'Research'?

The Aims of this Book

I have been teaching research methods to medical, nursing, and social sciences students, and in postgraduate medicine, for over 40 years. In that time, I have realised that the prospect of learning about doing research, or doing 'science', terrifies a lot of people. Many have a 'mental block' at the thought of it. 'Research is what scientists do and I'm not a scientist!' So, this is where I give my first, and possibly, most important piece of advice:

'Don't Panic!'

Can you think of the source? These words were written by Douglas Adams in 1979 . . . That's right! They are from his book, *The Hitch Hiker's Guide to the Galaxy,* and on the back of the Guide are found these immortal words. Remember them. You don't need to panic when you are learning about research. You can do it.

My goal is to de-mystify research. I aim to help you understand research, to be able to appraise research in scholarly articles, to be able to design a research project, and to believe that you could do research yourself. This book is not intended to impress my colleagues and bewilder students. I hope that, by explaining research in a straightforward and simple manner, I can make the process of learning about and understanding research easier. I shall try to explain jargon terms wherever possible and I shall use examples of classic research as well as some of my own and that of my students. (Over the past 10 years, I have supervised over 70 masters students' dissertations to completion.) I aim to illustrate the theoretical with examples of research in practice.

The other aspect of research which frightens the heck out of learners is . . . that's right – the 'S' word – *statistics*. Well, I guess I have to touch on the subject, but I shall leave it to those more able than myself to cover that subject in depth. I have included some parts on data analysis, but I shall try to make these as pain-free and understandable as possible.

Demystifying Research for Medical & Healthcare Students: An Essential Guide, First Edition. John L. Anderson.
© 2022 John Wiley & Sons Ltd. Published 2022 by John Wiley & Sons Ltd.
Companion website: www.wiley.com/go/Anderson/DemystifyingResearch

What is 'Research'?

If I were to ask you to come up with a definition of 'research', I guess that most people would aim for something which included words like 'rigorous', 'bias-free', 'academic', 'random', 'systematic', 'generalisable', and so on. They would probably be right . . . -ish. But I do not try to give a flowery, posh definition. The answer to the question is much simpler:

Research is about getting answers to questions.

And it is something which *we all engage in every* day of our lives. Let's consider what 'research' we do in our everyday lives. Think about it. What sort of things do you come up with?

- Planning your journey to work?
- Which car to buy?
- What house to buy?
- What to cook for dinner?
- Where to go on holiday?
- Etc., etc.

All of these involve us in some 'research'. Let's see . . . What are the options in travel to work? Walk, bicycle, bus/train, car, etc. So, we calculate how long each mode of transport might take – that is relatively easy. It has an answer in numbers. It is quantifiable – so it is what we call **quantitative** (sorry! There's an early bit of jargon!) data. So we know how much time each type of journey should take. Next, we work out the cost of each. Again, this is straightforward – we get a number in pounds and pence, and it is easy to say which costs more than another.

Now we are faced with a different form of question – which is the most convenient, and which is the most reliable? The answers to these are based upon personal choice and preferences – they have more to do with the quality of the experience and we can't measure these in numbers, so we are dealing with **qualitative** (sorry!) data and different types of information will guide our decisions.

The same sets of information can guide us when we buy a TV, a car, a house, or decide upon a meal. If you reflect on the last time you bought something, you may be aware of the sorts of 'research' you got involved in and how you found the information which informed your decision. Good old Google! Search engines have helped to make us all much more able to search for answers to questions – to do *research*.

So, research is something we do every day. But how did we learn to be researchers?

How Early Do we Start 'Researching'?

We start researching the moment we are born. Some scholars might insist that we explore our environment and learn whilst we are still in the womb. Maybe so. I know that as soon as we are born we start to explore out environment to learn more about it and to get answers to important questions such as 'What is food?' What is the first thing a newborn baby does? S/he will search for food. Can I eat this, or this, or that? It puts things in its mouth and lets the universe know it is looking for food by crying out. This early, trial and error learning (literally – suck it and see) **experimentation** is a fundamental type of research. The results will inform the baby's future actions.

That's how we learn. We are continually testing our environment (the world around us). So, when we give an infant a clock to play with and it ends up in pieces on the floor, be proud, not angry! That infant is trying to make sense of the thing we call 'clock' and is trying to answer the excellent research question 'how does this work?' Sometimes we are aware of it. Sometimes we are not. We do it in our physical world and in our social and psychological worlds. If we are lucky and don't stick our finger in a live electric socket, we live and learn and are all the wiser from it.

But What Makes our Research a Science?

We are all doing research every day, and we are all learning from it, but we are not all 'scientists'. For it to be scientific, we have to select a specific area (or field) to research and then we have to be **systematic** and **rigorous** in getting our answers to very specific questions. We may search a lot around a subject to find out what has already been researched, and we might, think about where the unanswered questions are and begin to plan our own study. Then we call it 'research', we write lots of scientific articles and become famous – I wish!

There are different types and levels of scientific research. I remember being interviewed for a job to do some research in learning difficulties and was surprised to hear the Chair of the interview panel say to me 'We want real, meaningful research. We are not setting out to *count angels on pinheads!*' What did he mean by that? Then I realised that his stereotype of researchers was of 'academics' who engaged in what is termed 'blue skies research'. That is, research which may advance our knowledge, but is of no practical benefit to people on an everyday level. Some people differentiate between 'applied research' and 'blue skies research'. To my mind there is no difference really. At some point and in some way, all research has an application and to try to differentiate which is which is like . . . trying to count angels on a pinhead!

OK – So we all Do 'Research' but I Am Not Good Enough to Do Meaningful Research

Many people are put off doing research because they don't think *they* can achieve the 'perfection' needed for good research. Don't panic! That is a myth. There are very few research projects which might be described as 'perfect'. Many are weak in some regard. But most are 'good enough' – good enough to provide us with answers which can advance our knowledge – at least by signposting us to other questions which still remain unanswered.

My dear friend Mick Bloor and I ran a brief research course together once in the Highlands of Scotland for senior service managers. They were all terrified of the prospect of learning about research, let alone doing it. So, in this course Mick described research thus:

Research is the art of the possible.

I always think that this is a very liberating and empowering statement. What he meant was that it is OK to do research that is as good as we can do – that is, it is good enough. Very few studies have the massive funding that is required in, for example, the testing of a potential new drug to treat cancer. We do what we can within the resources available to us. And we should do it with pride. We say what we have done, we alert people to the limitations of what we have done, and we do it. Do not be put off by thinking that 'my study is not as good as one I have read about'. Go ahead. Do it. Be thorough and systematic and you will likely succeed. The fact that you have picked up this book shows that you are trying to be systematic.

Always remember:

You are already a natural researcher.

By being thorough and systematic you will be a 'scientific' researcher.

'Research is the art of the possible.'

Overview of Research Methods

Introduction

As we have noted, some things which we can measure and attribute numerical values to fall into the category of **quantitative research.** Other things cannot be quantified and fall into the category of **qualitative research.** Some research incorporates elements of both and we refer to these approaches as **mixed methods.** In this chapter, we shall consider each of these in turn and then look at the different assumptions which underpin each of these approaches. So, to be crude, **quantitative approaches** are those which involve *numbers*. **Qualitative approaches** *do not* involve numbers. Remember that. It gets more complicated, but I'll explain that when we come to it in depth in later chapters. But, for now, here is a brief overview of what we will cover in the book.

All these approaches are shown in this figure and you can use this as a 'mind map' to negotiate the different topics covered in this book.

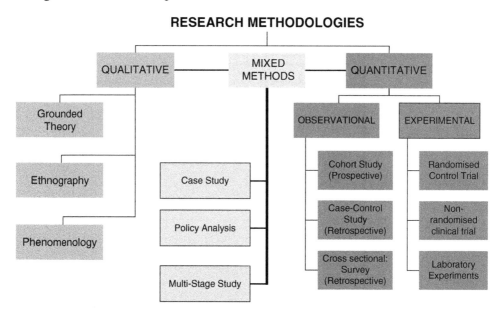

Quantitative Approaches

These are approaches in which we measure and count things. We use statistical methods to analyse the numerical date which we collect. These approaches fall into two categories – **experimental,** or interventional approaches, and **observational,** or non-experimental and non-interventional, approaches.

> **WARNING** – *Note the use of the term 'observational'. It does not refer to observation in the sense of observing something, but means that there is no experimentation or intervention. We do not manipulate any variables or make any experimental interventions.*

So, in **experimental** approaches, we introduce some change and then measure any effects which are thought to be 'caused' by that change. In **observational** approaches, there is no change – we measure things as they are. Let's look at the three main categories of these first.

Observational or Non-experimental Approaches

i. **Cross-sectional studies:** These are the commonest type of studies used in quantitative research. They involve taking a 'snapshot' of what is happening in a group or a population at a particular point in time. The most widely used approach is the **survey**. These are termed 'retrospective' studies, because what we are enquiring about has already happened – it is in the past. We shall look at these in depth later in Chapters 8 and 9.

ii. **Case-control studies:** Case-control studies are commonly used in epidemiological research when we want to check what factors cause a disease that we are concerned about. These are a pleasingly neat design. We identify and recruit a group of people with a disease, then we identify and recruit a group of people who are similar in almost every respect – except that they do not have that disease. Then we measure the extent to which each group have been exposed to a suspected causal factor and measure the difference between the two groups. If the 'Cases' score higher than the 'Controls', then we conclude that the factor we are comparing them on is indeed a suspected contributory factor for that disease or condition. Neat – eh? These are also termed 'retrospective' studies because what we are enquiring about has already happened – it is in the past. We shall look at these in depth later in Chapter 7.

iii. **Cohort studies:** The term **cohort** is a posh word for a group. It comes from the Latin 'cohors' which was a group of soldiers in a Roman Legion – a platoon, sort of. In cohort studies, we recruit a group of people and follow them up over a period of time. We may choose people for a specific reason or a wide range of reasons and record significant events as they arise. These are different to the last two approaches in that they are not 'retrospective' studies, because we are interested in what *will* happen – in the future. They are what we call 'prospective' studies. We shall look at these in depth in Chapter 6.

Experimental Approaches

i. **Laboratory experiments:** Most of us will remember our time in laboratories doing experiments. I remember tedious hours of work in the Chemistry labs doing titrations. You know, the sort of experiment where you have a measured amount of one chemical, A, in a beaker, and you painstakingly introduce into this – drip by boring drip – another chemical, B, from a burette . . . The rationale of these experimental studies is simple – you have almost complete control over the experimental environment, so that you can rule out **extraneous** (external) variables, such as spores that drift in the open window (as happened to Alexander Fleming – a sloppy researcher!) and you can reasonably confidently assume that any changes you record are due to the experimental variable that you have introduced. We can also use a **control situation** – for example, in culture studies, we would leave a petri dish with no culture for testing alongside the test dishes. Then we can identify the 'Fleming effect' if some external 'contaminant' gets in by chance and corrupts our findings.

Laboratory experiments can also be conducted with animal and human 'subjects' or 'participants' and I shall go into depth on these in the Chapters 2 and 3.

ii. **Non-randomised trials:** These are experimental approaches (often used in drug development) in which an experiment is conducted – but there is no control situation or control group. These are covered in depth in Chapter 4.

iii. **Randomised control trials (RCTs):** These are perhaps the most widely known and widely used experimental approach in medicine. Here we take the rationale of the laboratory experiment and take it beyond the laboratory. These are widely used to test the efficacy of new interventions or diagnostic tools. We recruit a group of participants and randomly allocate them to an **experimental group** or a **control group.** Those in the experimental group are given a new drug or treatment, whilst those in the control group get their standard treatment, usually with a **placebo** – an inert drug or treatment. If those in the experimental group do better than those in the control group, then we conclude that the new drug or treatment is better than the standard – or no treatment. There are many issues involved in RCTs and I shall discuss these in depth in Chapter 5.

Qualitative Approaches

These are approaches which do *not* involve numbers. Often the topic does not lend itself to quantifying – for example, when we are interested in studying people's belief-systems, or feelings. Sometimes the conventional approaches to sampling are not possible or do not make sense and therefore we chose a different approach from the ones described above. There are very many qualitative approaches, but for simplicity, I shall focus on the three most commonly used approaches.

i. **Grounded Theory:** Grounded Theory was developed by Barley Glaser and Anselm Strauss. Their book *The Discovery of Grounded Theory* was written at a time (1968) when there were very few academic books on qualitative research, other than ethnographic ones. Their aims in writing this book were to provide research students with a textbook to cite in defence of their qualitative approach, and to challenge the orthodox dominance of quantitative researchers in social sciences. They had conducted studies of death and dying in US hospitals – which is where I came into contact with them (I was working on the *Life Before Death* study and we wrote to ask them for any advice they could give – see Chapter 8). They describe an approach in which theory arises from and develops from the data as it is collected – for example, from observations, interviews, etc. I shall go into depth in these in the Chapter 14.

ii. **Ethnographic approaches:** Ethnographic approaches have their roots in **Anthropology.** In particular, the work of early anthropologists to document and analyse societies and cultures in the developing world. The most common practice in this sort of research was for the researcher to go to a particular society and study it – as a **participant observer.** This meant living with and being part of the system that they are studying. By immersing themselves into and observing the life of that group of people and the events which happened to them – including the sense, or meaning that they attributed to them – they were able to try to make sense of that social system, So, what's this got to do with modern healthcare? Well, this approach has been adapted to researchers getting involved with particular social groups or situations – such as being admitted to hospital, working in care homes, etc., in order to get an 'insider' view of the experience and what is going on (see Chapter 11).

More common, now, is to try to make sense of the **cultural** aspects of a group or situation by interviewing people – either individually or in focus groups – to capture their beliefs and practices. I shall go into depth and provide some rich examples of these in the Chapter 12.

iii. **Phenomenological approaches:** Note how we are progressing to bigger and more difficult to pronounce terms! Sorry about that, but we need to be able to understand what others are saying, so I shall try to explain their meanings. First, let's try pronouncing the term:

Phen – om – en – ol – ogy

That's right. Try practising it a few times to get the hang of it. (I still stumble over this one occasionally!)

Phenomenology is the study of people's 'lived experiences'. So, if we want to understand what people's experiences of an aspect of healthcare are, and the sense, or meaning, they attribute to these, then we are in the business of doing **phenomenology**. We usually do this using in-depth interviews to access people's experiences. There are two schools of phenomenology – **descriptive** and **interpretive** phenomenology, but we'll wait until Chapter 13 before getting into the detail.

There are more variations of qualitative research, but I don't pretend to understand them all – and you don't have to.

Mixed-Methods Approaches

I shall limit this section to discussing three of the most important of these approaches.

i. **Case study approaches:** In these, our aim is to focus on a single event or 'case' and by doing this we are able to provide a very detailed analysis of this case. Usually, we will combine quantitative and qualitative data in our examination of the case. For example, if we are looking at the impact of change in a GP practice, we would probably collect statistical data on the hours worked, the numbers of patients seen, etc., and we might interview a small number of staff and/or patients to find out what their views and experiences have been. Or we might take an individual patient and analyse them as a case, looking at numbers such as blood pressure, viral counts, etc., as well as qualitative data on the thoughts and feelings of the patient and those around her/him. Thus, we can obtain a full and detailed view of what is going on in this 'case'. I shall go into depth in these in Chapter 15.

ii. **Policy analysis:** In a policy analysis we are usually concerned with one (or both) of the following questions:

   a. What are the forces or pressures which led to the introduction of a new policy?

   b. What are the likely, or actual, effects of the introduction of a new policy?

   As you can imagine these are important issues for the development of health services and take us into more political issues, such as what interest groups might influence a country's decision about whether or not to introduce a new vaccination campaign, etc. Again, we usually deal with both types of data in considering these. I shall go into depth in these in Chapter 16.

iii. **Multi-stage studies:** There is an increasing trend towards mixing quantitative and qualitative approaches. For example, small-scale, qualitative studies are often used as pilot studies or feasibility studies to test methodologies and to identify the issues to be addressed in the main, quantitative study. This is very common in **survey research.** Often, clinical trials will incorporate the collection of qualitative data alongside the quantitative data. For example, the statistics about the effectiveness of a new treatment may be complemented by gathering data about patients' experiences and their feelings about their experiences of it. These are covered in Chapter 17.

The 'Sciences' of Research

It might seem odd to you that I have said 'SCIENCES'. First of all isn't there just 'science', so why have I put it in the plural 'sciences'? To tell you the truth, I was a bit nervous about putting this section in. In a book titled *De-Mystifying Research Methods,* my aim is to make things as simple, as understandable as possible. Yet here I am with the most complex sets of ideas that there are in research and I am struggling to make it simple! Anyway, here goes. I shall try to make it simple and to keep it brief.

I want to introduce you to four terms which are inter-related, and to show you how they are related. There are: **ontology, epistemology, methodology, and methods**.

Ontology

Ontology is the study of 'being' and what constitutes 'reality'. Now this is complex, so don't even go to Wikipedia and hope to find a simple version. There is none. The main philosophical debate is about whether there is one absolute reality or whether there are multiple realities. I have struggled with this for years and still do. I have reached these conclusions:

- In some cases, *there is only one reality.* If someone points a gun at me and threatens to pull the trigger, I am not going to get into a discussion about how he defines a gun. I am not going to argue that his faith in his gun is determined by a questionable philosophical stance and . . . **BANG!** I have lost the argument. He has proved his point. So, for a lot of things — for example, the 'realities' of the physical world – I am not going to question most of it. I believe in bricks and walls and roofs etc. I depend on these every day to live in. And whilst I might debate the qualities of bricks and walls and roofs with you, at the end of the day we would probably agree that they are there and that we can reach out and touch them. They are hard, and if one falls on your foot it will hurt. Facts. We share a common **physical universe** which we can live in and experience and we can check that out with other people. You could say that they were **objective** in that they exist whether we believe in them or not.

- But in some things, there is more than one *interpretation of reality.* And there are some things which are more negotiable in terms of their 'reality'. People's thoughts, feelings, senses, and experiences are definitely **subjective.** These belong to the individual who owns them and, although we can find out what they are, we may never be able (at least, at this point in our 'scientific' development) to fully understand the other's experiencing of life. Furthermore, our ability to understand – to get as near as possible to 'knowing' – the experiences of others, will be determined by our own situation in the **social world.**

One of the examples that I have used in teaching this, is that of *pain.* If you look up 'measuring pain' in Wikipedia (not my favourite source, but an interesting one), you will find the following story:

> *In 1940, James D. Hardy, Harold G. Wolff and Helen Goodell of Cornell University introduced the first dolorimeter as a method for evaluating the effectiveness of analgesic medications. They did their work at New York Hospital. They focused the light of a 100 watt projection lamp with a lens on an area of skin that had been blackened to minimize reflection. They found that most people expressed a pain sensation when the skin temperature reached 113°F (45°C). They also found that after the skin temperature reached 152°F (67°C), the pain sensations did not intensify even if the heat were increased. They developed a pain scale, called the 'Hardy–Wolff-Goodell' scale, with 10 gradations, or 10 levels. They assigned the name of 'dols' to these levels. Other researchers were not able to reproduce the results of Hardy, Wolff and Goodell, and the device and the approach were abandoned . . . In 1945, Time magazine reported that Cleveland's Dr. Lorand Julius Bela Gluzek had developed a dolorimeter that measured pain in grams. Dr. Gluzek claimed that his dolorimeter was 97% accurate.*

Sounds a bit far-fetched to me! Some of the approaches to develop 'pain-ometers' were bizarre and reminded me of the experiments in Nazi Germany (I deal with these in Chapter 18).

In the 1970s, pain was initially 'measured' as 'mild, moderate or severe'. Then people began to tinker with it to make it more sophisticated. They introduced 10-point scales, some of which are accompanied by faces smiling to crying. (See Figure 1.1.)

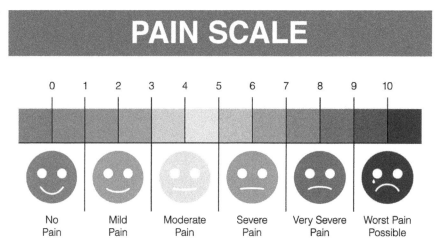

FIGURE 1.1   The 10-point pain scale (Harvard Men's Health Watch, 2018).
Source: Image: © EgudinKa/Getty Images.

Can you imagine, one patient says to another:

P1: How're you feeling today?
P2: Not great – I've got a *grade 8 pain!*
P1: Gee, I'm sorry to hear that! What axis are you measuring it on?

Those who believe that there is only one reality and that this reality exists independently of our knowledge of it are called **positivists.** Those who believe that all reality is subjective are called **relativists** or **interpretivists.** To me it does not make sense to say, 'I believe that all of "reality" is **subjective**', any more that it makes sense to me to say 'I believe that all of reality is **objective**'. But, I acknowledge that other people have different views. For me, life is too short to bother with them. And that's all I want to say about that.

Epistemology

Epistemology is the study of what constitutes 'knowledge'. It is concerned with defining the nature of what knowledge is and how we know things. So, the epistemologist will be concerned about different views on knowledge, beliefs, truth, justification, and internalism/externalism. (Don't even ask!)

In relation to research methods, if you hold a **positivist** belief (note my use of the term 'belief') then you are likely to want to have proof for your knowledge in the form of things you can see, touch, and get confirmation from others that they see and touch them too. You are likely then to favour methods which measure things and count things and to use statistics to analyse your data. One criticism is that they reduce everything to a number:

NRS: What's your depression like today?
PTNT: It's a *seven.*
NRS: Oh my, that's bad, I'd better get you some more pills!

If you hold an **interpretivist** belief, then you will not search for absolute proof for your knowledge, because you don't think that that exists. Therefore, you will be inclined to use inductive methods and qualitative approaches, because you recognise the subjectivity of your unique location in time (history) and society (class, gender, race, culture, etc.). You won't try to measure pain, or depression just by numbers. You might say ask questions like:

NRS: Can you describe your pain to me?

A third paradigm (way of thinking) is a **pragmatist** belief. This accepts aspects of both positivist and interpretivist beliefs and can adapt to the most realistic means of addressing an issue using either positivist or interpretivist approaches.

Methodology

Methodology refers to the broad approach which we take to guide our collection of data. The three main categories are quantitative (numbers), qualitative (no numbers), and mixed-methods (whatever you want).

Methods

Methods refers to the actual means of collecting your data – for example by measurements, surveys, interviews, questionnaires, focus groups, and so on.

They are linked, and I have tried to show a relatively simple way of thinking about it in Table 1.1. (I was inspired By Salma Patel's 2015 model which I have adapted here.)

To Sum Up

The main distinctions we tend to make in research are about:

- positivist vs interpretivist
- quantitative vs qualitative
- hypothetico-deductive vs hypothetico-inductive.

And if you bear those distinctions in mind, you'll get by!

Final Word

Research can exist outside of our knowledge of ontology and epistemology. Don't fret too much over these complex ideas. As you might end up debating whether it is positivist or relativist to decide how to count the number of angels you can get on a pinhead . . .

TABLE 1.1   Ontology, epistemology. Theoretical perspective, methodology, and methods.

Research Paradigm	Ontology	Epistemology	Theoretical Perspective	Methodology	Methods
Positivist	There is a single reality	Reality can be measured using the best scientific methods	Positivism	Quantitative methods – experimental and observational hypothetico-deductive	Sampling, measuring Numbers and statistics
Interpretivist	No single reality. Reality depends on the researcher's location in time and society	Everything is subject to interpretation. We need to discover how people experience their worlds	Interpretivism	Qualitative methods: phenomenology ethnography grounded theory Etc. Hypothetico-inductive	Participant observation Interviews Focus groups Etc.
Pragmatism	Reality is constantly being re-negotiated and interpreted	You can choose the best method for solving the problem	Pragmatism	Mixed methods	Any methods which will answer the question

Source: Adapted from Patel (2015).

For further reading, if you have the mental stamina to be confused further, you might look at: Devaux and Lamanna (2009), Griswold (2001), Heidegger (1971), Sturm (2011), Descartes (1985), and Haack (1993).

References

Descartes R. (1985). *The Philosophical Writings of Rene Descartes I*. Cambridge University Press.

Devaux M and Lamanna M. (2009). The rise and early history of the term ontology (1606–1730). *Quaestio* 9(173–208), 197–198.

Griswold CL. (2001). *Platonic Writings/Platonic Readings*. Penn State Press, p. 237.

Haack S. (1993). *Evidence and Inquiry: Towards Reconstruction in Epistemology*. Wiley-Blackwell.

Harvard Men's Health Watch. (2018). The pain of measuring pain: Doctors and patients use the 10-point pain scale to gauge the severity of pain, but there may be a better way.' Available at: https://www.health.harvard.edu/pain/the-pain-of-measuring-pain (accessed 25 September 2020).

Heidegger M. (1971). *On the Way to Language*. Harper & Row: New Yor, (original: 1959).

Patel S. (2015). The research paradigm – methodology, epistemology and ontology – explained in simple language. Available at: http://salmapatel.co.uk/academia/the-research-paradigm-methodology-epistemology-and-ontology-explained-in-simple-language (accessed 25 September 2020).

Sturm T. (2011). Historical epistemology or history of epistemology? The case of the relation between perception and judgment. *Erkenntnis* 75(3), 303–324.

CHAPTER 2

Experimental Quantitative Approaches

Laboratory Experiments

Introduction

I guess that most of us can remember laboratory experiments from our school days – unless, as some do, you have blanked this out! Laboratory experiments are:

- In the **quantitative** domain – we measure and count, we use **numbers.**
- They are usually **hypothetico-deductive** – we have a clear purpose and set of expectations in mind before we begin.
- They are in the **interventional** domain – we introduce an experimental variable which was not there at the start.
- They are **prospective** – we have a start point where we make our initial measurements, we have our interventions, and we have an end point when we make our final measurements.
- They are best suited to answering questions like: 'If I add/change this, will that happen?'

(None of my science teachers at school or university explained anything of the methodological science behind what we were doing – and that was a great pity. Over the years I have had to explain to undergraduate and postgraduate students the principles which underpin the 'sciences' of research – because most of them did not understand it either! Well, now, *you* do!)

Demystifying Research for Medical & Healthcare Students: An Essential Guide, First Edition. John L. Anderson.
© 2022 John Wiley & Sons Ltd. Published 2022 by John Wiley & Sons Ltd.
Companion website: www.wiley.com/go/Anderson/DemystifyingResearch

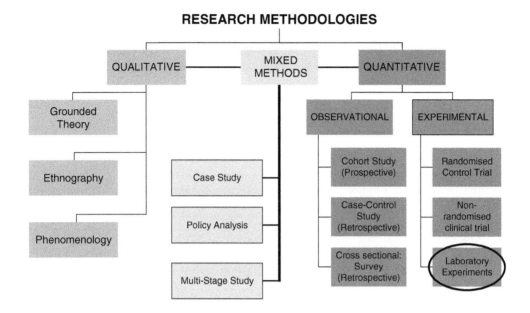

The 'Logic' of the Experimental Approach

How often do we, and others, ask the question, 'I wonder what happens if I . . . remove this thing here/do this instead of that/etc.' Famous last words. How many of us, when we see a sign saying **WET PAINT,** instead of avoiding the painted surface, touch it to see if it is really wet?! (Some of us never really shed those childhood rebellious behaviours!) So we or they touch the paint, and end up with sticky fingers! 'Yup. I guess it IS wet paint!' is the conclusion!

This may sound like a banal example, but it illustrates the first level of experimentation. We begin with a hypothesis – 'the paint is not wet' – and we test our hypothesis – by touching the wood (or better still, by encouraging someone else to touch it) – using the tried and tested approach of 'touch it and see'. This act of experimentation then either confirms our hypothesis – 'Yes, the paint is wet! Now where do I clean my hands?!' – or it refutes (denies) our hypothesis – 'No, the paint is not wet. Phew!'

So, the process is simple:

- We have a **question** – 'Is that paint wet?'
- We state our **hypothesis** – 'My hunch is that the paint is not wet' – this implies the **nul hypothesis** – 'My hunch is that the paint is wet'.
- We carry out our **experimentation** – we touch the paint.
- We note the **result** – the paint is wet!
- We **conclude** that this has refuted our hypothesis – it has confirmed the nul hypothesis – the paint is wet.
- We **disseminate** our findings – 'Look out – that paint really is wet!'

Easy! Now go on and think of a few examples on your own – if you send your ideas to me, I shall include the ones I like best and acknowledge you in the next edition of this book!

As an experiment, the hypothesis would have been 'Touching the paint will not dirty my hand – the paint is dry'. And the nul hypothesis (the opposite of the hypothesis) would have been . . .? Yes, that's right, 'Touching the paint will dirty my hand – the paint is *not* dry'. And the intervention would have been – touching the paint. The outcomes would have been:

    i. my hand will remain clean – the paint was dry; or
   ii. my hand will be messy – the paint was not dry.

Now, some of you might argue that this is not a true experiment – the act of touching the paint was not a true intervention, it was an 'interrogation' or 'questioning' or 'testing' of the paint. I'm not going to argue – you could take it either way, but I hope it shows the point I am trying to make – *experimentation is a part of our daily lives!* We are born researchers and experimenters.

One more thing to note is that not all experimental approaches are truly hypothetico-deductive, some are **hypothetico-inductive** – we don't have a clue about what might happen when we press the button to set off the atom bomb, but we want to find out . . .

A Basic Experiment

In a basic experiment, we set up a situation where we introduce one thing – a substance or a variable – to another thing (substance/variable) and observe the effects – the outcomes of doing this.

In a laboratory we can **control** the situation, the experiment, and the environment within which the experiment is done. So, if Substance A is zinc, and Substance B is hydrochloric acid, we should observe a fizzing as the acid meets the zinc and the gas hydrogen will be given off, leaving a residual substance (hydrogen chloride) behind. We can do the experiment with different concentrations of the acid, at different temperatures, at different atmospheric pressures, and at different levels of humidity – and measure the results in each condition. That is, we can take **external variables** into account to measure the extent to which they interfere with, or contaminate, our results. We can repeat the experiment as often as we want to check our results. And, most importantly, by keeping our equipment squeaky-clean, we can make sure that there are no substances on/in the equipment that can interfere with the experiment – 'Cleanliness *is* next to Godliness!' And to avoid the 'Fleming effect' we can conduct our work in sealed laboratories so that no dirt can blow in through a window and give us unexpected results!

Safety is most important! As laboratory researchers, we have to take precautions to ensure our own safety, the safety of other people in the lab, and the safety of everyone in society. So, we use appropriate protective clothing. We follow lab rules and protocols for conducting research in them. We follow appropriate guidelines and protocols for disposing of waste materials. Gone are the days when you could do lab experiments at night and, when no one was looking, just pour your materials down the drain! Before you begin to work in any lab, make sure that you have had safety protocols explained to you and that you understand them. If no one offers you an explanation, then ask your boss to explain them. Then, make sure that you stick to them!

I have included some examples of lab safety rules in the Appendix C to remind you of the sorts of things you should be aware of. Remember – if in doubt, ask.

Experimental Designs

The simplest experimental design is what we call a **single arm** experiment – see Figure 2.1. Most science lab experiments probably fall into this category. However, most experiments involving humans are **twin',** or **'double-arm** experiments (Figure 2.2). Some are **triple** or more (Figure 2.3). Single-arm experiments do not have a **control group,** whereas twin-arm and triple (or greater) experiments do have a control group. Some experimental designs have more than two groups, but more of this later. There was a tradition in the nineteenth century for scientists to try things out on themselves first of all. There is still an element of this 'gung-ho' culture in modern science – which ethics committees try to keep in check.

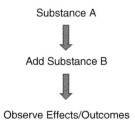

FIGURE 2.1   Single arm experiment.

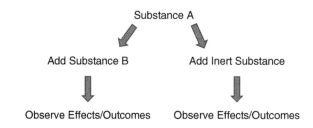

FIGURE 2.2   Twin arm experiment.

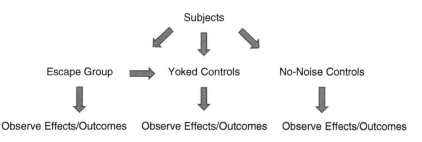

FIGURE 2.3   Triadic design with yoked controls.

Using Yourself as a Guinea-Pig

In 1882, the German physician and microbiologist identified the bacteria which caused tuberculosis and cholera. Renee Dubos, a microbiologist who specialised in the study of tuberculosis, and one of my favourite 'Great Thinkers' about health and medicine, described how Koch injected tuberculin into his own arm and suffered a very serious reaction which showed that he had himself been infected with TB in the past, but had never had clinical tuberculosis. He later discovered the causative agent of cholera – Vibrio cholerae. Max Joseph von Pettenkoffer was a Bavarian chemist and hygienist who was an anti-contagionist – he did not believe that (very new) idea that bacteria caused diseases like cholera (Figure 2.4). As Dubos recounts:

> *Around 1900 Pettenkoffer in Germany and Metchinoff in France, with several of their associates, drank tumblerfuls of cultures isolated from fatal cases of cholera. Enormous numbers of cholera vibrios could be recovered from their stools; some of the self-infected experimenters developed mild diarrhea, but the infection did not result in true cholera. More recently human volunteers were made to ingest billions of dysentery bacilli under conditions assumed to be optimal for the establishment of infection. Enteric capsules full of feces obtained directly from acute cases of bacillary dysentery in man were used as additional experimental refinements to increase the chances of establishing the disease. Yet only a few of the volunteers developed symptoms referable to dysentery and most of them remained unaffected by the experimental infection.*

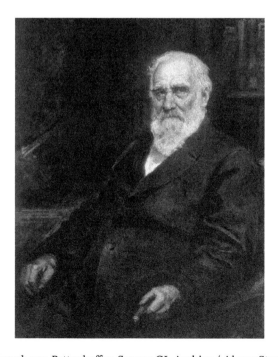

FIGURE 2.4   Max Joseph von Pettenkoffer. *Source*: GL Archive / Alamy Stock Photo.

The fact of the matter is that Pasteur and Koch did not deal with natural events, but with experimental artifacts. The experimenter does not reproduce nature in the laboratory. He could not if he tried, for the experiment imposes limiting conditions on nature; its aims are to force nature to give answers to questions devised by man. Every answer of nature is therefore more or less influenced by the kind of questions asked.

The art of the experimenter is to create models in which he can observe some properties and activities of a factor in which he happens to be interested. Koch and Pasteur wanted to show that microorganisms could cause certain manifestations of disease. Their genius was to invent experimental situations that lent themselves to an unequivocal illustration of their hypothesis – situations in which it was sufficient to bring the host and parasite together to reproduce the disease. By trial and error, they selected the species of animals, the dose of the infectious agent, and the route of inoculation, which permitted the infection to evolve without fail into progressive disease. Guinea pigs always develop tuberculosis if tubercle bacilli are injected into them under the proper conditions; introduction of sufficient rabies virus under the dura of dogs always gives rise to paralytic symptoms. Thus, by the skilful selection of experimental systems, Pasteur, Koch, and their followers succeeded in minimising in their tests the influence of factors that might have obscured the activity of the infectious agents they wanted to study. This experimental approach has been extremely effective for the recovery of agents of disease and for the study of some of their properties. But it has led by necessity to the neglect, and indeed has often delayed the recognition, of the many other factors that play a part in the causation of disease under conditions prevailing in the natural world – for example, the physiological status of the infected individual and the impact of the environment in which he lives.

(Dubos 1959)

DO NOT TRY THIS AT HOME! What Dubos has very eloquently illustrated is the difference between the **necessary** factors which need to be present to cause a disease – the bacilli and the host – and the **sufficient** factors required to lead to the onset of the disease – such as personal, physiological, nutritional, environmental factors, etc.

Why Have a Control Group?

Why indeed? Have a guess . . .!

That's right – we need to check that the 'Fleming Effect' has not happened. That is, we need to check that any changes we observe after introducing the experimental 'variable' are, in fact, due to the experimental variable and not to some outside variable, like, for example, dirt blown in through an open window which might contaminate our results!

Another reason is that the very act of *doing research* has, itself, an effect on what we are researching. Let me illustrate this.

The 'Hawthorne Effect'

The 'Hawthorne Effect' took its name from a series of studies on workers' productivity between 1922 and 1932 in the Western Electric Factory in Chicago – in the 'Hawthorne' works. At this period of time in American history, there was a near obsession with finding ways of making factory production more efficient. 'Time and motion' studies were rife. An early pioneer in this was Henry Ford who, in 1913, introduced the 'assembly line' in his car factories in which the work – cars being assembled – was brought to the workers in assembly lines rather that the workers having to move from car to car, thus cutting the time it took to complete the assembly of a Model T Ford car from 12 hours to 2.5 hours. As Henry Ford said, 'Walking is not a paying operation' (cited in Tuckett 1976). So, the initial experiments in the Hawthorne works were aimed at finding things which improved workers' productivity. A special production room – the *bank-wiring room* – was set up so that workers could do their work in 'laboratory' conditions. Observers sat in and watched what was going on. The work involved wiring boards of electrical circuits. The finished circuit boards were then placed in a tub. These could be counted as a measure of productivity and workers could be paid according to the numbers of circuit boards they completed.

The first variable to be studied was the lighting – would workers be more productive in higher/lower levels of light? So, the lighting level was increased. And productivity increased. Lighting levels were lowered; productivity increased. Cleaning the workplace, removing obstacles, and changing the working positions all seemed to increase productivity. Shortening the working day increased output. Returning to the original hours increased output. Other variables were experimented with. The results were that changing a variable usually resulted in increases in production – even when the change was back to the original condition! Output seemed to slump when the experiment was ended. Note that there is some controversy about this – no one has been able to identify the original data. Thus, Richard Nisbett has described the Hawthorne effect as 'a glorified anecdote'. But, if that is what it is, I think it is an illustrative one. However, it is still used in Social Psychology as an example of compliant behaviours during experimental situations. The most controversial of these were the experiments conducted by Milgram where experimental participants were instructed to carry on giving electric shocks to supposed 'subjects' in a phoney experiment, even though the gauges showed lethally high levels of electric shocks! And Zimbardo, who set up a mock prison setting then allocated roles of 'guards' and 'prisoners' to participants – with astounding results! (Read these – you will be shocked [no pun intended] and amazed at what people will do when they think they are taking part in an experiment!)

So, the 'Hawthorne Effect' is a term we use to describe a tendency in some people to try to do their best when they are taking part in experiments. It may be that the whole experimental situation, and the attention that they receive from the researchers, results in changes in their behaviour.

I first came across the term in 1971 at a conference in Aberdeen on research into doctor–patient communication. One presenter mentioned in her work that she had taken steps to avoid the 'Hawthorne Effect'. This stunned everybody there – 'What's that?' 'Have you heard of it?' Then, after some considerable digging, someone came up with the answer, 'It's the bank wiring room experiments!' All of us had read about them in our undergraduate psychology or sociology courses and referred to them as 'the bank wiring room experiments'. This immediately prompted a tendency for conference participants to refer to spurious jargon terms to try to catch each other out! (I sometimes wonder if we ever grow up!) Of course, in medicine, the 'Hawthorne Effect' is known as and is referred to as . . . that's right, the **'Placebo Effect'**.

And that is why we tend to expect experiments involving humans to have at least two arms, one of which will involve a 'control situation' or a 'placebo group' who do not receive an active intervention or treatment.

For further reading on this topic, try Fox, Brennan, and Chasen (2008), Kolata (1998), Landsberger (1958), Levitt and List (2011), and McCarney, Warner, and Iliffe, et al. (2007).

Example 1: Martin Seligman's Learned Helplessness Experiments

Martin Seligman is one of my psychology heroes. In his early research, he was doing some experiments involving Pavlovian conditioning in dogs. These involved restraining dogs in a 'Pavlovian hammock' and giving them conditioning in which tones (sounds) were followed by electric shocks which were painful but not damaging. These shocks could not be avoided – no matter what the dog did. They were inescapable – uncontrollable. Afterwards the dogs were put in a 'shuttle box' (Figure 2.5). This was a large box divided into two sections with a dog-shoulder high barrier in the middle. The floor had a grid which could be electrified on either or both sides. Seligman (1975) eloquently describes his initial results.

> *When placed in a shuttle box, an experimentally naïve dog, at the onset of the first electric shock, runs frantically about until it accidentally scrambles over the barrier and escapes the shock. On the next trial, the dog, running frantically, crosses the barrier more quickly than on the preceding trial; within a few trials it becomes very efficient at escaping, and soon learns to avoid shock altogether. After about fifty trials the dog becomes nonchalant and stands in front of the barrier; at the onset of the signal for shock it leaps gracefully across and never gets shocked again.*
>
> *A dog that had first been given inescapable shock showed a strikingly different pattern. This dog's first reactions to shock in the shuttle box were much the same*

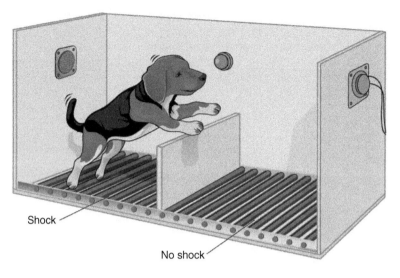

Shock

No shock

FIGURE 2.5 Shuttlebox design.

as of a naïve dog; it ran about frantically for about thirty seconds. But then
it stopped moving; to our surprise, it lay down and quietly whined. After one
minute of this we turned the shock off; the dog had failed to cross the barrier
and had not escaped from shock. On the next trial, the dog did it again; at first it
struggled a bit, and then, after a few seconds, it seemed to give up and to accept
the shock passively. On all succeeding trials, the dog failed to escape. This is the
paradigmatic learned-helplessness finding. (Seligman, 1975).

Seligman demonstrated from this and later work on human subject that learned
helplessness saps the motivation to initiate responses; disrupts the ability to learn; and
produces emotional disturbance. That is, it has three levels of effect:

- motivational
- cognitive
- emotional.

He went on to show how this effected people in real life and that this could even be
implicated in depression and death. Read his book *Learned Helplessness: On Depression,*
Development, and Death (1975); in addition to being educational, it is a thoroughly
good read!

Don Hiroto (Hiroto 1974; Hiroto and Seligman 1974) worked on learned helplessness research in humans – using the universally accepted subjects: university
students. Now, you can't put humans into shuttle-boxes, they are too unwieldy and
dangerous. But they designed a 'finger shuttle box'. This was a small box with two
compartments into which the research subject could insert her/his finger. There was
a low barrier in the middle and the subjects could move their fingers from one side
to the other. Another approach was to use a four-button board. This was a simple
board with four buttons, a green light (to indicate success), and a red light (to indicate

failure). Pushing any button four times made the noise stop immediately in the 'control' group, but not if they were in the 'helpless' group when no amount of button pushing could stop the noise. He used a **triadic** design – with subjects being **randomly assigned** to one of three groups. An **escape group** were given loud noise which could be turned off by pushing a button. A **yoked group** got the same loud noise as the escape group, but they had no control over it. The third group got **no noise.** Subjects in a yoked group are linked to the subjects in the experimental group, but have *no* control over the stimuli they are given. Next, all were taken to a finger shuttle box and were exposed to loud noise. They could escape the noise by moving their finger from one compartment of the box to the other. The escape group and the no-noise groups easily learned to escape the noise by 'shuttling' their fingers. The yoked group, however, failed to escape and avoid the noise: 'Most sat passively and accepted the adverse noise'.

Note the sophistication of this design. Both the experimental group and the yoked group got exactly the same amount of the stressor (noise). The only difference was that the experimental group could control the situation – the yoked group could not. And the control group were not exposed to the stressor at all. Thus, any differences between the experimental group and the yoked control group could not be attributed to different exposures to the stressor. And the no-noise control group acted as a group who received no stressor – that is, they acted as a group to check for any Hawthorne Effect!

Note about Giving Electric Shocks to Student Subjects in Research

It used to be widely accepted that low-level electrical shocks which were painful, but did not cause actual damage, were permissible in research studies. When I started studying Psychology at Aberdeen, the former professor had been very much into research on learning. Legend has it that he gave his research subjects higher and higher levels of electric shocks in his experiments, until they began to refuse to take part in his research – even though it meant having to fail to meet the course requirements to take part in at least three experiments! So research which involved giving electric shocks to subjects was stopped.

Seligman's work developed further to use the four-button board with a green light and a red light. The green light signalled success and the red light signalled failure after each burst of the noise. Twenty sets of white noise at 110 dB in 30 second bursts were the aversive stimuli. Students were allocated to an experimental group and a control group. All subjects were instructed that by pushing the buttons in the correct sequence they might stop the noise. If they got it right, the noise would stop and the green light would come on. If they did not get it right, the noise would not stop and the red light would come on. In the experimental group, pushing any button four times would stop the noise and the green light would come on to signal success. In the (helpless) control group, no matter which button was pushed in any sequence or in any number of times, the noise would not stop and the red light would come on to signal failure. After the trial, subjects were tested on simple cognitive tests – anagram solving and arithmetic tasks. Those in the experimental group did better than those in the helpless/control group at solving the tasks. In addition, those in the helpless/control group seemed to lose heart and give up trying to solve the tasks more than those in the experimental situation. He noted that learned helplessness, sapped the motivation to try; it had cognitive impairments, and it had affective (emotional) impairments.

Example 2: My Own Experiment

I have always been very impressed by Martin Seligman's work and was eager to do my own research on helplessness. So, when I was at the University of Hong Kong in the 1980s, I informed my staff in the Behavioural Sciences Unit in the Faculty of Medicine of my interests. Within a month, half of them had started doing their own work to replicate Seligman and Hiroto's work! My interests were in people's lifelong exposures to helplessness and how these might contribute to helpless characteristics – with the possible implications for survival from cardiovascular diseases and cancers. So, I set out on my quest. I was on 'long leave' in London. I had the necessary equipment built – a computerised control box, a set of headphones, and a four-button board. I made announcements to medical students and asked for volunteers for my pilot study. I vividly remember my first two subjects.

The first was in the **control group** – no matter what buttons he pressed, or in what order, or how many times, the noise could not be turned off and the red light would come on to signify failure. I remember him on the last of the 20 trials; he was bashing away at the buttons, frantically trying to find the correct sequence. Afterwards, I interviewed him about his life history of feeling in control or helpless. He was what you could call a 'straight A student'. He had five As or A*s in his A levels. He had never failed an exam in his life. He could never recall or imagine a situation in which he would not succeed. He said to me, 'Gosh, John, that was a really interesting trial. I know I didn't get it right in the time, but, I reckon that, with a few more goes, I could have got it right!' I de-briefed him about the experiment.

The second subject was in the **experimental group.** By pressing any button four times he could stop the noise immediately. He learned very quickly how he could stop the noise. I remember him on the last of the 20 trials; he looked fed up. As soon as the noise started be quickly pushed a button four times and the noise stopped. Afterwards, I interviewed him about his life history of feeling in control or helpless. He was also what you could call a 'straight A student'. He had five As or A*s in his A levels. He had never failed an exam in his life. He could never recall or imagine a situation in which he would not succeed. He said to me, 'I'm sorry, John, that was a real disappointment. I know that I could stop the noise by pushing a button four time. But it can't be as simple as that, so I don't feel that I really got it right – I didn't understand it!' I de-briefed him about the experiment.

This confirmed to me the importance of checking with experimental subjects *what they think is going on in the experiment.* The first subject felt that he was in control – even though he was in the 'helpless' group. The second subject thought he was helpless – even though he was in the 'control' group! The difference between them was *the sense they made of the trial* – how they **attributed** their part in the trial. Interesting, isn't it? But before I could complete my study, two things happened: (i) my equipment broke down and could not be repaired; and, more disappointingly to me, (ii) Martin Seligman and Judy Garber published their book *Human Helplessness: Theory and Applications,* in which they expounded in great detail an **attributional analysis** of learned helplessness – just the sort of thing I believed I had discovered!

Randomisation

Randomisation in experimental designs refers to the process by which your research participants are allocated to one group or another. (It does not, as some people think, refer to the recruitment of the sample.) The idea is that, by assigning participants to groups entirely by chance, this will avoid any **bias** or preference by the researchers. It is a means of ensuring equity, or fairness, in the distribution of participants to groups. Successful randomisation will ensure that each group of participants is roughly equal in characteristics, and should be roughly equal in their chances of performing in any tasks or tests they are given. When I started out as a researcher, we used to have 'tables of random numbers' which we had to refer to for allocations. Nowadays it is all done by computer, and quite rightly so. Never trust any method of randomisation which a human being can control or influence!

To Sum Up

First: you state clearly what you intend to do and why – including your hypotheses – if any. At this point, consider whether your study will be a single-arm experiment or whether it will have more arms?

1. Then you decide who, or what, you want to include in your research, and how you will recruit them.
2. Next, if you have more than one arm, you should randomly allocate your research participants, or 'subjects' to the different groups.
3. You conduct the experiment and you note the results.
4. You analyse your results.
5. You disseminate your results by presenting the findings at conferences, or by publishing them in a book or in professional journals.

So, in Hiroto's and Seligman's work, their goals were clearly stated and linked to earlier work. They recruited an appropriate number (96) of psychology students and randomly allocated them to one of the three groups – the 'control', the 'yoked control', and the 'helpless' groups. They began the experiments by the 'pre-treatment' helplessness testing/treatment. Then they tested the subjects' abilities to perform physical or cognitive tasks (performance on a shuttle-box scenario, anagram testing, or discrimination testing). They measured the final performances of the three groups of subjects and finally they compared them. Then they published their findings and toured the world giving talks about their work before moving on to develop their work further. Nice work if you can get it!

Research is the art of the possible!

References

Fox NS, Brennan JS, Chasen ST. (2008). Clinical estimation of fetal weight and the Hawthorne effect. *European Journal of Obstetrics, Gynecology, and Reproductive Biology* 141 (2): 111.

Hiroto DS. (1974). Locus of control and learned helplessness. *Journal of Experimental Psychology* 102: 187–193.

Hiroto DS and Seligman MEP. (1974). Generality of learned helplessness. *Journal of Personality and Social Psychology* 31(2): 311–327.

Kolata G. (1998). *Scientific myths that are too good to die*. New York Times (6 December).

Landsberger HA. (1958). *Hawthorne Revisited*. The New York State School of Industrial and Labor Relations: Ithaca.

Levitt SD and John AL. (2011). Was There Really a Hawthorne Effect at the Hawthorne Plant? An Analysis of the Original Illumination Experiments. *American Economic Journal: Applied Economics* 3(1): 224–238.

McCarney R, Warner J, Iliffe S, et al. (2007). The Hawthorne effect: a randomised, controlled trial. *BMC Medical Research Methodology* 7: 30.

Renee D. (1959). *Mirage of Health*. Harper & Row Publishers: New York.

Seligman M. (1975). *Learned Helplessness: On Depression, Development, and Death*. WH Freeman and Company: San Francisco.

Tuckett D. (1976) *An Introduction to Medical Sociology*. Tavistock Publications: London.

CHAPTER 3

Experimental Quantitative Approaches
Real-Life (Field) Experiments

Introduction

It is time now for us to move out of the laboratory. Let's consider some experiments which have been done in **real-life situations.** There have been experimental studies which have been set up in real-life situations – in everyday settings.

They tend to involve work which could not be conducted in laboratories – they are **naturalistic** – i.e., they are done in real-life situations. In many, it may not be possible to introduce experimental variables, or to randomise participants to experimental and control groups. However, at times situations may arise which result in there being an 'experimental-like' situation, or a **quasi-experimental** situation, which allows us to make observations and measurements – as though it were a laboratory experiment. In this chapter we shall have a look at them and the issues that come up in them.

So, real-life experiments:

- Are still in the **quantitative** domain – we measure and count, we use numbers.
- They are usually **hypothetico-deductive** – we have a clear purpose and set of expectations in mind before we begin.
- They are in the **interventional** sector – we introduce an experimental variable which was not there at the start.
- They are **prospective** – we have a start point where we make our initial measurements, we have our interventions, and we have an end point when we make our final measurements.
- They are useful for answering questions about what would happen in a real-life situation if we changed one or more of the factors in that situation.

We have less control over them because they are being conducted in a natural setting – often like the 'Candid Camera' or 'You've Been Framed' TV programmes

Demystifying Research for Medical & Healthcare Students: An Essential Guide, First Edition. John L. Anderson.
© 2022 John Wiley & Sons Ltd. Published 2022 by John Wiley & Sons Ltd.
Companion website: www.wiley.com/go/Anderson/DemystifyingResearch

where hidden cameras or observers record what happens. Sometimes situations occur when an experiment is not being conducted deliberately, but the circumstances are such that we can make comparisons between two different approaches to tackling the same issue and we can compare the findings – insofar as we can – for the different results. Let's begin with a classic case study.

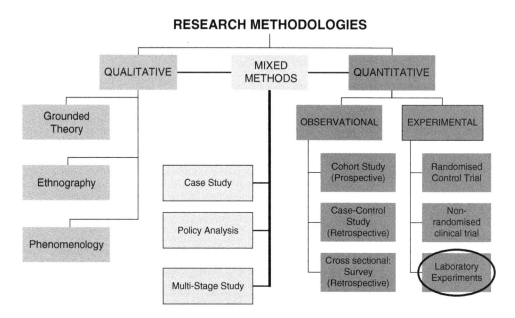

Example 1: The Nineteenth-Century Cholera Epidemic in London

At the time of the cholera outbreak in London in 1854, the prevailing medical view was that it, like some other diseases, such as plague and malaria, were caused by a 'miasma' or 'bad air' which emanated from the ground. John Snow was a sceptic of this theory (Figure 3.1). So, during the outbreak of cholera in the Soho area of London, he talked to local residents and mapped the pattern of the disease. As a result, he identified what he thought to be the source of the outbreak as the public water pump on Broad Street, and his 'experiment' was *to remove the handle of the pump!* This controlled the outbreak and demonstrated to his satisfaction the role of water in the transmission of cholera (Snow 1849).

After the outbreak had passed, the authorities replaced the pump handle. They rejected Snow's explanation that faecal contamination of the water supply was responsible for the cholera outbreak, as it was too unpleasant at that time to accept the faecal–oral route of transmission (Chapelle 2005). How times have changed!

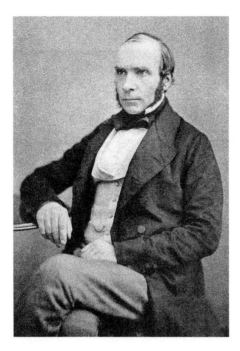

FIGURE 3.1   John Snow – being very smart and learned. *Source*: Unknown author / Wikimedia Commons / Public domain.

Example 2: The Paddington Station Experiment

Mary Sissons conducted her classic study of interactions between people of different social classes in Paddington Station in London (Sissons, 1971). Thinking of all the happy hours I have spent waiting for trains there between 1967 and now makes me realise how much it has changed. It used to be much larger inside before the shops and restaurants were added, and therefore there were many more offices overlooking the vast station concourse. It was the perfect place for 'people watching'. So, Mary was able to set up her cameras in the offices overlooking the station concourse. Of course, this sort of study raises many more ethical issues now than it did then – see Reece and Siegal's (1991) book on the ethics of social research.

She hired an actor who dressed up in one of two different roles. In his 'middle-class' role he dressed up in manual worker's clothes and spoke and behaved as though he was 'working-class'. In his 'middle-class' role, he was dressed like a businessman and talked and behaved as though he was 'middle-class'. He approached 80 people and asked them if they could tell him the way to Hyde Park (which is a five-minute walk from the station). For half, he was in his 'middle-class' role and for half, he was in his 'working-class' role. The interactions were filmed from the offices and audio-recorded by a hidden microphone carried by the actor. Once the interactions had ended, a researcher approached the 'subjects', explained the study to them, interviewed them and obtained their consent for their participation in the study.

She found that middle-class to middle-class interactions went more smoothly than any others. Instant rapport was more likely, the interactions lasted longer, there was more smiling and there was a definite ending. This experiment was used by the Open University and the BBC as a featured example of Field Research. Google it! Watch the video.

Example 3: Urban Sound Planning in Brighton and Hove

A colleague at BSMS, Harry Witchell, worked with Brighton and Hove City Council to help solve a common urban problem – that of safety in tunnels, or underpasses, specifically the Brighton Beach Tunnel. In the past, there were problems with public safety because of anti-social behaviours which led to the tunnel's closure. In an attempt to try to make this a 'more inviting and safer' environment, due to increases in its use, an experiment was carried out. Video cameras and a sound system were installed in the tunnel.

> *The music interventions were played between the hours of 07:00 pm and 07:00 am on Thursday nights, Friday nights, and Saturday nights; for the duration of the pilot study, the tunnel was left open all night on these nights. Playlists of traditional, archetypal representatives of classical, jazz, and contemporary dance music (and silence) were cycled repeatedly to tunnel users, most of whom passed through the music intervention in approximately 30 seconds; the music was chosen to be non-aversive, and the played sound level was measured to have a LAeq ranging from 68 to 81 dB(A).*

> *Extensive data were gathered in the form of video files; based on motion sensing, over 15,000 filmed episodes were recorded, with almost all of these having one or more individuals moving in the tunnel (Easteal et al., 2015).*

So, in this natural space, it was possible to introduce one of four **sound interventions:**

- classical music;
- jazz;
- contemporary dance music; and
- silence.

> *'Participants' were naïve members of the public who were passing through the tunnel. There was no randomisation as such, but the four conditions (classical music; jazz; contemporary dance music; and silence) were equally cycled, so there was a 'random' effect in terms of exposure to each of these. All participants were unknown – they were anonymous. The results were interesting.*

Classical music seemed to lessen loitering when compared to silence or other music. Music with a faster tempo led to faster walking speeds. The researchers also noted an unexpected effect of music – dancing in the tunnel. Also, in a daytime experiment, 'brief exposure to music led to an increase in charitable donations to collectors for the Martlets Hospice'.

They concluded that 'At the end of the experiment, no vandalism or weather damage occurred to any of the equipment, suggesting that this intervention strategy can work in an open public space at night.'

I like this experiment. It's nice to have an experiment which notes an unexpected result – dancing! It demonstrated a good partnership between the Local Authority and the University; and it gave meaningful results which had an immediate practical application.

Note: There is no requirement for REC approval for studies which are 'naturalistic observations' of people. Filming in public – as long as no individuals can be identified in any publications or presentations of the results – does not raise any untoward ethical issues.

Example 4: An Experiment to Examine T2DM Decision Making

John McKinlay is an old teacher, friend, and mentor of mine. We met in Aberdeen in 1966, and he left there to go to MIT in Boston (USA) where he established the New England Research Institute and has become one of the most prolific and successful sociologists of all time. Along with others in his Institute, he conducted a series of studies of diabetes – including some very interesting and innovative experiments. In one (McKinley et al. 2012), they were interested in finding out if there were race/ethnic differences in the diagnosis of diabetes when physicians are experimentally presented with signs and symptoms of diabetes.

Previous work in the USA had found that Type-2 Diabetes Mellitus (T2DM) varied considerably by race/ethnicity. They noted that:

Both the National Institutes of Health (NIH) and the American Diabetes Association (ADA) report race/ethnicity to be a major independent contributor to T2DM. Assuming the race/ethnic disparity in T2DM to be real, researchers seek its explanation in either: (a) social and behavioral risk factors or life styles; or increasingly, (b) genetic contributions and family history. We consider a third possible contributor to race/ethnic disparities in T2DM – the racial/ethnic patterning resulting from diagnostic decisions, principally by primary care providers. Notwithstanding the possibility of a modest race/ethnic contribution, we question whether the reported wide race/ethnic variation in the prevalence of physician diagnosed T2DM accurately reflects its actual distribution in the general population. We hypothesize the actual prevalence of signs and symptoms of T2DM, when undiagnosed in the community, is patterned far more strongly by SES (than by race/ethnicity), but when eventually diagnosed by physicians it is patterned more by race/ethnicity (than by SES).

To investigate the size and distribution of undiagnosed T2DM in the community, they designed and conducted a **random sample survey** in the general population in the Boston area – The Boston Area Community Health (BACH) Survey. This was an epidemiological survey of Boston residents aged between 30 and 79 years. A 'stratified two-stage cluster sample was used to recruit residents of Boston with approximately equal numbers of participants by gender, race/ethnicity (non-Hispanic black, Hispanic, non-Hispanic white), and age group (30–39, 40–49, 50–59, 60–79)'. Altogether, 5503 adults participated (1767 black, 1877 Hispanic, 1859 white; 2301 men and 3202 women) – a response rate of 63.3% of eligible participants. Anyone who reported five of the six cardinal symptoms – fatigue; being overweight; frequent urination; thirst; not feeling well; hypertension – was considered to be highly likely to have undiagnosed T2DM.

This part of the study showed 'no significant race/ethnic differences in the prevalence of the (undiagnosed) signs and symptoms indicative of diabetes within a socioeconomic level (lower class $\chi2$ $p = 0.79$, middle class $\chi2$ $p = 0.34$, upper class $\chi2$ $p = 0.40$). However, significant differences are evident by SES ($\chi2$ $p < 0.0001$), and they are consistent within each race/ethnic category'. So – *no racial differences* in the prevalence of T2DM, but there were differences according to *socio-economic status*. This set the scene for the experimental study.

In the **experimental** part of the study, they used video scenarios of real clinical cases, with professional actors and actresses, trained to realistically simulate a 'patient' presenting to a primary care doctor. There were 24 identical versions of the clinical scenario. These varied only with the patients' age, gender, socio-economic status, and race. The vignettes simulated an initial consultation of five to seven minutes.

The 'subjects' were 192 primary care doctors who viewed the vignettes and were asked to give the most likely diagnosis and their degree of certainty. They were then interviewed and asked to say how they would manage the case in their practice.

As they describe:

A factorial experiment is a research design consisting of two or more factors (e.g. race/ethnicity, gender, and socioeconomic status) each with discrete values (or 'levels'). All possible combinations of these levels across the factors are then randomly assigned to subjects. Such experiments permit estimation of the effect of each factor on the response variable, as well as the effects of interactions between factors and the response variable. This approach permits estimation of the unconfounded effect of a 'patient's' race/ethnicity (also age, gender and SES) on diagnostic decision making when primary care physicians encounter different randomly assigned patients presenting with exactly the same signs and symptoms strongly suggesting undiagnosed diabetes.

An ordered version of a clinical vignette varying only the 'patient's' race/ethnicity (non-Hispanic black, Hispanic, or non-Hispanic white), age (35 or 65 years), gender, and SES (as depicted by their dress and occupation as a janitor or a lawyer) was shown to each of 192 licensed internists, family physicians, or general practitioners practicing in New Jersey, New York, or Pennsylvania. Physicians were also required to be graduates of an accredited medical school in the US and to be providing clinical care at least half time. Since this study was part of a larger international study concerning the management of T2DM in different countries (health care systems) it was not possible to include international medical graduates (IMGs). We stratified physician subjects according to gender and level of clinical experience (graduated from medical school between 1993–1999 (less experience) or between 1969–1983 (more experience)) (there were 2 × 2 = 4 strata) and recruited eligible physicians until each of the 4 strata was complete. Each of 24 vignette pairs was viewed twice in each of the 4 strata for a total of (24 × 2 × 4=) 192 physicians.

Sampling of physicians was done using a **purposive sample** to fill each design cells (male/female; more/less experienced) – rather than a straight random sample of physicians. In this way, they were more quickly able to get the required numbers to fit the profiles they needed for the study.

Thus, the permutations were as shown in Table 3.1:

Their results showed that doctors were significantly more likely to diagnose diabetes in the black and the Hispanic 'patients', 73.4% of the physicians' diagnosed T2DM when the 'patient' was black, 60.9% when Hispanic and 48.4% when white ($p = 0.009$) – when fully adjusted for the 'patient's' age, gender, and SES, the percentage of physicians giving a diabetes diagnosis was 64.5% for lower SES patients (janitor) versus 57.3% for upper SES patients (lawyer) ($p = 0.265$) and the corresponding level of certainty for lower SES patients was 24.4 compared to 20.4 for upper SES patients ($p = 0.241$). In other words, in making an initial diagnosis, physicians focus more on the 'patient's' race/ethnicity rather than their SES.

They concluded: 'this paper suggests that the signs and symptoms of T2DM, when undiagnosed in the general community, are patterned by SES and not race/ethnicity and that following diagnosis by a physician they are patterned by race/ethnicity'.

Don't you think that is interesting? It raised, for them, the question about whether the higher rates of black and Hispanic persons diagnosed with T2DM was a result of a **racially-skewed stereotype** rather than a true profile of the population in need of care.

Remember Mick Bloor's saying: 'Research is the art of the possible'? John's study was well-funded. Thus, they were able to hire and train actresses. They were able to develop the scenarios of the 'patients'. They were able to conduct the sampling in a very professional manner. They were able to get the physicians to spend their time taking part in the experiment. Thus, they were able to go beyond the laboratory. They were able to do the experiment with real, practising physicians, rather than with medical students. And they had the expert statistical expertise required for their very complex analyses within their organisation. Well done them!

Example 5: Reduction of Postoperative Pain by Encouragement and Instruction of Patients

This is one of my favourite field experiments. It is halfway between being an experiment and a randomised control trial (RCT) (see next chapter). It was conducted in 1964, so it is a classic, both in the temporal (time) sense and in its importance. A group of

TABLE 3.1 Patient and physician characteristics in each vignette.

'Patient' Characteristics in each Vignette											
Male						Female					
Age 35						Age 35					
Low SES			High SES			Low SES			High SES		
B	H	W	B	H	W	B	H	W	B	H	W

Male						Female					
Age 65						Age 65					
Low SES			High SES			Low SES			High SES		
B	H	W	B	H	W	B	H	W	B	H	W

Physician Characteristics

Less Experienced	More Experienced
Male	Female

anaesthetists and surgeons in Boston (USA) were concerned about the problems of treating postoperative pain (Egbert et al. 1964). So, they devised a study to test a theory about how postop pain might be better managed.

They recruited 97 patients who were admitted to their hospital for abdominal operations (appendicectomy, cholycystectomy, etc.). These were randomly allocated to a 'special care' (experimental) group or a 'normal care' (control) group. The **control group** all received their normal treatment – no more and no less. Throughout their hospital stay.

Those in the special care group received their normal care, plus:

1. When the anaesthetist visited them the evening before the operation, they were told that they would experience pain after the operation, how severe it would be, and how long it would last. They were reassured that this pain was normal after an operation.
2. They were told that they would receive pain killing drugs.
3. They were given advice about how to minimise the pain – by relaxing the abdominal muscles. They were given instructions on how to turn over in bed, and they were told that they should request medication if they needed it.
4. On the afternoon, after the operation, the anaesthetist visited them again. He went over what he had told them the evening before; reassured them that their pain was normal; and they were again told to ask for medication if they wanted it.
5. This was repeated the next morning, and once or twice a day until they did not need any more analgesic medication.

The control group received their normal care throughout.

An independent observer (an anaesthetist who the patients had not met) visited 57 of them to record the patients' evaluations about their pain, as well as noting his own impressions about their appearance.

This was a **double-blind** experiment. The patients were not told that they were part of an experiment – **first blind.** The nursing staff, who administered the medications, and the surgical staff who made decisions about the patients' discharge, did not know that there was an experiment in progress – **second blind.** In this way, they avoided the. . . what? That's right . . . the **Hawthorne Effect,** or in this case, the **placebo effect.** The researchers were well aware of the potential for a placebo effect – enhanced by patients trying to please them and nursing staff trying to please the surgeons – or vice versa. So by using the double-blind design, they minimised, to the best of their ability, the potential for this.

The results were interesting. Remember, the special care group were warned that they would experience pain and were encouraged to ask for as much medication as they wanted. You might think that this would have made them super-vigilant and sensitive about their pain and, along with the invitation to dip into the analgesic jar as often as they wanted, their medication use might be high. The researchers were able to calculate the use of pain killers for each patient, and then to compare the two groups. The results showed that the special care group used *half as much* analgesic as the control group. (See Figure 3.2.) The independent observer noted that the special care group patients 'appeared to be more comfortable and in better physical and emotional condition than the control group". The surgeons discharged patients in the special care group on average *2.7 days* earlier than those in the control group.

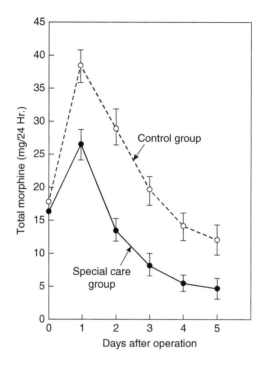

FIGURE 3.2 Postoperative treatment with narcotics (Means for each day + Standard error of the mean).

Don't you just love this study? It was a relatively inexpensive one to conduct. And its findings were clear. The study design was a dream (Figure 3.3).

1. They identified a problem– post-operative pain in surgical patients.

2. They developed an intervention based upon current theory and knowledge – the psychology of fear and stress. They took from that the fact that if we know in advance that something stressful or unpleasant is about to happen, then we are better able to prepare ourselves to deal with it. And, if we have a sense of control, we are more likely to be able to cope with it.

3. Their interventions were based upon theory - aspects of the of the psychology of fear and stress (Janis, 1958). These were: (i) **anticipation** – warning the patients in advance that they would experience pain; and (ii) giving them a **sense of control** – 'you can do this to help avoid the pain' and 'you can ask for as much pain-killing medication as you want'. They worked!

4. They engaged an appropriate methodology – a twin-arm, double-blind, experimental approach, and chose a consecutive series of patients to participate in it.

5. They carried out the study and analysed their results.

6. They published their results for all the world to see!

This study could be called an RCT. But the researchers described it as an **experiment.** So, I have included it in this chapter as a fine example of what can be achieved when experimental design is applied in a real-life situation. In the next chapter I shall discuss RCTs.

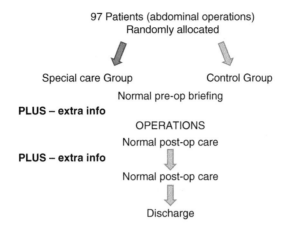

FIGURE 3.3   Egbert et al.'s research design.

Let me tell you something about this study and its findings. I have taught about it since 1974. I have lectured about it to medical and nursing students, to psychology students, to sociology students, to healthcare administrators, undergraduates and postgraduates, and to members of the public. All but one of these groups either said something like, 'Oh, that's interesting'. (yawn), or 'We already know that' (not!). The one group who sat up and started taking notes were . . . Guess who? . . .Yes – the *healthcare administrators!* I could almost see them doing the calculations, Half our analgesics budget, that's about £xxx,000! And 2.7 hospital bed days in a surgical ward – that about £5000–6000 per patient! Meanwhile, those who should have been thinking, 'How can I use this study to improve my patients' care?' (medical and nursing students) were yawning or dismissing it! Sometimes, it's a hard job being a teacher!

To Sum Up

You can see clearly that these real-life experiments we have looked at above are **quantitative** – they all use numerical data! They are clearly **hypothetico-deductive** – they had a clear purpose and set of expectations in mind before they began. They are in the **interventional** domain – they introduced an experimental variable which was not there at the start; from Snow removing the handle of the water pump to Egbert et al. providing additional information to surgical patients. They are **prospective** – they all had a start point where they made their initial measurements, they had their interventions, and they had an end point when they made their final measurements. And they were all conducted outside of the lab!

- You can see that Snow's 'experiment' was a single-arm one – He believed that if he removed the pump handle, then people would not be able to drink contaminated water. He did it and the cases reduced.
- The Paddington Station and the Brighton Tunnel experiments were good examples of testing behaviour in public places. Their 'interventions' – an actor in different

roles in Paddington, and different music, in Brighton, evoked different behaviours which were filmed, noted, and measured.

- Egbert used the everyday practice of preparing patients for operations as an opportunity to add an intervention – special briefing – and then to note and measure the impact of this in comparison with no special briefing.
- McKinley, in Boston, used actors as the 'interventions' and by noting physician's responses to different actors was able to determine how actors from different ethnic/racial backgrounds were treated in different ways.

Research is the art of the possible!

References

Chapelle F. (2005). *Wellsprings*. Rutgers University Press: *New Brunswick*. New Jersey, p. 82.

Easteal M, Bannister S, Francesco JK, et al. (2015). Urban sound planning in Brighton and Hove. *Conference paper presented at Forum Acusticum*, 7–12 September, Krakow.

Egbert LD, Battit GE, Welch CE, et al. (1964). Reduction of postoperative pain by encouragement and instruction of patients: a study of doctor-patient rapport. *New England Journal of Medicine* 20(16): 825–827.

Janis IL. (1958). *Psychological Stress: Psychoanalytic and Behavioural Studies of Surgical Patients*. Wiley: New York.

John S. (1849). *On the Mode of Communication of Cholera*. John Churchill: London.

John BM, Lisa DM, and Rebecca JP. (2012). Do doctors contribute to the social patterning of disease? The case of race/ethnic disparities in diabetes mellitus. *Medical Care Research* 69(2): 176–193.

Reece RD and Siegal HA. (1991). *Studying People: A Primer in the Ethics of Social Research*. Mercer University Press: Georgia.

Sissons M. (1971). *The psychology of social class in Money, Wealth and Class*. Open University Press: Milton Keynes.

CHAPTER 4

Experimental Quantitative Approaches

Non-randomised Clinical Trials

Introduction

Clinical trials of new forms of tests or treatment begin with **Phase I** trials then **Phase II** Trials. (**Phase III** trials or **Randomised Control Trials** (RCTs) are covered in the next chapter.)

These early trials to test new forms of assessing or treating patients are:

- Still in the **quantitative** domain – we measure and quantify what we are observing.
- They are usually **hypothetico-deductive** – we test a hypothesis.
- They are **interventional** – the new forms of testing or treating patients form our interventions.
- And they are **prospective** – we recruit a group of participants, and we give them our new test or treatment and we measure the outcomes.

The difference between these and the experimental approaches we have discussed so far, is that **these do not include a control group.**

Before we test new medicines on people, we usually test them in the laboratory first. The *ABPI Handbook* states this:

> *. . . before an IMP can be given to humans, sponsors must first test it thoroughly in animals. The main aims of these pre-clinical studies are:*
>
> - *to find out the effects of the IMP on body systems (pharmacodynamics)*
> - *to study the blood levels of the IMP, and how it is absorbed, distributed, metabolised and eliminated after dosing (pharmacokinetics)*
> - *to find out if a range of doses of the IMP, up to many times higher than those intended for use in humans, are toxic to animals and if so, to identify the target organs and the margin of safety in terms of (a) the*

*no-observed-adverse-effect dose level (NOAEL) relative to body weight and
(b) IMP exposure – the concentration of IMP in the bloodstream over 24
hours (toxicokinetics), and*

- *to make a formulation of the IMP, such as a capsule or injection, suitable for
early studies in humans.*

*After the pre-clinical studies, there are four phases of trials in humans, which
in practice often overlap. Phases 1 to 3 are done before a licence is granted and
Phase 4 is done after authorisation to market the drug. The phases are different
in terms of the number and types of subject studied, and the questions asked.
The numbers in the table are indicative only and can vary.*

(ABPI 2014)

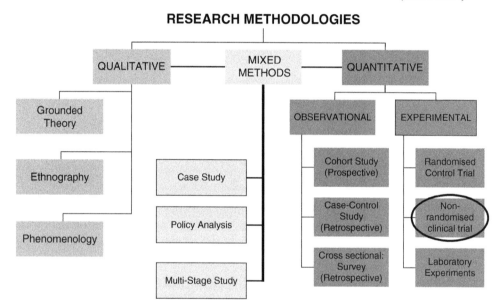

Phase 0 Clinical Trials

These are sometimes the first tests of a new drug or treatment in humans. I say 'sometimes', because it is more often the case that we start with Phase 1 trials. Phase 0 trials usually involve very small numbers of subjects and involve giving them very low doses of the trial substance to make sure there are no harmful effects.

Phase I Clinical Trials

Phase I clinical trials are those studies where we are testing a diagnostic procedure or a treatment *for the first time in humans*. Previous studies will have been done on potential new medicines in laboratories on chemical, biological specimens, and animals. Now it is time to try these out in 'real life' on human subjects. And the first issue to be addresses is: 'How safe are they?' The second issue relates to 'How much can we safely give?' So Phase I clinical trials *used* to be designed to test:

1. The *safety* of the new drug – what are the **side effects** if any?
2. What is a *safe dose range* we can give – what is the *Maximum Tolerable Dose* (MTD)?

They *did not use to be* concerned with effectiveness. However, there has been a gradual shift over the past years (in my view to help accelerate the process for the drug companies) to include wider goals for these trials, and the Health Research Authority (**HRA**) defines them as such:

> *A Phase 1 trial is usually the first time that an IMP is tested in humans and so it will usually investigate the safe dose range and potential side effects, how it is metabolised and whether it might work in patients.*

> *(My italics, HRA 2020)*

The HRA website is one of my favourites! I can spend days browsing it. In 2016, when it was first being set up, I used to spend hours and hours going round and round in circles trying to find out what approvals were needed for which kinds of research and trying out the decision-making tools. I used to joke, rather bitterly then, that there were lots of tools in the HRA; but things have greatly improved and now it really is a useful website!

The shift in focus to include 'whether it might work in patients' reflects increasing pressure to streamline the process of developing new drugs. This has led to concerns in some circles that corners are being cut and participants' welfare may be at risk. Such trials can impose quite a burden on participants. They may have to spend considerable time as residents in the test centre. They may be subjected to many tests – often invasive such as endoscopies and lumbar punctures. Healthy volunteers are normally paid a fee. (Many students do this in their holidays to earn money.) Matt Lamkin and Carl Elliot give an account of a strange situation in the 1960, when two comedy presenters approached a naïve man on the street and made him a bizarre offer:

> *Posing as the hosts of a radio program called 'Job Opportunities', Jim Coyle and Mal Sharpe explained that they needed an employee for a new tourist attraction. In this attraction, the employee would be confined to a flame-filled pit where he would try to fight off bats, snakes, and maniacs. 'What we're trying to do, really, is create a living hell', Coyle explained. 'Have people pay admission; they look down in the pit; they see you down there; the flames are all around you. There will be four maniacs with you and you've got to control them'. Then Sharpe asked the prospective employee, 'Have you ever worked with maniacs before?' 'No, never', the man said. In exchange for spending twelve hours a day fighting maniacs, the employee would be paid $46 a week, plus one meal a day – bat meat, which the employee would be expected to grill in the flames. The job would carry some risks, Coyle explained. 'I had an employee before, and I will tell you this directly and honestly, he was a little careless and incautious – I gave him specific instructions – and he perished', Coyle says. 'Now I want you to understand this before we get any further. He did perish'. The man was undeterred. 'Yeah, I'd like to try it', he said, sticking with his decision even when*

Sharpe reminded him that the death index for the job was 98%. 'In other words', Sharpe said, 'if you took this job the odds would be 98% in favor of your perishing'. The man replied, 'It's a chance. I like to take chances'.

(Lamkin and Elliot 2018)

I think the point they are making is that some people will volunteer for, or take very low pay for, dangerous work which has a risk of them not surviving it – very much like Phase 1 trials.

Phase I Clinical Trials in Oncology

Cancer Research UK (who funded the unit I used to work in) give the following information about Phase 1 Oncology trials:

Patients are recruited very slowly onto phase 1 trials. So even though they don't recruit many people, they can take a long time to complete.

They are often dose escalation studies. This means that the first few patients that take part (called a cohort or group) are given a very small dose of the drug. If all goes well, the next group have a slightly higher dose. The dose is gradually increased with each group. The researchers monitor the side effects people have and how they feel, until they find the best dose.

In a phase 1 trial you may have lots of blood tests because the researchers look at how your body copes with and gets rid of the drug. They carefully record any side effects you may have and when you have them.

The main aim of phase 1 trials is to find out about doses and side effects. They need to do this first, before testing the potential new treatment to see if it works. Some people taking part may benefit from the new treatment, but many won't.

(CRUK 2020)

Phase 1 **oncology trials** are usually conducted using people who have cancer, and who have had all the treatments that are available, but which do not help anymore. They usually have to have a life expectancy of at least three months – so that they can be complete the trial (Arkenau et al. 2008). They are not usually paid for taking part, unlike non-cancer clinical trial participants. The trials can involve a large commitment, both in terms of time, travel, and discomfort.

One of the dangers of taking part in a Phase 1 trial in the hope of finding a last-minute, miracle cure is the **therapeutic misconception** – the belief that they are receiving treatment to help 'cure' their cancer. Thus, the way in which trial doctors explain the purpose of the trial and what they will go through has been subject of concern and they has been subjected to a lot of scrutiny. People with such advanced cancers have little hope of a miraculous cure. Sure, there is always that one grain of hope that there will be a trial of a new wonder drug which might save their lives – and no one would want to take any hope away. But we should not raise their expectations unduly. On the plus side, participants do get a lot of attention when they are on the trials. They are monitored carefully and anything significant can be communicated to their GP or Oncologist. They have something to hope for – and this can be very important to some people. However, like many of the chemotherapies which many participants would have been on in the past, there can be quite serious, even life-threatening, side effects of the agents they are given. It is a big commitment and I have every respect for those who say 'I am doing it for the benefit of others'.

One team published a paper in 2008, summarising the results of 29 Phase 1 trials at the Marsden Hospital in London. They analysed the outcomes of 212 patients who took part in these trials. Arkenau et al. describe them thus:

> *A total of 148* **patients** *(70%)* **were treated** *in 'first in human trials' involving biological agents (132* **patients***) or new cytotoxic compounds (16* **patients***) alone and 64* **patients** *(30%) received chemotherapy-based regimens with or without biological agents.*

I have highlighted their use of the terms 'patients' and 'treated'. (This type of terminology was common when Rachel Ballinger and I did our analysis of communication between trial doctors and potential trial participants – I shall describe this later in Chapter 14) These terms perpetuate the therapeutic misconception – 'I am still a patient being treated'.

Arkenau et al. evaluated the tumours before the third cycle of the trial – between weeks 6 and 8. They reported a 'partial response' in 19 people (9.4%), stable disease in 88 people (44%), and progression of disease in 95 (47%). 'The 30- and 90-day mortality was 1.9% (4 out of 212) and 18.3% (39 out of 212), respectively. Treatment related mortality was 0.47% (1 out of 212) and 11.8% (25 out of 212) of the patients have been withdrawn from an ongoing study due to toxicity' (Arkenau et al. 2008). So, half a percent of people died because of the effects of the trial agents (or 'treatments' as they were described). They concluded:

> *This analysis demonstrated that treatment within the context of a phase I trial could be considered as a valuable therapeutic option. Interestingly, those trials incorporating classical cytotoxics were associated with a better outcome. Clearly, this relates to patient selection, particularly when the trial may involve the use of a cytotoxic in chemonaive cases. The treatment in our cohort was generally well tolerated and treatment-related deaths and toxicities were low. Moreover, a significant number of patients achieved disease control for a significant duration. However, the challenge remains in appropriate patient selection and for this, the use of an objective clinical score could be a helpful tool.*
>
> *(Arkenau et al. 2008)*

Now, here is a challenge for you: (i) What sense do you make of these findings? (ii) What is missing from these trials? (My thoughts are given at the end of the chapter.)

Phase II Clinical Trials

If Phase I trials show that a new agent is relatively safe, the next step in the development of a new drug is a **Phase II trial.** These specifically check *effectiveness* – to see if it does what we want it to do. But these trials continue to monitor the safety and side effects of the developing treatment. Larger numbers are recruited into these trials. The CRUK literature defines them like this:

> *Phase II trials aim to find out:*
>
> - *if the new treatment works well enough to be tested in a larger Phase III trial;*
> - *which types of cancer the treatment works for;*
> - *more about side effects and how to manage them;*
> - *more about the best dose to use.*
>
> *These treatments have been tested in Phase I trials, but may still have side effects that the doctors don't know about. Treatments can affect people in different ways.*
>
> *Phase II trials are usually larger than phase I. There may be up to 100 or so people taking part. Sometimes in a phase II trial, a new treatment is compared with another treatment already in use, or with a dummy drug (placebo).*
>
> *Some Phase II trials are randomised. This means the researchers put the people taking part into treatment groups at random.*
>
> (CRUK 2020)

Again, the principles are the same for cancer drug trials as for other drug trials except that cancer drug trials usually recruit people with cancer and do not pay them; whereas, in other drug trials, healthy volunteers are recruited to take part and they are paid.

Safety in Clinical Trials

There have been some tragic events during Phase I and Phase II trials. Some have been noted above in relation to Phase I oncology trials. But other trials involving heathy volunteers have ended in tragedy. I have selected a few to illustrate this.

TGN 1412 Trial

Six healthy young male volunteers at a contract research organisation were enrolled in the first Phase I clinical trial of TGN1412, a novel superagonist anti-CD28 monoclonal antibody that directly stimulates T cells. Within 90 minutes after receiving a single intravenous dose of the drug, all six volunteers had a systemic inflammatory response characterised by a rapid induction of proinflammatory cytokines and accompanied by headache, myalgias, nausea, diarrhoea, erythema, vasodilatation, and hypotension. Within 12–16 hours after infusion, they became critically ill, with pulmonary infiltrates and lung injury, renal failure, and disseminated intravascular coagulation. Severe and unexpected depletion of lymphocytes and monocytes occurred within 24 hours after infusion. All six patients were transferred to the care of the authors at an intensive care unit at a public hospital, where they received intensive cardiopulmonary support (including dialysis), high-dose methylprednisolone, and an anti-interleukin-2 receptor antagonist antibody. Prolonged cardiovascular shock and acute respiratory distress syndrome developed in two patients, who required intensive organ support for 8 and 16 days. Despite evidence of the multiple cytokine-release syndrome, all six patients survived. Documentation of the clinical course occurring over the 30 days after infusion offers insight into the systemic inflammatory response syndrome in the absence of contaminating pathogens, endotoxin, or underlying disease. (Suntharalingam et al. 2006)

Fialuridine

Before it was trialled on human subjects, **Fialuridine** was tested on animals, including mice, rats, dogs, monkeys, and woodchucks. Those tests found that animals could survive doses which were a hundred times more than those given to humans without any toxic reactions. A Phase II trial on human subjects was conducted. In week 13 one of the subjects suddenly developed hepatic toxicity and lactic acidosis. The trial was stopped. But seven more subjects became ill and five died. Two had to have liver transplants. These totally unforeseen consequences led to a review of protocols for testing potent biological molecules on human subjects. Attarwala (2010) concluded, 'Though there is always a risk involved with clinical trials, these risks can be potentially reduced if more scientific research toward development of animal models closely mimicking drug behavior in humans can be developed.'

BIA 10–2474 Trial

In one phase trial, **BIA 10-2474** (an orally administered reversible FAAH inhibitor) was given to healthy volunteers with a view to assessing its safety.

> *'Single doses (0.25 to 100 mg) and repeated oral doses (2.5 to 20 mg for 10 days) of BIA 10-2474 had been administered to 84 healthy volunteers in sequential cohorts; no severe adverse events had been reported. Another cohort of participants was then assigned to placebo (2 participants) or 50 mg of BIA 10-2474 per day (6 participants)'. 'They had received the highest cumulative dose (250 to 300 mg) administered to humans' (Kerbrat et al. 2016). In this final cohort, four of the six participants developed an acute, rapidly progressing neurological reaction. This included headaches, memory impairment and altered consciousness. Magnetic Resonance Imaging (MRI) scans showed symmetric, bilateral cerebral lesions 'including microhemorrhages and hyperintensities on fluid-attenuated inversion recovery and diffusion-weighted imaging sequences predominantly involving the pons and hippocampi'. 'One became brain dead. Two recovered. One person had memory impairment and one had a residual cerebellar syndrome.'*

Two of the four had previously taken part in other Phase I trials. Kerbrat et al. (2016) suggest that the adverse reactions were related to an accumulation of the drug. They conclude:

> *severe toxic effects in the central nervous system as a result of an increased level of endocannabinoids have not been reported previously; this suggests the possibility of an offtarget effect of the drug, owing to the low specificity of BIA*

10-2474 for FAAH, or an effect of a metabolite.4 These unanticipated severe adverse events were caused by the drug and reflect the complexities of clinical drug research.

(Kerbrat et al. 2016)

Why Do People Take Part in these Trials?

Chen and her colleagues (2017) carried out a survey of 654 healthy volunteers who had taken part in a Phase I trial in USA, Belgium, and Singapore. The asked them about their willingness to enrol in such trials. They found that their participants were willing to take part in many kinds of Phase I trials – including those involving diverse side effects and procedures. They were keener to participate in trials with low risk, familiar procedures. Their willingness did not vary with their income. They were least likely to agree to invasive procedures like lumbar punctures and bone marrow biopsy, or where there was a risk of irreversible damage – such as kidney damage or death – or where there might be a chance of effects on their minds. 'In addition, respondents reported that more money, fewer total procedures, the importance of a study, and the doctor performing the procedure would influence their willingness to participate in a given study. Money is an important factor in healthy volunteers' decisions to participate in phase 1 clinical trials, thus it is not surprising that more money might influence their decisions' (Chen et al. 2017). Not surprisingly, those with lowest incomes express desire to take part in clinical trials. Chen et al. (2017) reported that there was a relatively high proportion of participants with incomes of less than half the national average income in the three countries in their study.

So, there may be a potential to *exploit* people who are financially disadvantaged in clinical trials – as in all types of research – and I shall discuss later when considering ethical issues.

To Sum Up

- Phase I and Phase II clinical trials are the earliest tests of new treatments on human volunteers. The examples shown demonstrate that they are quantitative, hypothetico-deductive. and experimental.
- The difference between these and the majority of experimental approaches we have discussed so far, is that these **do not** include a control group. They are all tightly controlled and usually conducted under close clinical supervision. They are part of the progression to the next step – Phase III Clinical Trials or Randomised Control Trials.

So, remember, earlier I asked you to consider two questions about Arkenau et al.'s work (2008): (i) What sense do you make of these findings? (ii) What is missing from these trials? In answer to my questions:

1. There is the possibility of their results being due, in a large part, to a placebo effect. There are a lot of negative side effects – including the occasional death.

2. How do we rule out the placebo effect? **We use a control group.** That is what is missing in the studies they included in their review.

Clinical trials have to be done if we are to develop new medicines. The challenge for us is to make them fair and ethical.

Remember: 'Research is the art of the possible!'

References

ABPI. (2014). *Guidelines for phase 1 clinical trials: 2012 edition.* (Updated in 2014 by Arnold & Porter LLP on behalf of the ABPI.)

Arkenau H-T, Olmos D, Ang JE, et al. (2008). Clinical outcome and prognostic factors for patients treated within the context of a phase I study: the Royal Marsden Hospital experience. *British Journal of Cancer* 98, 1029–1033.

Attarwala H. (2010). TGN1412: from discovery to disaster. *Journal of Young Pharmacists* 2(3), 332–336.

Cancer Research UK. (2020). *Phase 1 trial.* Available at https://www.cancerresearchuk.org/about-cancer/find-a-clinical-trial/what-clinical-trials-are/phases-of-clinical-trials (accessed 6 May 2020).

Chen SC, Sinai N, Bedarida G, et al. (2017). *Phase 1 healthy volunteer willingness to participate and enrollment preferences.* Clinical Trials 14(5), 537–546.

Health Research Authority. (2020). *Phase 1 clinical trials.* Available at https://www.hra.nhs.uk/planning-and-improving-research/policies-standards-legislation/phase-1-clinical-trials (accessed 6 May 2020).

Kerbrat A, Ferre JC, Fillatre P, et al. (2016). Acute neurologic disorder from an inhibitor of fatty acid amide hydrolase. *The New England Journal of Medicine* 375, 1717–1725.

Matt L and Carl E. (2018). Avoiding exploitation in phase I clinical trials: more than (un)just compensation. *The Journal of Law, Medicine & Ethics* 46, 52–63.

Suntharalingam G, Perry MR, Ward S, et al. (2006). Cytokine storm in a phase 1 trial of the anti-CD28 monoclonal antibody TGN1412. *The New England Journal of Medicine* 355(10), 1018–1028.

CHAPTER 5

Experimental Quantitative Approaches
Randomised Control Trials

Introduction

There are three things you already know about **Randomised Control Trials** (**RCT**): (i) they are trials; (ii) they have controls; and (iii) they are randomised!

- We are still in the **quantitative** domain (measuring, counting, and numbers).
- They are **hypothetico-deductive** – we begin with a clear, specific hypothesis and we test that hypothesis.
- They are **interventional** – we introduce a variable which we want to test – our new treatment.
- They are **prospective** – we follow our participants over a period of time to measure the effects of our interventions.

These follow the classic experimental designs for two-arm or multiple-arm experiments. Only in these cases they are used to test our new interventions – usually against an existing 'gold standard' or a practice which is currently believed to be the best practice.

My epidemiological hero, Archie Cochrane, is acclaimed as the 'champion of the RCT' as a means of eliminating quackery in medicine and promoting **evidence-based-practice.** He is probably best remembered in his legacy of Cochrane Centres which have been set up around the world to promote the development of evidence-based-practice by conducting systematic reviews of RCTs. He also had a wicked sense of humour – but more of that later.

Demystifying Research for Medical & Healthcare Students: An Essential Guide, First Edition. John L. Anderson.
© 2022 John Wiley & Sons Ltd. Published 2022 by John Wiley & Sons Ltd.
Companion website: www.wiley.com/go/Anderson/DemystifyingResearch

RESEARCH METHODOLOGIES

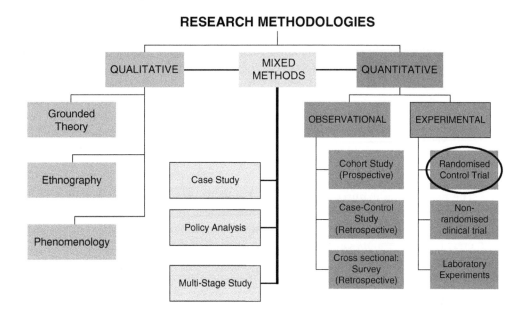

Equipoise

One of the conditions which is considered necessary for the conduct of an RCT is that of **equipoise.** This refers to a state where there is divided belief in the medical community about whether or not one treatment is better than another. For example, if there are two forms of surgery for a cancer – A and B – and opinion is divided about which is best, and both sides provide roughly equal levels of evidence for the benefits of their preferred treatment, then we can say that a state of 'equipoise' exists. If there is convincing evidence that A is the better treatment, then, naturally we should use A. However, if there is convincing evidence that B is the better treatment, then, naturally we should use B. And when opinion is divided, then we should conduct an RCT to find out which is best. In its purest form, equipoise suggests a state where opinion is more or less evenly divided. But then new treatments are developed, and then we need to use RCTs to test them. You should be aware that in medical practice, past custom and practice is a very strong incentive for continuing to do the same thing – even though it may not have been properly evaluated against alternative treatments. This was the situation in relation to treatment for breast cancer when Ted Chesser and I were doing our study of psycho-social aspects of breast cancer and its treatment (see Chapter 6). We noticed that one of the leading surgeons who we were working with was conducting radical mastectomies because his father had developed the technique and he had devised a way of extending the surgery to remove the lymph nodes in the patient's armpit – an extended radical mastectomy. Fisher et al.'s (1985a, b) study comparing the results of radical mastectomy with alternative treatments for primary breast cancer was the first UK study to break with the surgical convention – the surgical 'mantra' that 'radical mastectomy was the only way to properly treat breast cancer'. Ironically, this study, which had concerns about women's welfare at its heart, received a lot of criticism over the ethics of randomly allocating women to a mastectomy vs a lumpectomy group! It was the first to show that 'more conservative' forms of treating breast cancer could be equally effective in terms of survival rates and years of tumour-free life as the more radical and mutilating forms of treatment.

In 1977, Archie Cochrane featured in a BBC programme called 'The Trouble With Medicine' in the *Horizon* series. He stated that there were a lot of treatments used within the NHS which had never been fully evaluated or tested, and that a lot of the medicines that patients were given were counteracting one another, which resulted in a great deal of people being hospitalised because of the *adverse effects of previous treatments*. The programme went on to talk about ways to rationalise medicine – by means of **randomised controlled trials.**

The programme featured a specific RCT which Archie had been involved in. It looked at the treatment of patients after a heart attack. At that time, there were about 200,000 heart attacks every year. Many of these patients were brought into hospitals and ended up in coronary care units (**CCU**). About half of the patients who had heart attacks died, and it was hoped that these CCU would reduce this appalling death rate. They were set up as a result of a number of medical advances, particularly monitoring apparatus and defibrillation. Defibrillators – machines which could restore normal rhythm to the heart by giving an electric charge through two paddles placed on a patient's chest – changed the situation dramatically. Before their introduction, patients were regularly dying from ventricular fibrillation. This became a rare event after their introduction.

So, CCUs were set up in many hospitals, but there had not been any proper attempt to *evaluate* them. It was not known if they would save more lives than if, for example, patients were treated **at home**. When a randomised control trial of CCUs was proposed, there was a great deal of opposition. One of the experts who had suggested it was Archie Cochrane. In his words:

> *We realised there would be very severe ethical problems and a great resistance from the consultants for doing it. So we asked the DHSS and the Medical Research Council to set up an independent ethical enquiry into the ethics of carrying out such a trial.*

The trial went ahead on the condition that it reported regularly. In four centres in south-west England, 450 patients were randomly allocated to receive either **home care** by their family doctor, or **hospital care**, initially in an intensive care unit. The early results showed a small number of deaths – six in the **home treatment group** and slightly more, eight, in the **hospital group.** But this wasn't how Archie Cochrane presented them:

> *Well, just for fun I reversed the table and showing more deaths, 8 at home, as opposed to 6 in hospital. And I showed that to some of the consultants before the meeting, and there was a massive uproar. All said at once, 'Archie, that trial is unethical! It must be stopped at once!' So, I let them go on a bit, blow their tops, but then as they were calming down, I apologised humbly, that I'd shown the wrong table and showed them the correct table – with fewer deaths at home than in hospital – and said didn't they think it was* unethical to continue with coronary care units – *which was entirely logical after what they had been saying about the ethics of the trial. But I was unable to convince them, I'm*

afraid. But it does make the point that there's an enormous amount of emotion about coronary care units!

The final report showed that by the end of nearly a year, 80% of patients treated at home were still alive, compared to 73% in hospital. But for older patients without complications, 78% survived at home, compared to 66% in hospital – a difference of 12%. The report concluded that there was 'a significant difference in favour of home treatment for patients aged 60 years and over without initial hypotension' (Mather et al. 1976).

RCT Research Design

There are several stages in an RCT:

1. We recruit a group of participants or patients to try out the new intervention (treatment) on.
2. We randomly allocate them to a treatment and a control group.
3. We establish baseline measures of important variables.
4. We give the treatment to the treatment group and a placebo (i.e., no active or their current treatment) to the control group.
5. We follow them up and make final measures both groups for the 'effects' we are anticipating.
6. We analyse our data and publish our results.

Please Note: The **randomisation** in an RCT does *not* refer to the **sampling**. It refers to the **allocation** to the different arms of the trial. The most common method of sampling is to recruit a **consecutive series** of patients with the condition we are hoping to improve by our new intervention/new treatment. Some trials recruit whoever they can, from whatever source they can. Some recruit healthy volunteers by advertising. Others recruit patients with conditions which may benefit from the new treatment being tested. This often means that a trial will begin and snowball as it gets under way. One of Sod's Laws in research is that, when you start to recruit for a study, the patients disappear! So, you are usually unaware of who will be in your trial until the end of it. Then the first thing you do is to check that your randomisation has worked – you want to get roughly equal types of participants in each group. If there are major differences – e.g. by age-group – then you can **purposively sample** to increase the numbers in the hope that this will help balance the profiles of your experimental and control groups. See Figure 5.1.

Blinding

Blinding refers to keeping the participants and/or the staff looking after the participants in the dark about which group the participants are in – and thus avoiding any Hawthorne Effect. In a **double-blind RCT** (the gold standard), the *participants* in the trial are unaware of which group they are in, and the *staff* caring for them are unaware

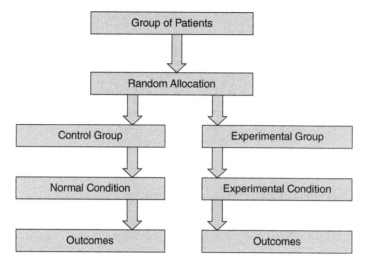

FIGURE 5.1 RCT experimental design.

of which group the participants are in. By 'blinding' the participants, you hope to overcome the placebo effect. By 'blinding' the staff, you hope to avoid any bias in the endpoint measurements which they make. See Figure 5.2. The important issues are: a) by blocking the patient's/participant's knowledge of which group they are in, you cut down on the extent to which attempts on their part to 'help' the researchers are cancelled by the randomisation; and b) by blocking the staff's knowledge of which group the patients/participants are in, you reduce the propensity for them to exert any bias in the way they treat the patients/participants.

But *blinding is not always possible.* For example, in the mastectomy/lumpectomy RCT mentioned above it was impossible to disguise the operation the patients had.

In a **single-blind RCT,** *either* the staff *or* the participants are unaware of which group the participants are in. In an **open trial,** *both* the staff *and* the participants are aware of which group the participants are in.

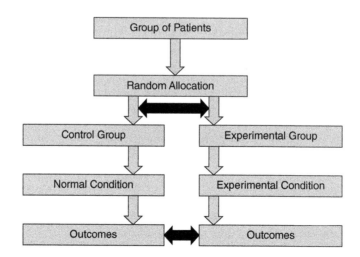

FIGURE 5.2 RCT experimental design showing double blinding.

Because blinding is so important for avoiding bias, we may have to go to great lengths to ensure blinding is successful. But often staff have their own agendas in RCTs and there have been accounts of staff going to great lengths to discover which groups patients are in. Archie Cochrane in his book *Effectiveness and Efficiency: Random Reflections on Health Services* (Cochrane 1999), gives accounts of doctors holding up to the light the envelopes with the randomisation details in the hope of finding out which group patients were in. And he mentions one doctor who tried to access the confidential files containing information about the randomisation by trying to force open a locked filing cabinet with a paper knife!

Now, why would people want to know what group patients are in? I think you can answer that yourself. Think about the story which Archie told about the RCT of CCUs (above). . . some people may want to influence the results of research studies! I know this may be difficult to accept, but not all healthcare professionals are squeaky clean – either unintentionally or intentionally.

Some of the methods we use to conceal the randomisation in RCTs include:

- Always get a computer-generated random sequence for the allocation of participants to groups in an RCT.
- Better still, also get the computer to generate the labels for any medicines and any letters to be used in informing trial staff about treatments.
- Keep confidential material in locked filing cabinets.

I shall return to issues of blinding and fraud in research later. Now let's have a look at some examples of RCTs.

Example 1: Streptomycin treatment of pulmonary tuberculosis

We know about Fleming's discovery of penicillin. During the Second World War it was used primarily for the treatment of wounds. In 1946, the Medical Research Council (MRC) planned to investigate the use of Streptomycin, which was showing promise, in the treatment of pulmonary tuberculosis. The drug was in short supply but the MRC decided that 'a part of the small supply of streptomycin allocated to it for research purposes would be best employed in a rigorously planned investigation with concurrent controls' (MRC 1948).

One problem which can beset researchers is that sometimes there are different types of a disease. The MRC teams had to make a decision about who to include and who to exclude from the study. So, they defined cases to be included as: 'acute progressive bilateral pulmonary tuberculosis of presumably recent origin, bacteriologically proved, unsuitable for collapse therapy, age group 15 to 25 (later extended to 30)'. The decision to 'deny' the experimental treatment to those in the control group (they were 'treated' only with bed rest) was justified on the grounds that: (i) bed rest was the only treatment available up to that point in time; and (ii) there were insufficient amounts of the drug to give it to every participant in the trial.

They elicited the support of three hospitals – the Brompton Hospital, Colindale Hospital, and Harefield Hospital. The London County Council and the Middlesex County Council gave their full support enabling access to the area which served a population of almost six million. They wrote to the TB departments of the hospitals, to TB officers, and to medical superintendents of general hospitals, explaining the trial and asking them to cooperate by sending x-ray films of potentially suitable patients for inclusion in the trial. They visited clinics and hospitals to explain the trial and show the type of case they were after. Suitable cases were discussed by the Committee's Selection Panel and, when someone was identified as suitable, they made a request to the local authority concerned for that patient to be given absolute priority for admission to one of the trial centres. Most were admitted within a week. Although they had thought that this type of case was common, they were not. (One of Sod's Laws of research!) After three months not enough cases had been found, so the team had to widen their recruitment net to include other hospitals from Wales, Scotland, Leeds, and another London hospital. Six months later they had recruited 109. Two had died and were excluded. The remaining 107 were randomly allocated to the treatment (Streptomycin) group (55) or the control (bed rest) group (52). The allocation to groups was done according to a predetermined list drawn from random numbers by Bradford-Hill.

> *The details of the series were unknown to any of the investigators or to the co-ordinator and were contained in a set of sealed envelopes, each bearing on the outside only the name of the hospital and a number. After acceptance of a patient by the panel, and before admission to the streptomycin centre, the appropriate numbered envelope was opened at the central office the card inside told if the patient was to be an S or a C case, and this information was then given to the medical officer of the centre. Patients were not told before admission that they were to get special treatment. C patients did not know throughout their stay in hospital that they were control patients in a special study; they were in fact treated as they would have been in the past, the sole difference being that they had been admitted to the centre more rapidly than was normal. Usually they were not in the same wards as S patients, but the same regime was maintained.*

> *(MRC 1948)*

The Committee noted:

> *It was important for the success of the trial that the details of the control scheme should remain confidential. It is a matter of great credit to the many doctors concerned that this information was not made public throughout the 15 months of the trial, and the Committee is much indebted to them for their co-operation.*

Patients were admitted to the centres a week before the trial started. This allowed for pre-trial observations. The data showed that the randomisation had equalised the two groups. All patients were required to stay in bed at the centre for at least six months so that the results could be measured then. Members of the research and clinical teams met regularly to discuss the trial and any problems which arose. They also obtained independent checking of tests of tubercle bacilli and streptomycin levels. Each centre submitted monthly reports from standard records and x-rays for each patient. The x-rays were independently reviewed by two radiologists and a clinician. One of the radiologists and the clinician were not connected with the trial in any way. All three met to discuss x-rays, where there had been any difference of interpretation, and agreement was reached without difficulty in all cases.

All of the treatment group were given 2 g per day of streptomycin by four six-hourly i/v injections. Although the original intention was to give streptomycin for six months, results from studies in other centres suggested that the maximum effect was reached within the first three to four months. So, it was agreed to treat patients for four months but to observe them for the complete six-month period. Both groups of patients were on bed rest throughout the trial.

> *The supply of streptomycin available during the investigation was limited. The type of disease selected was one considered hitherto unsuitable for any form of treatment other than bed-rest. Bed-rest accordingly was the treatment given to one group of 52 patients (C), while 55 patients were treated with bed-rest plus streptomycin (S).*

> *(MRC 1948)*

The results after six months are shown in Table 5.1.

To quote the MRC report:

> *The overall results given in [Table 5.1] show differences between the two series that leave no room for doubt. The most outstanding difference is in the numbers who showed 'considerable improvement' in the radiological picture – i.e. those for whom at the end of the six-months period there was a reasonable prospect of recovery. Twenty-eight of the S patients (51%) and only four of the C patients (8%) were considerably improved (the probability of such a difference occurring by chance is less than one in a million).*

> *(MRC 1948)*

TABLE 5.1   Assessment of radiological appearance at six months as compared with appearance on admission.

Radiological Assessment	Treatment (Streptomycin) Group		Control Group	
Considerable improvement	28	51%	4	8%
Moderate or slight improvement	10	18%	13	25%
No material change	2	4%	3	6%
Moderate or slight deterioration	5	9%	12	23%
Considerable deterioration	6	11%	6	11%
Deaths	4	7%	14	27%
Total	55	100%	52	100%

Source: Adapted from MRC (1948).

TABLE 5.2 Condition at 12 months in relation to condition on admission.

Group	Improvement		No Change		Deterioration		Death		Total	
Treatment Group	31	56%	4	7%	8	15%	12	22%	55	100%
Control Group	16	31%	5	10%	7	13%	24	46%	52	100%

The results at 12 months follow-up, compared to the patients' conditions at the start of the trial, are shown in Table 5.2.

This classic study demonstrated, for the first time, the value of treating patients with TB by streptomycin injections.

> *The investigation reported here has demonstrated the value of streptomycin in one not very common form of tuberculosis . . . much organized work is yet required to determine the precise indications of streptomycin and the best schemes of dosage in pulmonary tuberculosis.*

> *(MRC 1948)*

Alan Yoshioka, in a paper commemorating the original study, points out that the mode of randomisation used in the MRC trial – allocation using **random numbers and sealed envelopes** – was notably different from previous methods of randomisation in which patients were alternately (i.e., the first one in the experimental group, the second one in the control group, and so on . . .) allocated to the trial groups. He alludes to previous 'favouritism in selection of participants' and Bradford-Hill's avoidance of any suggestion of this in the trial.

> *In the era of the slogan, 'fair shares for all,' suspicion of favouritism was to be avoided. Under Bradford Hill's scheme, there could be no such worries, as the decision whether to include the patient in the trial was made in complete ignorance of which group the patient would join. The new method of random allocation 'removed personal responsibility from the clinician,' the BMJ noted. Hart's secretary once advised about a patient with pulmonary disease whose physician was seeking to enrol him in the trial, 'the strongest point against any possible acceptance of his case is that with the control system we dare not take isolated cases of this kind – we don't decide whether the case is to be a treated one or a control case'. When one senior physician contracted tuberculosis, the MRC obtained supplies for him outside the trial, rather than compromise the integrity of this admission system.*

> *(Yoshioka 1998)*

A *BMJ* editorial in the same issue commented on the rigour of the study:

> *In such trials it is often tempting to add little groups of patients of differing types here, there, and everywhere with the object of learning rather more. Though with a statistical design it will certainly sometimes pay to do so, very often the*

rather more becomes the rather less. Such a trial gives doubtful answers to the many points but no decisive answer to any. This temptation the Committee, and the clinicians co-operating with it, resisted.

. . . the Committee set up a selection panel. This panel conceivably might have been influenced in selecting or rejecting a patient if it had known beforehand whether the patient was to be allocated to the streptomycin or to the controlled group – e.g., if alternate patients had been taken. It was relieved of any such worries by an ingenious system of sealed envelopes. Once a patient had been accepted an appropriate numbered envelope was opened, and not till then was the patient's group revealed. The allocation to 'S' or 'C' in this form had been made at random by the statistician.

To remove all possibility of bias the Committee had the films assessed independently by two radiologists and a clinician, each of whom had no knowledge whatever whether the film they saw related to a streptomycin or to a control case. Such a method vastly increases confidence in the results, and it is important to realize that it in no way questions the intellectual honesty of the investigator who is thus asked to work 'blind'. It guards not only against unconscious bias but, equally important, against any honest attempt in the assessor to allow for a possible bias.

(BMJ 1948)

Now let us look at other studies which have shown imagination and originality in achieving blinding as a means of overcoming bias in the treatments to patients in experimental and control groups.

Example 2: Randomised, prospective, single-blind comparison of laparoscopic versus small-incision cholecystectomy

This study was first brought to my attention by Professor Malcom Reed, the Dean of Brighton and Sussex Medical School. Malcolm, a surgeon, was one of the research team in this study. The issue which they were addressing was to evaluate two types of operating procedures for removing the gall bladder (cholecystectomy) – *small incision cholecystectomy* versus *laparoscopic cholecystectomy*. Many years ago, large incisions were used and the size of incisions used in the operation have gradually become smaller and smaller. Let's allow the researchers to describe the situation:

Before small-incision procedures could be established in surgical practice, laparoscopically assisted removal of the gallbladder was introduced and rapidly became popular despite early concerns about its safety. These concerns were later confirmed by a rise in common bile-duct injury and other injuries not hitherto associated with cholecystectomy. Such complications prompted calls for careful evaluation of laparoscopic cholecystectomy as well as the establishment of training programmes in the new technique. Unfortunately, many surgeons deemed such evaluation as 'ethically unjustified' and 'very difficult if not impossible to conduct' due to the 'obvious advantages' of the laparoscopic procedure. Investment by instrument manufacturers in new laparoscopic instruments and imaging systems may have helped establish these new techniques as part of surgical practice before safety and cost-effectiveness had been established. Indeed, when our trial began in January, 1992, there had been no reports of a randomised comparison of conventional and laparoscopic cholecystectomy.

Trials which have been published since do not take account of the effect of beliefs of patients and carers which may have affected the results. We did a prospective, randomised, single-blind trial comparing laparoscopic and small-incision cholecystectomy in which we have minimised bias by standardising the two procedures and blinding patients and their carers during the preoperative and early postoperative period.

(Majeed et al. 1996)

So, here the issue was one of vested interests and personal preferences for the mode of surgery to be adopted. This made the **blinding of staff** a vitally important issue for the successful conduct of the trial. Patients were screened for suitability before they were admitted to hospital. They were admitted on the day before their surgery. They were randomly allocated to either the laparoscopic or the small-incision procedure. A sealed envelope containing the randomisation details was opened in the theatre – after anaesthesia had begun. Four surgeons, who had received training on simulators and had taken part in at least 40 laparoscopic cholecystectomies before the trial. They were considered to be 'over the learning curve for both the laparoscopic and small-incision approaches' (Majeed et al. 1996).

The blinding procedures involved all patients having *two sets of dressings* after the operation (Figure 5.3). 'To help ensure that ward nurses could not guess which operation had been performed, each dressing was stained with bloodstained fluid or aqueous iodine solution. These dressings were not disturbed unless there was a problem (wound pain or pyrexia), in which case they were replaced after examination of the wound.' After the operation, both groups of patients received their normal care. They were assessed in the daily ward rounds and were given pain-killing medication as required via patient-controlled analgesia and oral analgesia as appropriate. Patients were assessed throughout their hospital stay and followed up after three weeks, when a research nurse (blind) interviewed the patients, to assess time off work and return to full activity. A surgeon examined them in a separate room. Questionnaires were sent to patients after eight weeks and six months to collect this information if they had still not returned to full activity.

They screened out 42 patients and invited 205 to participate; 200 were eventually included and randomised in the trial – 100 in each group. There were no significant differences between the two groups. In presenting the results, the authors do a very good job at describing in detail and explaining exceptional cases. They explain very

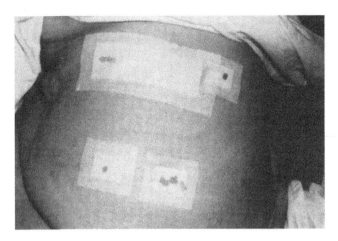

FIGURE 5.3   Majeed et al. – twin sets of dressings used in 'blinding'. *Source*: Majeed et al. (1996), with permission of Elsevier.

well how, at each stage of their patients' care, the blinding was maintained. This, they explain, was necessary to combat potential bias amongst staff as a result of their beliefs and feelings about the two procedures, which might have influenced carers' decision about when patients should have been discharged. 'Blinding of ward staff and removal of carer control over discharge from hospital is therefore an important aspect of our trial.' They encouraged patients to mobilise early, but allowed patients to determine when they should be discharged. Prior experience and stereotypes amongst medical practitioners had been shown to influence their views on how long patients should stay in hospital and how long they should be kept off work – 'A poll by Majeed et al. (1995) confirms that surgeons and general practitioners would tend to keep patients undergoing open cholecystectomy off work longer than those undergoing the laparoscopic operation. It is interesting, in this study, in which patients decided their own time off work, that those undergoing the small-incision operation returned to work at the same time or earlier than those who had the laparoscopic operation.'

They concluded:

> *This study shows that a prospective randomised trial of laparoscopic cholecys-*
> *tectomy can be done and that it is possible to eliminate bias for or against the*
> *procedure from carers and patients. Once such bias is removed, we found that*
> *laparoscopic cholecystectomy takes longer to do and offers no benefit over small-*
> *incision cholecystectomy in terms of postoperative recovery, hospital stay, and*
> *time back to work or full activity.*

(Majeed et al. 1996)

So, you can see in this case how vital HCPs' expectations and beliefs were in potentially influencing the outcomes of the study, and therefore why blinding was so important. They went to great lengths to keep the HCP carers naïve as to the operations which had been performed on individual patients. This, and the fact that they allowed the patients to decide when to go home and when to resume their full activity after the operation, made sure that any HCPs' biases could not affect the outcomes of the trial. Obviously, this took a lot of effort and commitment from a lot of people, but it was worth it because they were able to conclude with a great degree of certainty: 'We believe that, due to the small number of refusals, our results may be applicable to all patients suitable for elective cholecystectomy.'

Example 3: Arthroscopic Partial Meniscectomy versus Sham Surgery for a Degenerative Meniscal Tear

The meniscus is a piece of cartilage between the thighbone (femur) and the shinbone (tibia). There are two in each knee. A torn meniscus happens when a knee injury involves a forceful twisting of the knee joint, resulting in pain, swelling, and giving way of the knee joint. They are one of the most common injuries and are often referred to as 'torn cartilages'. An arthroscopic partial meniscectomy is the one of the most common orthopaedic procedures performed in the United States. The procedure aims to 'relieve symptoms attributed to a meniscal tear by removing torn meniscal fragments and trimming the meniscus back to a stable rim'. But Sihvonen et al. point out that 'rigorous evidence of its efficacy is lacking'. So, in the true spirit of Archie Cochrane, they conducted a 'multicenter, randomized, double-blind, sham-controlled trial to assess the efficacy of arthroscopic partial meniscectomy in patients who have a degenerative tear of the medial meniscus without knee osteoarthritis' (Sihvonen et al. 2013). It was a potentially very controversial and sensitive study. Fortunes could be made by orthopaedic surgeons performing this operation: 'the number of arthroscopic partial meniscectomies performed has concurrently increased by 50%. Approximately 700,000 arthroscopic partial meniscectomies are performed annually in the United States alone, with annual direct medical costs estimated at $4 billion' (Sihvonen et al. 2013). So, you can see that there might well be vested interests in the results of such a trial. The trial was a very rigorous one. It was carefully planned and executed and great care was taken in the blinding of both patients and staff. I shall try to explain it as fully and simply as possible.

The trial was conducted at five centres in Finland from which patients were recruited. Each of the sites had an established, reputable team, experienced in arthroscopic knee surgery. Patients who fitted the inclusion criteria of having knee pain consistent with a meniscus injury were assessed for eligibility. All were 35–65 years old who had had symptoms for at least three months of a degenerative medial meniscus injury which did not respond to non-surgical treatment. Surgeons examined each patient carefully to assess their suitability for the study and make baseline measurements. They were then put on the waiting list (approximately three months) for surgery. The trial was explained to the patients and it was made clear to all of them that they might be randomised to receive **placebo surgery** – a point that was repeated before the actual randomisation. After excluding unsuitable patients, 146 were included in the trial and were randomised into the arthroscopic partial meniscectomy group (70) and the sham surgery group (76) and their baseline characteristics were similar.

A nurse opened an envelope with the random allocation and showed it to the surgeon – but did not say it out loud so the patients were unaware of which group they had been allocated to. These allocations had been prepared by a statistician, who had no clinical involvement in the trial, using a computer-generated sequence. The envelopes were kept in a secure location at each centre. The two procedures are described in detail by the team:

Arthroscopic partial meniscectomy: *The damaged and loose part of the meniscus tissue was removed with arthroscopic instruments (mechanised shaver and meniscal punches) until solid meniscus tissue was reached. The meniscus was then propped to ensure that all loose and weak fragments and unstable meniscus tissue had been successfully resected, preserving as much of the meniscus tissue as possible. No other surgical procedure (synovectomy, debridement, excision of fragments of articular cartilage or chondral flaps, or abrasion and/or microfracture of chondral defects) was performed.*

Placebo surgery: *A standard arthroscopic partial meniscectomy (APM) procedure was simulated. The surgeon asked for all instruments and manipulated the knee as if APM was being performed. The mechanised shaver (without the blade) was also pushed firmly against the patella, outside of the knee, to mimic as closely as possible the feelings and sounds of the normal use of the arthroscopic shaver. Further, to simulate the sounds of normal APM, suction was also used to drain the joint and saline was splashed. The patient was kept in the operating room for the amount of time required to perform an actual APM.*

(Sihvonen et al. 2013b)

Postop care for both groups conformed to a specific protocol which maintained that all patients received the same walking aids and graduated exercise programme. Medications were given according to standard practice and patients were discharged after full recovery. All the staff delivering the patients' care were blind to the treatments. To that effect, the statement 'a procedure according to the degenerative meniscus trial was performed' was included in all patients' notes (Figure 5.4).

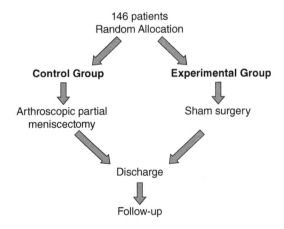

FIGURE 5.4 Sihvonen et al.: RCT design.

The three main outcome measures were **knee pain,** the **Lysholm Knee Score,** and the **Western Ontario Meniscal Evaluation Tool** (**WOMET**). Knee pain was rated on an 11-point scale which ranged from 0 (no pain) to 10 (extreme pain). Both the Lysholm Knee Score and the WOMET are validated instruments for this group of patients. These were assessed at baseline, and at 2, 6, and 12 months after surgery.

The results showed that there was an improvement in all three outcome measures from operation to 12 months, but there were no significant differences between the two groups. This meant that there was no clinically significant benefit of arthroscopic partial meniscectomy over the sham surgery. They concluded that:

> *These results argue against the current practice of performing arthroscopic partial meniscectomy in patients with a degenerative meniscal tear.*

> *(Sihvonen et al. 2013)*

Damn! There goes the profit in those operations.

Discussion

I hope you can now understand the importance of blinding, and the efforts which some study teams have gone to carry out a **double-blind randomised control trial** and to protect their blinding against people who might wish to expose the randomisation and thus sabotage the trial. Of course, trials, such as the three that I have discussed here, have been very well resourced. They have also been exposed to very high levels of ethical scrutiny – no organisation wants to be associated with a trial that goes wrong! Therefore, those institutions with risk-averse cultures will be very reluctant indeed to embark upon such trials.

One of my students, Kavi – a homoeopathic medicine practitioner – proposed a very well thought-out RCT to evaluate the impact of homoeopathic interventions as opposed to 'normal' approaches to combat the adverse effects of cancer chemotherapies. Wow! What a panic and negative approach it caused in his university before it was finally turned down! Although he is a homoeopathic practitioner and is registered with the UK body, although homoeopathic 'medicines' are not classified as 'medicines' (they are classified as inert substances), and although they were to be sourced from reputable suppliers, there were all sorts of questions and pejorative accusations levelled at him and myself – 'will these poison our patients?'; 'Where will these come from – India?' and on and on! The final argument was that Masters' students should not be conducting RCTs. Fair enough. We changed our study. (He is now a clinical trials manager in a UK university.)

But do not be disheartened. Remember in the last chapter we discussed Egbert et al.'s study? That was an example of a relatively inexpensive experiment to conduct, and it was of relatively low risk. You *can* conduct an experimental study if you plan it well and keep the costs down – research is the art of the possible!

Another consideration is that some trials have very *narrow inclusion criteria,* such that you might meet someone with those clinical characteristics very infrequently in normal clinical practice. It is important to bear in mind that the results of any trial should only be used as a guide for the treatment of patients who match the inclusion criteria of its participants. For example: depression is a very common mental illness. Most people who have depression also suffer from other symptoms – notably, anxiety. Yet many RCTs involving treatment for depression expressly exclude patients who also experience other symptoms. So, ask yourself, are their results generalisable to *all* patients with depression? The answer has to be *no*. They can only be generalised to and guide the treatment of patients who had only depression and no other symptoms. Check that out in RCTs in your line of work.

Another concern is the *acceptability* of the treatments to participants. Some drugs are unpleasant or difficult to take. Some interventions will not suit everybody. This is particularly true in trials of different diets. One of my students did a systematic review to examine the evidence for dietary interventions in the treatment of breast cancer. She found very few RCTs and the most promising one had to be abandoned because a high proportion of the women who took part in the trial could not sustain the *experimental diet*. So, we have to bear in mind the *feasibility* and *acceptability* of our interventions. Another study of patients with advanced metastatic melanoma and patients with metastatic breast cancer were asked to follow a 'low phe and tyr diet (10 mg kg^{-1} phe and tyr per day) for 1 month'. They found that 'only three of the 22 patients with metastatic melanoma and three of the 15 patients with metastatic breast cancer agreed to *start* the diet. All patients experienced problems and side-effects and increases in anxiety and depression.' And they concluded that 'Low phe and tyr diets do not appear to be a viable treatment option for patients with advanced cancer' (Harvie et al. 2002).

To Sum Up

So, we can see from the above examples of RCTs that they are clearly are in the **quantitative** domain. They all test the benefits of one treatment versus another. They are **interventional** –introducing an intervention to test – the new treatment. They are **prospective** and follow participants over a period of time to measure the effects of the interventions. They use the classic experimental designs for two-arm trials to test their interventions against an existing practice which is currently believed to be the best practice (see Figure 5.5).

The **'gold standard'** is to have an RCT which is **double-blind** – neither the patients/participants nor the staff providing their care know which group the patients/participants are in. In that way we exclude or minimise **placebo** effects and reduce the possibility of anyone's **bias** in favour of one treatment or the other. And in the examples above you can see the lengths some researchers have to go to in order to maintain their 'blinding'. Majeed et al. (1996), in order to keep the healthcare staff blind as to which operation had been performed (in order to avoid any bias creeping in to the care given and the assessments of how well or otherwise the patients were doing), put two sets of dressings on to each participating patient. Sihvonen et al (2013) went further and actually operated on the participating patients in both the experimental and the control groups – only the experimental group received 'sham' or fake, placebo operations. This

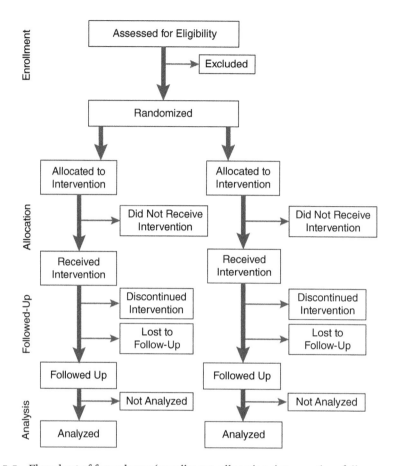

FIGURE 5.5 Flowchart of four phases (enrollment, allocation, intervention, follow-up, and data analysis) of a parallel randomized trial of two groups (in a controlled trial, one of the interventions serves as the control), modified from the CONSORT (Consolidated Standards of Reporting Trials) 2010 Statement

had the effect of ensuring that neither the patients who had the operations, nor the staff looking after them were aware of which group they were in and could not prejudice the results by their own biases.

Sampling, as you saw in the examples here, is usually by means of a **consecutive series** of appropriate participants – *not* by random sampling. **Randomisation** refers to the **allocation** of participants to the groups in the trial. However, because of the narrow inclusion criteria, you could say that they were: a) **purposive,** they selected participants who were suitable, then b) they were a **consecutive series** of appropriate people.

There is strict **regulation** and control of RCTs. This adds to the time taken to set one up, get all the necessary approvals, and conduct the trial.

It is worth noting that, in RCTs, it is important that the people in the sample are sufficiently similar to the population of patients to whom the results will be applied, and that the interventions tested are the same as the ones which will be used in real life – otherwise we cannot generalise the findings to the real world. You might do a piece of homework here and consider the discussions going on at an international level about a) the use of the Oxford/Astrazeneca vaccine and its use to immunize against COVID-19 in people over 65 years old, and b) the length of time which should be left between the first and second doses of this vaccine, etc.

Research is the art of the possible!

References

Alan Y. (1998). Use of randomisation in the Medical Research Council's clinical trial of streptomycin in pulmonary tuberculosis in the 1940s. *British Medical Journal* 317, 1220–1223.

BMJ Editorial. (1948). The controlled therapeutic trial. *British Medical Journal* 2, 791–792.

Cochrane A. (1999). *Effectiveness and Efficiency: Random Reflections on Health Services*. The Royal Society of Medicine Press: London.

Fisher B, Bauer M, Margolese R, et al. (1985a) Five-year results of a randomized clinical trial comparing total mastectomy and segmental mastectomy with or without radiation in the treatment of breast cancer. *The New England Journal of Medicine* 312, 665–673.

Fisher B, Redmond C, Fisher ER, et al. (1985b) Ten-year results of a randomized clinical trial comparing radical mastectomy and total mastectomy with or without radiation. *The New England Journal of Medicine* 312, 674–681.

Harvie MN, Campbell IT, and Thatcher N. (2002). Acceptability and tolerance of a low tyrosine and phenylalanine diet in patients with advanced cancer – a pilot study. DOI 10.1046/j.1365-277X.2002.00365.x

Majeed AW, Brown S, Hannay DR, et al. (1995). Variations in medical attitudes to postoperative recovery period. *British Medical Journal* 311, 296.

Majeed AW, Troy G, Nichol JP, et al. (1996). Randomised, prospective, single-blind comparison of laparoscopic versus small-incision cholecystectomy. *Lancet* 347, 989–994.

Mather HG, Morgan DC, Pearson NG, et al. (1976). Myocardial infarction: a comparison between home and hospital care for patients. *British Medical Journal* 1, 925–929.

Medical Research Council. (1948). Streptomycin treatment of pulmonary tuberculosis. A Medical Research Council investigation. *British Medical Journal* 2,769–782.

Sihvonen R, Paavola M, Malmivaara A. (2013a). Arthroscopic partial meniscectomy versus sham surgery for a degenerative meniscal tear. *The New England Journal of Medicine* 369(26), 2515–2524.

Sihvonen R, Paavola M, Malmivaara A. (2013b). Finnish Degenerative Meniscal Lesion Study (FIDELITY): a protocol fora randomised, placebo surgery controlled trial on the efficacy of arthroscopic partial meniscectomy for patients with degenerative meniscus injury with a novel 'RCT within-a-cohort' study design. *British Medical Journal Open* 3, e002510. doi:10.1136/bmjopen-2012 0025 10.

Schulz KF, Altman DG, (Moher D; for the CONSORT Group). (2010). CONSORT 2010 Statement: updated guidelines for reporting parallel group randomised trials. *British Medical Journal* 340, c332. doi: 10.1136/bmj.c332. PMC 2844940. PMID 20332509.

CHAPTER 6

Observational Quantitative Approaches

Cohort Studies

Introduction

You will remember that 'cohort' is a posh word for a 'group'. It comes from the Latin 'cohors' meaning a unit (or group) forming one tenth of a Roman Legion. (And those of you who know your Latin and your Roman history – or have seen the Monty Python film 'The Life of Brian' – will know how fearsome the Roman Legions were.)

So, a cohort is a **group** of people, and in a cohort study we recruit a group of people and *follow them up* over a period of time to record what happens to them, then use statistical analyses to describe the results. I could end this chapter there, but, out of a strong sense of duty, I shall go on to tell you a bit more about this kind of study and show you some examples, and the difficulties you might encounter in doing a **cohort study**.

So, to remind you:

- We are still in the **quantitative** domain – we are still very much concerned with gathering numerical data.
- It is still a **hypothetico-deductive** approach and we should have hypotheses in mind when we set out on this sort of endeavour.
- This is still an **observational** type of study – there is no intervention or experimentation involved.
- Again it is a **prospective** approach in that we make initial observations, or measurements, and then by following the group over time we can see how, if at all, these change.

Demystifying Research for Medical & Healthcare Students: An Essential Guide, First Edition. John L. Anderson.
© 2022 John Wiley & Sons Ltd. Published 2022 by John Wiley & Sons Ltd.
Companion website: www.wiley.com/go/Anderson/DemystifyingResearch

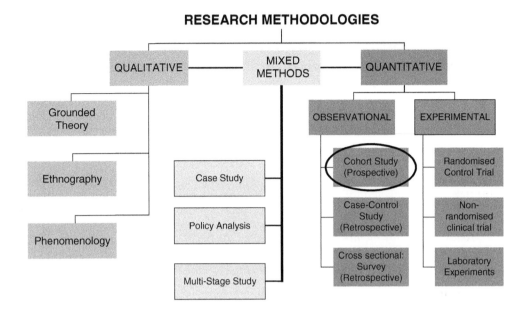

Example 1: The 1946 National Birth Cohort (MRC National Survey of Health and Development)

Note when this study was started – just after the end of the Second World War (WW2). This was a time of social change in the UK. Servicemen were returning home from the war and they wanted a better, fairer society to live in. The Labour Party led by Clement Attlee won a landslide victory, defeating Winston Churchill who had led the country so well to victory during the war. The Welfare State was created – introducing free education for all, welfare benefits, housing, etc., and, of course, in 1948 the NHS was established. In this period of reform, the fairer society ethos also heralded renewed research interests to investigate inequalities in health care and in 1946, the National Study of Health and Development (NSHD) was established.

The NSHD, under the directorship of James W.B. Douglas, began with a survey of *all* births in the week of 3–9 March in 1946. (NB – I was **NOT** included in the sample – I was not born until September of that year!) In that week, there were 15,130 births in England, Wales, and Scotland. Of these 13 687 (91%) took part in the 'Maternity Survey' which aimed to investigate two issues: (i) whether or not the high costs of having a baby might put people off having one – thus explaining why the national fertility rate had been falling; and (ii) what was the distribution and the use made of obstetric and maternity services, and how effective were they in preventing infant deaths and protecting the health of infants and mothers. A class-stratified sample of 5362 single births was selected for inclusion and follow-up in the cohort study. That is a lot! It is the oldest and the longest running study of its kind in the UK. It aimed to be representative of British society, and it was. By selecting ALL births within one week in the initial survey, they ensured a total representation of births. The sub-sample for the cohort study used the sophisticated sampling procedure of stratifying; that is, selecting numbers to appropriately represent the social class structure of British society at the time – thus making sure of **equity** – equal representation – in the study. For a full account of the set up of the study and the rational for the approach used, see Mike Wadsworth's detailed accounts (2006 and 2010). He points out that the *survey* was meant to be the only part of the research, but that it showed itself to be so useful that they decided to conduct follow-ups into social class differences in child health and development.

Data collection was mainly done by health professionals. Health visitors gathered the data at the first two follow-ups. Then doctors and school nurses carried out examinations to collect later data for the study. When any child was hospitalised, the hospitals were contacted for details. Mike Wadsworth summarises the study nicely in his article (2010):

> *Today, with study members in their seventies, the NSHD is a leading source of evidence on the long-term biological and social processes of ageing and how ageing is affected by factors acting across the whole of life.*

> *The participants have been followed up in the course of 24 data collections. Regular interviews with the mothers were conducted by health visitors, with additional assessments by school doctors and teachers. In adult life, research nurses conducted home visits at ages 26, 36, 43, 53 and 69, a detailed clinic visit took place between ages 60–64, and there have been a number of postal questionnaires, including annual questionnaires to women (47–54 years) to capture the menopause transition. At the latest home visit at age 69, the participation rate was 80% (N = 2149).*

> *During childhood, the main aim of the NSHD was to investigate how the environment at home and at school affected physical and mental development and educational attainment. During adulthood, the main aim has been to investigate how childhood development and lifetime social circumstances and lifestyle affected adult health and function and how these change with age. Now that participants have reached their seventies, the NSHD has developed into a life course study of ageing.*

> *(Wadsworth, 2010)*

You can see how extensive their data collection has been and how they have kept up contact with their participants over the years. The mind boggles at how the huge amount of data was that was stored and analysed. Remember that computers did not come into common use until the 1980s and that, until then, all of the data was in paper form. This had to be stored somewhere! This is a big practical issue with large-scale cohort studies, although nowadays computerised record-keeping does save space! As Wadsworth acknowledges:

> *These years preceded the introduction of computers, and analysis was undertaken using a counter-sorter. This often involved abstracting data from the original cards to make new sets of cards that contained only the information required for the analysis. Since the original coded data about each of the 5,362 sample members was stored on many cards, and several cards of data were usually required for an analysis, this was a cumbersome and time-consuming*

process. Methods of analysis were greatly constrained by the counter-sorting method of handling punched cards.

(2010)

(Oh, how I miss the old **counter-sorter**! We used it throughout the *Life Before Death* study – see Chapter 8). He acknowledges that the difficulties in managing such data contributed to the decision to follow up only a sample of 5362 of the 13 687 initially recruited to the study. In their 2006 paper, Wadsworth et al. give a detailed account of the cohort and attrition (drop-outs). By 1999, 469 had died, 640 had withdrawn completely, 119 were living abroad, 461 had emigrated, 330 were untraceable ('lost'), 280 declined to participate on that occasion and 28 more withdrew from the study. **But 3035 were successfully contacted**!

Example 2: The mortality of doctors in relation to their smoking habits – a preliminary report

Following on from their **case-control study** (see next chapter), **Doll and Hill** carried out a cohort study of British doctors. In October 1951, they sent questionnaires to *all* 59,600 registered members of the Medical Profession to ask about their smoking habits. A total of 41,024 (69%) replied and 40,564 (68%) were complete enough to be included. They excluded women and men under 35 who replied because lung cancers were relatively rare in both of these groups. The **Registrars General** in the UK provided details of the cause of deaths of every individual in the cohort who died in the 29 months following the distribution of the questionnaire. They also wrote to the doctors who had certified the deaths of 36 people in whom lung cancer was a main or contributory cause, to ask for more information. Thus, it was possible to compare the death rates for different causes of death and compare that data with the deceased's smoking behaviours. This is shown below (Table 6.1).

They concluded:

Though the numbers of deaths at present available are small the resulting rates reveal a significant and steadily rising mortality from deaths due to cancer of the lung as the amount of tobacco smoked increases. There is also a rise in the mortality from deaths attributed to coronary thrombosis as the amount smoked increases, but the gradient is much less steep than that revealed by cancer of the lung.

Again, this was a massive endeavour – to recruit and record smoking and death data for *41,024 doctors*. They were followed up for *two and a quarter years* in this preliminary report – a relatively short period of time – but enough to give more incriminating data for the case against smoking tobacco. The full study ran from *1951 to 2001*. Their 1956 report provided convincing evidence that smoking tobacco increased the risk of lung cancer.

Causes of Death	No of Deaths Recorded	Death Rates of Non-Smokers	Death Rates of Men Smoking a Daily Average of:			Death Rate of All Men
			1–14.99 g	15–24.99 g	25 g +	
Lung Cancer	36	0.00	0.48	0.67	1.14	0.66
Other Cancer	92	2.32	1.41	1.50	1.91	1.65
Respiratory Disease	54	0.86	0.88	1.01	0.77	0.94
Coronary Thrombosis	235	3.89	3.91	4.71	5.15	4.27
Other Cardiovascular Disease	126	2.23	2.07	1.58	2.78	2.14
Other Diseases	247	4.27	4.67	3.91	4.52	4.36
All Causes	789	13.61	13.42	13.38	16.30	14.00

TABLE 6.1 Standardised death rate per annum per 1000 men aged 35 years and above in relation to the most recent amount of tobacco smoked.

Source: Adapted from Doll and Bradford Hill (1954a).

Example 3: The Framingham Heart Study

This is perhaps the most well-known cohort study in the field of **cardiology.** You can learn all about it by visiting its website – **www.framinghamheartstudy.org**. It is a collaboration between the US National Heart, Lung, & Blood Institute and Boston University. Its aims were:

> *to identify the common factors or characteristics that contribute to CVD by following its development over a long period of time in a large group of participants who had not yet developed overt symptoms of CVD or suffered a heart attack or stroke.*

The project began in 1948 when 5,209 men and women aged 32–62 were recruited in the town of **Framingham** in Massachusetts. They were people who had no signs of heart disease. They were monitored over the years using physical, physiological, and psychosocial measures in an attempt to identify risk factors for cardiovascular disease (**CVD**). Over the years there have been several cohorts recruited to the study. These include the **original cohort** (1948), an **offspring cohort** recruiting children of the original cohort (1971), the **omni cohort** looking at possible race risk factors (1994), a **third-generation cohort** (2002), a **new offspring spouse cohort** (2003), and a **second-generation omni cohort** (2003).

Initially, participants consented to give a detailed medical history, and have physical examinations and medical tests every three to five years in order to identify factors which might contribute to CVD. Then, with more generations being recruited, family patterns became accessible to identify previously unknown risk factors. In recent years genetic research has been a central theme of the study. The term **risk factor** is attributed to having its origin in this study.

Specific findings which have emerged from the study have included:

- Identifying high blood pressure and high blood cholesterol to be major risk factors for CVD (1957).
- 'Risk factor' was introduced to our vocabulary (1961).
- Physical activity found to reduce the risk of heart disease and obesity confirmed to increase the risk of heart disease (1967).
- High blood pressure found to increase the risk of stroke (1970).
- Psychosocial factors found to affect heart disease (1978).
- Progression from hypertension to heart failure described (1996).
- Obesity is a risk factor for heart failure (2002).
- Discovery that social networks exert key influences on decision to quit smoking (2008).
- Researchers contribute to discovering hundreds of new genes underlying major heart disease risk factors (2009–10).
- Associations between new metabolites (including the amino acids glutamate and glutamine) and adverse metabolic profiles that predispose to the risk of developing diabetes, heart disease, or stroke (2012).
- Discovery of genetic variants that may influence brain structure, which may help elucidate the genetic mechanisms contributing to neurodegenerative disease (2015).
- Researchers find that former smokers who quit smoking 25 or more years ago still have three times as much risk of developing lung cancer compared to people who have never smoked (2018).

The outputs from this study have been possible because, with the involvement of a community, they were able to measure and, therefore, test associations between many different factors and many different outcomes. It is a high-profile study which may explain its success in maintaining participations and recruitment. See Levy and Brink (2005) for more details.

Example 4: Psycho-Social Aspects of Breast Disease and Its Treatment

Not all cohort studies involve such large numbers or such long time periods as those we have looked at so far. The only cohort study I have been involved in was early on in my career, when I worked with (the late) Dr Ted Chesser at the Middlesex Hospital Medical School.

In our study, we were keen to document the psycho-social impacts of having and being treated for breast cancer. I was particularly interested in **communication**

issues – which I had recently taken an interest in whilst working on the *Life Before Death* study (1973). We got the co-operation of all the breast surgeons in the hospital, who agreed that we could approach and recruit new patients of their's who were admitted for breast surgery. So, we had the co-operation of the surgical teams and the ward staff. I approached a consecutive series of newly admitted patients the day before their operation. This was usually in the early evening after they had received all of the pre-operative briefings from the staff. I explained the purpose of the research and the interviews I would like to conduct and I got their informed consent. I would then interview them about their current problem, about what they had been told by various doctors and nurses, and about their feelings about the operation and the possible outcomes. These were usually: (i) would the operation be a lumpectomy (removal of the lump only) or a mastectomy (removal of the whole breast – with or without additional tissues); (ii) would it be a 'tumour'/'malignant lump'/cancer; and (iii) how would that affect their lives? Future interviews would be arranged for the day after the operation, the day before discharge, at three-monthly, six monthly, and one-year follow-ups (Anderson and Chesser 1973; Chesser and Anderson 1975).

In practice, the interviews during their initial hospital stay were easy to arrange and conduct. However, it proved very difficult to identify when patients were being invited back for the follow-up visits and letters were sent to those who were showed an interest in attending for the later interviews. In effect, there were two groups of patients within the cohort – those who had a mastectomy (the cancer group) and those who had a lumpectomy (the benign group). The latter group were, to all intents and purposes lost – they could not understand the reason for us asking all our questions and often did not attend any follow-ups. With the former group, there were other issues which made follow-up interviews problematic. These included reticence on the part of same staff to facilitate the follow up information – 'We're not sure when Mrs Smith is due back . . .'. As a result our work really focused on the data gathered in the 2/3 interviews held whilst patients were in-patients for their operations.

The main focus of the research was, therefore, shaped by this and focused very much on communication issues – we particularly highlighted the lack of open communication between doctors (and surgeons) and the women in the cancer group, which differed from the more open communications found after women were confirmed as being in the benign group. Our aim to highlight psycho-social effects of breast cancer and its treatment was therefore limited and, at the time, there were two other centres who were better resourced that we were and were being more successful in their recruitment – so we cut our losses and limited our work to the early stages of treatment and communication issues. Another difficulty was the measurement of **Quality of Life** (QOL). There were no **validated** (standard) measures of QOL and we were all having to try to make up our own assessments of impact upon QOL.

It is interesting – I presented a paper on this work at a conference in 1973. In it I emphasised the extent of obfuscation and avoidance amongst doctors when discussing breast cancer and cancer in general with patients. A friend who sat in on my presentation, had, unbeknown to me, contacts in the press who he fed interesting research news to. So, David informed a journalist about my 'interesting study'. This journalist then phoned me and interviewed me about the work. I was surprised to see his article 'Doctors are bad at communicating with cancer patients' on the front page of the *London Evening Standard!*

On reading his article, I was pleasantly surprised to find that it was accurate. So, you can imagine my surprise, when the next day I was summoned to the Dean of the Medical School's office and asked to explain myself. It turned out that a Professor of Pathology had taken offence at the article and complained to the Dean about 'some jumped-up social worker claiming that Middlesex doctors were bad at communication with their patients'! I pointed out to the Dean that I had not made such a claim – I had criticised *doctors in general* for lacking communication skills – and I pointed out that I was a Medical Sociologist not a social worker! The Dean eventually calmed down and cautioned me to be more careful in the future and check that there were no journalists in the room when I was giving a conference paper. I have done so ever since!

Sampling in Cohort Studies

Like all quantitative studies, a wide variety of sampling methods can be used in cohort studies. The aim is always the same – to get a sample which *best represents the population* from which we are sampling and from which we can *generalise to the whole population* (within certain confidence intervals).

In the example of the NSHD, above, we saw that the first step in their sampling was to choose *one week in 1946*. You might like to think about the issues of selecting your whole sample from one week out of the 52 weeks in the year. Might there be any advantages or disadvantages? An advantage could be simplicity – a pragmatic decision to lessen the complications of taking parts of your sample from other weeks. Are there any reasons to think that some bias may be introduced by the selected method? Next, they aimed to recruit *all people born in that week* – a *total sample of that week*. But that was for the initial survey (a cross-sectional approach) and a **class stratified sample** from the births in that week was decided upon. This is more sophisticated, but adds complications to the process. (Remember they were working in the pre-computer age!) However, it ensures fairness in representing participants from all social classes. So, the end result is both do-able and ensures **representativeness** (equity), and, therefore, they are able to generalise to the population from which their sample was drawn. They had the resources to do that.

In the second example – The British Doctors Study – Doll and Hill tried to recruit *all* practising doctors in the UK. There was no sampling – it was a *total* sample. And 68% took part – an amazing result in terms of recruiting British doctors to a research project! That part was relatively straightforward, but the fact that they were able to get the co-operation of the Registrars General throughout the UK to tag their medical records and follow-up to gather the second set of data when doctors died is a very impressive feat. Again, this was a very well-resourced study. They had the resources to do it.

The third example – The Framingham Heart Study – was also very well resourced. Their first question was 'Where to conduct the study?' As Dawber, Meadors and Moore (1951) stated, the ideal would have been to 'set up in a number of widely separated areas simultaneously, so that the various radical and ethnic groups will be represented, and a variety of geographic, socioeconomic and other environmental factors can be considered'. In 1948, Framingham was essentially middle-class white, however: 'it was a place where such a study could be done, and it was not grossly atypical in any respect that appeared relevant' (Dawber and Moore 1952, p. 242). The official website gives a clear account of the selection of participants.

The official sampling frame was the population aged 30 to 59 as of January 1, 1950, according to the town census. A separate list was drawn up for each of the 8 precincts in the town. Within each precinct, the lists were arranged by family size and then in serial order by address. Two of every 3 families were then selected for the sample. The sample was a systematic sample. In each family all residents in the eligible age range were invited to have an examination. The recruitment effort was organized with 6 committees set up (Arrangements, Publicity, Industry, Business, Civic Organizations and Neighborhood Organizations) to organize the logistical and publicity aspects of the effort. The Neighborhood Organizations committee developed a network where every selected individual was contacted by someone he knew personally and urged to participate in the study.

The formal sampling generated a list of 6,507 individuals (following de-duplication). Of these, 4,469 (69%) were recruited, but this was not felt to be a high enough response rate. So, the researchers included an additional 740 volunteers to bring the total number in the sample up to 5,209.

However, it was recognised that the sample *did not represent US society as a whole*. Their website clearly states: 'the Framingham investigators have always been aware that the site may not be representative of the United States and have made repeatedly comparisons with other regions to test its generalizability'. Because of the changing nature of the Framingham community, the need to diversify the study participants was recognised – hence the omni cohorts. The first of these in 1994 recruited 507 men and women 'of African-American, Hispanic, Asian, Indian, Pacific Islander and Native American origins, who at the time of enrolment were residents of Framingham and the surrounding towns' – thus giving a more balanced racial profile to the study.

In the final example – Psycho-social aspects of breast disease and its treatment – a consecutive series of admissions for breast surgery to one London hospital were recruited. Thus, it was a single-centre study of relatively low numbers. Nowadays, the trend for such research is for people from different centres to collaborate or for the research centre to get other centres to co-operate in supplying access to participants – as in Doll and Hill's case control study. We had no outside funding for our study and I devoted up to half of my time to it and Ted about 10% of his time to it (he was the senior investigator after all!), so it was low in resources. Ted and I took who we could get from those admitted to our hospital.

Data collection

Wherever possible in research, we use **validated tools** (i.e., tried and tested measures) of collecting data, such as validated questionnaires. However, in all of the examples given here, all had to develop their own measures at some points to collect the information they wanted. These were all piloted – and tested and refined – before actually being used. However, most new research will probably have to rely upon developing their own data gathering tools at some point. Sure, we can rely on validated questionnaires, etc., *when they are appropriate and available* . . . But sometimes we have to innovate and/or compromise: research is the art of the possible!

Issues around Recruitment and Retention

All cohort studies lose participants for various reasons. People die, they move away, they get fed up, they forget to reply, etc. one of the key points to bear in mind when embarking on a cohort study is to motivate your participants from the very beginning. Here are some ways to help improve cooperation:

- Help them to understand the importance of the research – *convince them that this research is worthwhile.*
- Make them feel valued – *their part in the research is important.*
- Make it easy for the participants to take part – *make it convenient for them.*
- Show them you appreciate their cooperation – *personalise your appreciation.*
- Keep them informed of the study progress – *show that the study is producing results.*

In the NSHD, The British Doctors Study, and the Framingham Heart Study, the importance was obvious and appreciated by most people – hence the high participation rates. In the NSHD and the Framingham study, people were proud to be a part of it. The Framingham study created and nurtured a sense of *community* – this was *their* study, being done in *their* community. In our study of psycho-social aspects of breast disease, for sure, everyone thought it was an important issue, but there seemed to be a slight sense of 'stigma' about it. Women were not keen to be associated with a study whose focus was *cancer* – particularly those in the 'benign' group. So, the sooner their involvement was over, the better. It might be worth pointing out that in the early 1970s 'cancer' was a **taboo** word – like 'death' and 'dying'. Few practitioners realise that now.

The Framingham study was conducted in a single town – Framingham. It involved that community – and it involved the spouses and children of initial participants. When participants could not visit the clinics for follow-ups, the clinic staff travelled to them! There were also regular questionnaires sent out and phone calls, all of which maintained contact with the cohorts. So successful were they that Tsao and Vasan (2015) refer to 'the superb follow-up of nearly the entire sample'. They praise the study 'The 99% retention rate of participants regularly returning for scheduled examinations at FHS is a testament to the dedication of the participants to the study and contributes to the high quality of the study.'

The NSHD participants are sent a birthday card (with special celebrations of their 65th and 70th birthdays!). Data was collected by home visits if necessary. The study developed **duty of care protocols** to help advise participants in whom clinical problems were identified during the study screening – for example by advising them to see their GP. 'If scientists subject volunteers to clinical research investigations, there is an imperative to do no harm, just as there is in a clinical consultation. The duty of care protocols required at least 1 day a week of a survey doctor on the fieldwork team to deal with resulting queries raised by participants or their GPs. The survey doctor ensured that participants were appropriately referred to their GP (rather than offering advice on individual clinical care), reassured participants, facilitated their retention in the study, ensured appropriate clinical follow-up where necessary, avoided unnecessary work for the GP and avoided leaving GPs uncertain as to what to do as a consequence of tests that they had not ordered' (Kuh et al. 2011).

Pros and Cons of Cohort Studies

One of the first things to note about cohort studies is the *complexity* of them and the issues that can arise from maintaining records and results over a period of time. Large-scale cohort studies such as the first two examples shown here are *costly* – they need a lot of funding and *time* to manage. They can, therefore, be very expensive to set up and to run. The difficulties involved in the data analysis – such as how to deal with missing data in your analyses – can make them tricky to handle.

There is a danger, when a large cohort has been set up, for the initial aims and hypotheses to change – a sort of **purpose creep.** This can be seen to an extent in the NSHD study which set out to examine factors related to child development, and now, because of its success, is able to look at factors which affect how people die. I have noticed in other cohort studies for additional measures to be included as they became interesting or 'fashionable' to research. This should be carefully justified.

Physical Activity and Risk of Ovarian Cancer: A Prospective Cohort Study in the United States

One of my postgraduate students – Dr Aalya Al-Assaf – who was studying on our MSc in Public Health was interested in the role of physical exercise on the onset of ovarian cancer. She chose a **systematic review** to study this topic. This example is a cohort study which was identified in her systematic review.

Hannan et al. (2004) began a cohort study of women recruited to the Breast Cancer Detection Demonstration Project (BCDDP) which aimed to detect breast cancer. Originally this project had 283,222 participants who were 'given breast examinations between 1973 and 1980 in 1 of 29 screening centers in 27 U.S. cities'. In 1979 the National Cancer Institute started a follow-up study.

> *These individuals were all women diagnosed with breast cancer during BCDDP screening (n = 4275), all women who had biopsies indicating benign breast disease (n = 25,114), all women who had been recommended for a biopsy or surgery but for whom the procedure was not performed (n = 9628), and an additional sample of women selected from those who did not undergo nor were recommended for biopsy and who were matched to the women in the above categories on age, time of entry into the screening program, length of participation, ethnicity, and location (n = 25,165).*
>
> (Hannan et al. 2004)

The follow-up had four phases. In Phase I, in 1979, 61 431 participants returned a baseline questionnaire. Those who completed the questionnaire were sent further questionnaires in Phase II, between 1987 and 1989; Phase III, in 1993–95; and Phase IV, in 1995–98. The Phase II questionnaires had questions about *physical activity*. These were completed by 51,690 participants and were taken as the start of the follow-ups for this (2004) study. Women who were diagnosed with ovarian cancer before Phase II were excluded, as were those diagnosed with breast cancer before Phase II, along with any who had had both ovaries removed and any who did not give adequate information about physical activity. This left 27,365 women of whom 23,798 (87%) completed the Phase III (1993–95) questionnaire and 23,058 (84%) who completed the Phase IV questionnaire (in 1996–98).

During follow-ups, *121 cases of ovarian cancer were identified.* These were identified from self-reporting (as long as the diagnosis was confirmed by pathology results or by the participant being included in a cancer registry) and from official sources.

There was a rigorous assessment of the physical activity reported in the Phase II questionnaires in 1987–1989.

> *The number of hours spent in vigorous activity was used as an additional measure of physical activity. The methods used to calculate the physical activity variables are based on previous work in this cohort.*
>
> *(Hannan et al. 2004)*

They concluded that: 'In this cohort of U.S. women, we found no overall significant association between physical activity and risk of ovarian cancer.'

Critique

This is an example of a very large cohort study which had a goal-shift during the period of the study. It started as a study investigating the detection of breast cancer in 1979 and underwent a change in focus to include assessment of physical examination in the 1987–89 follow-up. Changing your goals or adding to them is a strength in cohort studies – *as long as the baseline measurements have been included appropriately.*

In this study, physical activity was only measured on *one occasion* – in 1987–89. The study ran until 1998. Thus, the question we have to ask is this: 'Is the single assessment of physical activity – however thorough – sufficient to give an indication of lifelong physical activity before onset of ovarian cancer?' What were women's levels of physical activity before the Phase II assessment? And was a single point of assessment in 1987–89 sufficient as a measure of physical activity all the way up to 1998? My thinking is that it wasn't.

Beware!

In Aalya's review, studies fell into two categories – case-control studies and cohort studies. As an exercise, I asked Aalya to design a 'perfect' cohort study. The numbers she came up with were astonishing! Ovarian cancer is a relatively rare cancer – it has an incidence rate of 17 per 1000 women. So, to end up with 300 cases, you need to recruit how many women into your cohort? . . . That's right 17,647 women. Now if we decide to recruit them to the cohort at the age of 25, how long should we run the study – 25/30/40/50/60 years? Can you imagine the amount of data you would need to gather for the specific purpose of investigating the relationship between physical exercise and ovarian cancer? How often should you assess their physical exercise? To my mind, this should be done every year because people's physical exercise behaviours can change a lot over time. Do you see the problem? In fact, there were some studies (names not mentioned) which recorded the level of physical activity at the beginning of the study – then never again. One can only assume that the research teams in those studies had also measured a lot of other things and were interested in any outcomes!

To Sum Up

So, to summarise. . . The examples I have chosen here of cohort studies all demonstrate the following characteristics:

- They gather numerical data. **They are quantitative.**
- We should have hypotheses in mind when we conduct this sort of research – we should be **hypothetico-deductive.**
- There is no intervention or experimentation involved, these are **observational studies.**
- We recruit a group to our study and follow the group over time to see what changes – they are **prospective.**

These have their pros and cons. Large-scale cohort studies tend to be complex, involving vast amounts of data with complex analyses. They are therefore expensive and require careful planning and management. So, as in the case of assessing a relatively rare condition such as ovarian cancer, a case-control study is a more efficient option. However, with adequate resources, studies like the National Study of Health and Development and the Framingham Study, can yield valuable data and convincing results. However, not all cohort studies have to be large scale. For example, the relatively small study which Ted Chesser and I started, did not require massive resources – it was small, and very specifically focused. But, like all cohort studies, they require good planning and attention to detail. I think we let ourselves down by underestimating some of the challenges involved. But don't be put off: smaller studies can be done, and they can also generate some really interesting findings.

Research is the art of the possible!

References

Anderson JL and Chesser ES. (1973). Doctor-patient interaction: briefing patients for breast surgery. Paper presented at the British Sociological Association Medical Sociology Conference.

Bernstein L, Ross RK, Lobo RA, et al. (1987). The effects of moderate physical activity on menstrual cycle patterns in adolescence: implications for breast cancer prevention. *British Journal of Cancer* 55, 681–685.

Biesma RG, Schouten LJ, Dirx MJ, et al. (2006) Physical activity and risk of ovarian cancer: results from the Netherlands cohort study (the Netherlands). *Cancer Causes Control* [serial online]. 17(1), 109–115. http://search.proquest.com/docview/213060802?accountid=9727 (accessed 12 May 2012).

Chesser ES and Anderson JL (1975). Treatment of breast cancer: doctor-patient communication and psychosocial implications. *Proceedings of the Royal Society of Medicine* (68), 793–795.

Dawber, Thomas R., Meadors GF, et al. (1951). Epidemiological approaches to heart disease: The Framingham Study. *American Journal of Public Health* 41, 279–286.

Dawber TR and Moore FE. (1952). Longitudinal study of heart disease in Framingham, Massachusetts: an interim report. Presented at the 1951 Annual Conference of the Milbank Memorial Fund.

Doll R and Bradford HA. (1954a). The mortality of doctors in relation to their smoking habits – a preliminary report. *British Medical Journal* 1(4877), 1451–1455.

Doll R and Bradford HA. (1954b). Lung cancer and other causes of death in relation to smoking – a second report on the mortality of British doctors. *British Medical Journal* 2(5001), 1071–1081.

Dosemeci M, Hayes RB, Vetter R, et al. (1993). Occupational physical activity, socioeconomic status, and risks of 15 cancer sites in Turkey. *Cancer Causes Control* 4(4), 313–321; CASE-CONTROL STUDY.

Gordon T and Kannel William WB. (1968). The Framingham Study: introduction and general background. In: *The Framingham Study: An Epidemiological Investigation of Cardiovascular Disease, Section 1*, (Kannel WB and Gordon T, Eds.). National Heart Institute: Bethesda (pp. 1a–1).

Hannan LM, Leitzmann MF, Lacey JV, Jr, et al. (2004). Physical activity and risk of ovarian cancer: a prospective cohort study in the United States. *Cancer Epidemiol Biomarkers Prev* [serial online] 13(5), 765–770.

Hannan LM, Leitzmann MF, Lacey JV, Jr, et al. (2004) Physical activity and risk of ovarian cancer: a prospective cohort study in the United States. *Cancer Epidemiol Biomarkers Prev* [serial online] 13(5), 765–770. http://cebp.aacrjournals.org/content/13/5/765.full.pdf+html (accessed 12 May 2012).

Kuh D, Pierce M, Adams J, et al. (2011). Cohort profile: updating the cohort profile for the MRC National Survey of Health and Development: a new clinic-based data collection for ageing research. *International Journal of Epidemiology* 40, e2–e9.

Levy D and Brink S. (2005). *A Change of Heart: How the People of Framingham, Massachusetts, Helped Unravel the Mysteries of Cardiovascular Disease*. Alfred A Knopf: New York.

Tsao CW and Vasan RS. (2015). Cohort profile: the Framingham Heart Study (FHS): overview of milestones in cardiovascular epidemiology. *International Journal of Epidemiology* 44(6), 1800–1813.

Wadsworth M, Kuh D, Richards M, et al. (2006). Cohort profile: the 1946 National Birth Cohort (MRC National Survey of Health and Development). *International Journal of Epidemiology* 35, 49–54.

Wadsworth M. (2010). The origins and innovatory nature of the 1946 British national birth cohort study. *Longitudinal and Life Course Studies* 1(2), 121–136.

CHAPTER 7

Observational Quantitative Approaches
Case-Control Studies

Introduction

This type of study is one of my favourites. It is a very focused approach which tests a specific hypothesis and thus it is an efficient methodology. It uses the logic of experimental methodologies to answer the question 'Is it likely that X is involved in the aetiology of Y?'

Case-control studies:

- Are in the **quantitative** domain (we measure things).
- They are in the **observational** arm of the quantitative domain (there is no experimentation or intervention).
- They are **hypothetico-deductive** (we are testing a hunch or hypothesis);
- And they are **retrospective** (the data that is collected is about things that have already happened).

Now, as you are aware, in order to 'prove' a causal link between two things – in the first example I shall discuss below, we shall look at a study investigating the link between smoking and lung cancer – we really need to do experimental work to see if smoking is really linked to the onset of lung cancer. However, I am sure you can imagine the methodological and ethical issues involved in recruiting a group of human subjects, randomly dividing them into two groups, then asking the experimental group to smoke 40 cigarettes a day for 20 plus years – and asking the control group not to smoke at all – then measuring how many of them developed lung cancer . . .!

But what we *can* do is . . . Carry on with the logic of the experimental method, but instead of starting with a group of healthy people and randomly allocating them to smoking/non-smoking groups, then seeing how many in each group develop lung cancer, we start with the **end-points** – people with lung cancer/people without lung cancer – and compare these two groups to see if they differ in respect of our **suspect**

Demystifying Research for Medical & Healthcare Students: An Essential Guide, First Edition. John L. Anderson.
© 2022 John Wiley & Sons Ltd. Published 2022 by John Wiley & Sons Ltd.
Companion website: www.wiley.com/go/Anderson/DemystifyingResearch

variable: smoking. Don't you think that this is an ingenious way of **reversing the experimental design** to test the hypothesis? I certainly do!

And that is exactly the approach which was adopted in the classic study 'Smoking and carcinoma of the lung', conducted by Richard Doll and Austin Bradford Hill which was published in the *British Medical Journal* on Saturday 30 September 1950. This was another history-making and life-changing study which was so important in setting the trend for the future of healthcare around the world. So, I shall describe it in more detail now as an illustration of the methodology.

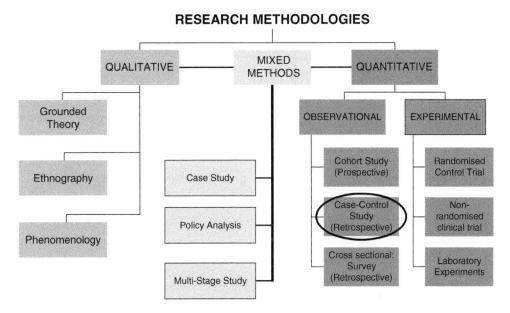

Example 1: Smoking and Lung Cancer

Lung cancer used to be the main cause of cancer deaths in men and women. There was concern to find what caused it, and if possible to reduce the death rates from it. There were, at that time, many factors which were suspected of being involved in the **aetiology** (cause) of lung cancer – air pollution, occupational exposure to cancer-inducing substances, alcohol, and smoking. So, Doll and Hill used a case-control approach to test their hunch (**hypothesis**) that smoking might be involved as a contributory factor in the onset of lung cancer. Let's follow their steps.

1. Bradford Hill at that time was Professor of Medical Statistics at the London School of Hygiene and Tropical Medicine (LSHTM) in the centre of London, and London is where the study was conducted. They got 20 London hospitals to agree to take part.

2. These hospitals all agreed to let them know when a new case of lung cancer was identified.

3. So, when a hospital phoned to let them know that a new case of lung cancer was diagnosed, a researcher (an **almoner**) went to the hospital to interview the new patient and take a history of their smoking behaviours.

ED: do you know what an almoner was? I guessed you might not! Almoners – often called 'lady almoners' – were responsible for ensuring that when patients were discharged from hospitals, they had a roof over their head and had enough money to feed themselves. They were the forerunner of the hospital social worker. The name 'almoner' comes from the term 'alms' as in 'alms for the poor' – a charitable donation.

4. Then they would identify and interview a non-cancer patient in the same five-year age group and of the same sex and take a history of their smoking behaviours.

5. The interview data were then analysed to identify any differences between the lung cancer patients – the **cases** – and the non-lung cancer patients – the **controls.**

6. The results were published in the *British Medical Journal (BMJ)* on 30 September 1950 (Figure 7.1). They concluded:

The figures obtained are admittedly speculative, but suggest that, above the age of 45, the risk of developing the disease increases in simple proportion with the amount smoked, and that it may be approximately 50 times as great among those who smoke 25 or more cigarettes a day as among non-smokers.

This was the first UK study to find such convincing evidence for the link between smoking and lung cancer and prompted other studies (see Chapter 6) to confirm the link between smoking and cancer.

The Case-Control Study Approach

OK, let's look at the methodology. It is simple. First: identify and recruit a group of people with the condition (or characteristic) that you want to explain (your **cases**) and interview them in-depth about the factor that you suspect might lead to the condition or characteristic. Next, identify and recruit a group of people – as similar in all respects to your cases as possible – but who do not have that condition or

BRITISH MEDICAL JOURNAL

LONDON SATURDAY SEPTEMBER 30 1950

SMOKING AND CARCINOMA OF THE LUNG
PRELIMINARY REPORT

BY

RICHARD DOLL, M.D., M.R.C.P.
Member of the Statistical Research Unit of the Medical Research Council

AND

A. BRADFORD HILL, Ph.D., D.Sc.
Professor of Medical Statistics, London School of Hygiene and Tropical Medicine; Honorary Director of the Statistical Research Unit of the Medical Research Council

FIGURE 7.1 Doll and Bradford-Hill's *BMJ* article.

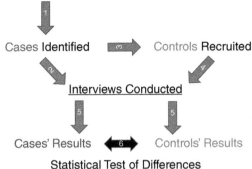

FIGURE 7.2   Outline of the case-control method.

characteristic (your **controls**) and interview them in-depth about the factor that you suspect might lead to the condition or characteristic. Analyse your data and, hey presto! (See Figure 7.2.)

Example 2: Depression and disability in people with podoconiosis

A *modified* case-control approach was used by Bartlett et al. (2015) in their study of depression and disability in people with podoconiosis in Ethiopia. Although this was, strictly speaking, a cross-sectional study, it included case-control *methods* in its design. (Podoconiosis is a very disabling and stigmatising condition with swelling of the lower legs and feet. It is caused by exposure to irritants in the clay soil – it is not a contagious condition. It affects an estimated four million people in Africa, and it is very common in Ethiopia.) If this had been a true case-control study, then depression (the outcome) would have been the basis for selecting cases.

In their study area, 86% of people lived in rural areas. There were about 30 000 households or housing units, and about 9% of households have people with podoconiosis. They recruited 271 new podoconiosis patients in a random sample of *cases*. These were identified through local clinics and doctors. As *controls,* they approached neighbours who lived in the next nearest household and recruited 268 of them. Both cases and controls were asked to complete validated questionnaires – the Patient Health Questionnaire (PHQ-9) and WHO Disability Assessment Schedule II (WHODAS II). Their results showed that 'elevated depressive symptoms' (a PHQ score of 5 or more) were significantly higher among the people with podoconiosis (cases) than healthy neighbours without podoconiosis (the controls) – 12.6 and 0.7% respectively. Also, the risk of suicide was estimated to have been much higher, 5.2% for 'cases', compared to 0.4% for 'controls'.

Thus, in this example, they had adapted the case-control methodology to recruit controls who were similar in terms of geographical location – to rule this out as a contributory factor to the depression they were measuring for. Quite a nice touch, don't you think?

Measuring Your 'Suspect Variable'

This is crucial to the success of your study. Doll and Hill used a very detailed and lengthy questionnaire to measure smoking behaviours.

> *The assessment of the relation between tobacco-smoking and disease is complicated by the fact that smoking habits change. A man who has been a light smoker for years may become a heavy smoker; a heavy smoker may cut down his consumption or give up smoking - and, indeed, may do so repeatedly. An acute respiratory disease may force the sufferer to stop smoking, or he may be advised to stop for one of many pathological conditions.*
>
> *The difficulties of a varying consumption can be largely overcome if a more detailed smoking history is taken than is customary in the course of an ordinary medical examination – for example, one man who was described in the hospital notes as being a non-smoker admitted to the almoner that he had been a very heavy smoker until a few years previously. In this investigation, therefore, the patients were closely questioned and asked (a) if they had smoked at any period of their lives; (b) the ages at which they had started and stopped; (c) the amount they were in the habit of smoking before the onset of the illness which had brought them into hospital; (d) the main changes in their smoking history and the maximum they had ever been in the habit of smoking; (e) the varying proportions smoked in pipes and cigarettes; and (f) whether or not they inhaled.*
>
> *Smoking histories obtained by this investigation are not, as would be expected, strictly accurate, they are reliable enough to indicate general trends and to substantiate material differences between groups.*
>
> *(Doll and Hill 1950)*

Uses

The case-control approach is mainly used in health research. I believe it is a much misunderstood and, therefore, a very under-used approach. It can be used in many more contexts. For example, if we were concerned about identifying factors which led to drug use and we suspected that one possible factor was, perhaps, early exposure to others using drugs, then we might use a case control study approach. In this example, our 'Cases' would be 'people who are drug users', and our 'Controls' would be 'people who are not drug users'. We would interview a sample of both groups and compare the 'exposure' rates in both groups. The main challenge for us in this example would be to find acceptable means of identifying and matching participants for the control group. Have a think about this approach and see what examples you can come up with.

Matching Cases and Controls

This can be tricky. Doll and Hill were pragmatic about it and confined their choice of controls to hospital in-patients. They made the judgement that the other two most important factors to control for were age group and gender. So, they recruited patients who were in the same five-year age group as the cases, and who were of the same gender. This may sound simple, but it was not always easy. Doll and Hill discuss some of the issues that they had to contend with, and they discussed in detail the extent to which the two groups might be 'representative' of cancer and non-cancer patients attending London Hospitals. (NB: this is an important consideration in any study.) The following extract shows something about their thinking about the matching:

> *There remains the possibility that the interviewers, in selecting the control patients, took for interview from among the patients available for selection a disproportionate number of light smokers. It is difficult to see how they could have done so, but the point can be tested indirectly by comparing the smoking habits of the patients whom they did select for interview with the habits of the other patients, other than those with carcinoma of the lung, whose names were notified by the hospitals. The comparison is made in Table XI and reveals no appreciable difference between the two groups.*

> *At two specialized hospitals (Brompton Hospital and Harefield Hospital) it was not always possible to secure a control patient by this method, and in such cases a control patient was taken from one of the two neighbouring hospitals.*

> *(Doll and Bradford 1950)*

You might wish to define the inclusion criteria for your controls in whatever way makes sense for *your* study. For example, factors such as ethnicity, sexuality, place of residence, etc., may be important things to think about. The point is to *make sure that your controls are as alike as possible to your cases in any important aspect which could be thought to influence the outcomes.*

It is possible to recruit controls as a *group* once all the cases have been recruited. This can sometimes make it easier to match controls to cases.

An overview of the process is shown in **Figure 7.2** above.

To Sum Up

The examples here, show that case-control studies are **quantitative** – we measure and use statistics to analyse the data. We use this approach to test a very specific hypothesis, (**hypothetico-deductive**) concerning a 'suspect' variable and its possible association with a specific outcome. The more specific we can be, the better. We measure things which have already happened and do not follow people over a period of time. These studies are **retrospective.** There is no experimentation or intervention – they are **observational**. A **consecutive series** of *cases* is usually recruited, but **purposive sampling** is used for *controls*.

The selection of 'controls' is one of the most important aspects of this approach. Controls should be as alike to cases as possible – except for the outcome – the condition you are studying. So, Doll and Hill (1950) selected controls from people who, like the lung cancer cases, were also in-patients in the same hospitals. They matched them for gender and for age-group, so that factors related to being ill, gender and age, were as similar in the two groups as possible. In that way, they 'controlled' for being ill, gender and age. Bartlett, Deribe, Kebede, et al. (2015) chose controls who were near neighbours of cases – a form of *'geographical sampling'*. This was appropriate because the two groups, living near one another, were likely to experience similar lifestyles and geographic or environmental conditions. This was a very pragmatic choice for sampling in the countryside in which their study was being conducted. In general, the more complex your matching criteria is, the more difficulties you will experience in your recruitment of participants, and the more difficulties you will experience when doing your statistical analysis – one problem being that you will require larger numbers in order to control for all the factors you take into account.

Research is the art of the possible!

References

Bartlett J, Deribe K, Tamiru A, et al. (2015). Depression and disability in people with podoconiosis: a comparative cross-sectional study in rural Northern Ethiopia. *International Health* 7(4), 1876–3405.

Doll R and Hill AB. (1950). Smoking and carcinoma of the lung. *British Medical Journal* 2(4682), 739–748.

CHAPTER 8

Observational Quantitative Approaches
Cross-Sectional Studies (Surveys)

Introduction

The term 'cross-sectional studies' is our way of saying that the study is being done at one point in time and we are taking a **snapshot** of the situation now and investigating things that might have led up to this point in time. They are perhaps the commonest type of study done in healthcare and social research. They have their advantages and disadvantages and I shall discuss these at the end of the chapter. In this section, I shall focus on **surveys** which are probably the most common of the cross-sectional approaches, and what I cut my teeth on as a researcher. In fact, I shall use that first piece of work as an example because it reflects a 'gold standard' approach to conducting a survey.

> NB – I am not being immodest here – the credit for the quality of the research goes to my old boss Ann Cartwright who conceived of and initiated the Life Before Death study (Cartwright et al. 1973).

So, to remind you:

- We are still in the **quantitative** domain – we are still very much concerned with gathering numerical data.
- It is still a **hypothetico-deductive** approach and we should have hypotheses in mind when we set out on this sort of endeavour.
- This is still an **observational** type of study – there is no intervention or experimentation involved.
- Again, it is a **retrospective** approach – we are investigating things which have already taken place.

Demystifying Research for Medical & Healthcare Students: An Essential Guide, First Edition. John L. Anderson.
© 2022 John Wiley & Sons Ltd. Published 2022 by John Wiley & Sons Ltd.
Companion website: www.wiley.com/go/Anderson/DemystifyingResearch

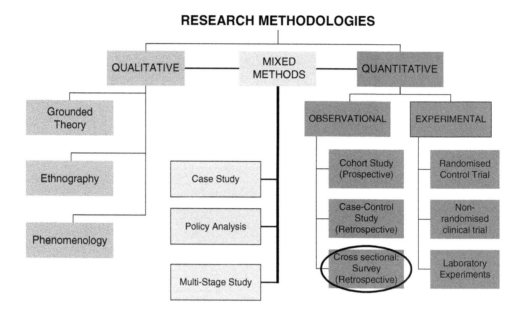

Again, one of the aspects of this type of research that I shall be focusing on is the selection of a sample to study – the **sampling.** Some studies are able to take a **total sample** of the population they are studying. Can you think of any examples of these? That's right – the **National Census.** That survey is a study which tries to collect data from *every* household in the country. And it does rather well. Of course, there are some groups of people who are missed for various reasons. Can you think of any examples? But very few researchers have access to the sorts of resources that are needed to do a total population sample.

Example 1: Life Before Death

When I first started work at the Institute for Social Studies in Medical Care in 1970, I was given the following essential pieces of equipment (see Figure 8.1):

- A **2B pencil (for ease of erasing – hard leads make indentations in the paper!).**
- An **eraser.**
- A 12-inch, clear, plastic **ruler.**
- A pair of **scissors.**
- A roll of clear **Sellotape** (in a dispenser).
- A **slide rule:** AKA a computer. This is the Western equivalent of an abacus in China and Japan. All of our calculations – yes **ALL** of our calculations – were done using the slide rule.

The scissors and Sellotape were for *cutting and pasting* – literally! We wrote our text in pencil, and when we wanted to change the order, or insert new text, we physically cut the page to remove the old text, and sellotaped in the new text.

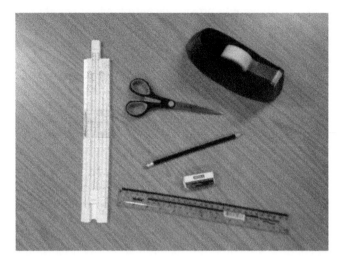

FIGURE 8.1   Essential research equipment 1970 – clockwise from left: slide rule, scissors, Sellotape, pencil (2B), eraser, clear ruler.

All of our data was put on 80-column **punched cards.** These could be fed into a **counter-sorter,** a machine the size of a large sideboard, which **counted** what was on any column you set it at, and which could **sort** the cards by any column you set it at. In this way you could do frequency counts and cross-tabulations. That's when the slide rule came in to its own – to calculate percentages and to calculate Chi-Square statistics!

The aim of this study was to document the lives and experiences of people who died in England and Wales (The Scottish had a slightly different way of organising care and were, therefore excluded.) No one except John Hinton (my next boss and a wonderful man!) had done any work on death and dying in the UK, and his were relatively small-scale studies. There had recently been a couple of books published in the USA by Anselm Strauss and Barney Glazer (who we shall meet again in the section on Qualitative Approaches). As we said in the introduction to our book, 'Death has become a taboo subject in modern society'. As a result, we only had anecdotal evidence of what was going on in providing care for people who had died and we only had hunches about some of the gaps in the care they received. This project aimed to get answers to these questions.

A survey seemed to be the most appropriate method to invoke for this study, because the aim was to make it **representative** of all adults who died and to be able to state – within a certain degree of confidence – how **generalisable** our findings would be to the total population of adults who died.

The first issue to be addressed was: *who could provide the information we needed –* about people's experiences in their last year of life? We couldn't identify in advance everyone who was going to die and follow them up for a year because (i) whilst some deaths are relatively easy to predict in the latter stages of their course, most are not; and (ii) there would be ethical objections raised about researchers behaving like vultures and hovering around people who were thought to be dying.

So, let's think . . . Who could provide us with the best possible information? GPs? Hospital doctors? Nurses? For sure, any HCP involved in the care of the person who died could provide us with some information – but it would be limited information, reflecting only what they had seen – and would only tell us about people who were receiving these services. Any other ideas? . . . OK, other carers you say. Sounds promising, but who? The husband or wife? Good – but what about those who were not married or had been widowed – remember that men have a shorter life expectancy than women (especially in the 1960s and 1970s) and there would be far fewer men available to tell us about their wives' experiences.

OK, let's cut to the chase! We opted to try to identify the individual (relative, friend, or neighbour) *who had been the one who had been the most involved in the person who died's care,* and to interview them. This was felt to be the most practical solution.

So, let's be clear about it and define the population that we are interested in. In this case it was *adults who died in England and Wales.* Now, because all deaths have to be registered, we have an advantage – we can get details of these from the local Registrars throughout the country. We could not include *all* deaths because there were about a half of a million (560,077) adult deaths per year at this time. The most obvious way to sample from these would be to take a **random sample** from all of the adult deaths. Random samples are the gold standard method of sampling. Nowadays, this can be done very simply by a computer. In those days this had to be done by hand using tables of random numbers. A **sample size calculation** (sometimes called a **power calculation**) can assist you in determining an appropriate size of sample to ensure that: (i) you have sufficient numbers in your sample to ensure that you can confidently predict from your sample what the 'real' results are likely to be in the population you drew your sample from – this avoids having too few and your study being 'under-powered'; and (ii) you do not have too many in your sample so that some results, which may be 'statistically significant' as a result of your high numbers, are not spurious. We estimated that a sample size of nearly one thousand (1000) would be appropriate.

Now we come to another problem – and this is a very practical one. At the time, the Institute for Social Studies in Social Care was still the Medical Research Unit in the Institute of Community Studies (**ICS**). The ICS had been founded by Michael Young and Peter Wilmott in Bethnal Green in East London. From there, they began their pioneering work on families and kinship (Young & Wilmott, 1957, 1973) and it was from there, in our offices in Bethnal Green Square, that this study was run. So, imagine the situation where you have identified a random sample of all deaths in England and Wales and you start your fieldwork (your interviews). You send one of your trained interviewers from London to Blackpool. She does the interview and takes the train back (Figure 8.2). The next in your list is in Plymouth, so she catches the train there, does the interview and comes back – and so on (Figure 8.3). This would be fine if you had unlimited time and money – but it would be wasteful of the researchers' time and costs – most of which would be spent on travelling around the country! So, what do we do?

That's right – we find a way of **clustering** our interviews so that a team of interviewers can focus on one area and then move on to the next. So, we first decide on a way of grouping our interviews. The obvious solution is to adopt a **multi-stage approach.** First, we sample a number of areas (we chose 12), then you *sample within those areas.* The obvious approach might seem to take a random sample of all of the areas and then a random sample of deaths within each. However, not all areas are equal in size. We were dealing with registration districts, and there were more smaller districts than larger districts. So, a straight random sample of districts would have

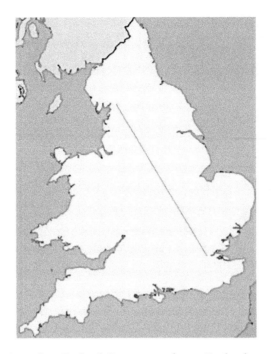

FIGURE 8.2   The first interview: Bethnal Green to northwest England.

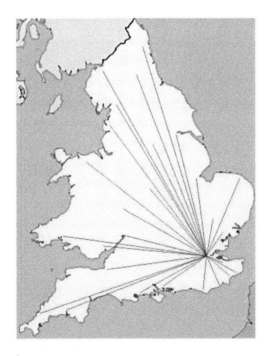

FIGURE 8.3   The interviews progress . . .

meant an over-representation of smaller (usually rural) districts. The way around this is to sample **with probability proportional to population.** The simple (!) way of doing this begins by making a list of all registration districts and number them from 1 to 50 million (or whatever the total population is). So, if the first district has 200,000 people in it – it is numbered 1–200,000; if the next has 150,000, it is numbered 200,001–350,000 and so on, up to . . . 50,000,000. Then you randomly select 12 numbers from 0 to 50,000,000, and the districts which contain those numbers are the districts you select. The next step is to take a straight **random sample** of all adult deaths from each of the districts (Figure 8.4).

The logic of this method is immaculate – from a statistical point of view. If you were to take a straight random sample of 1000 from all 560,077 deaths, then each person who died has an equal chance of being selected – 1/560,077. It you first sample districts with probability proportional to population, and sample randomly within each of your districts, then again (and this is true!) statistically each person who died in the country has an equal – 1/560,077 chance of being selected. So, this is a very useful method of sampling to avoid biases that you might get when the units (e.g., registration districts) are of different sizes.

So, we had our sample of districts. The General Register Office helped by taking a random sample of deaths registered during the relevant period of persons aged 15 and over who lived in the study area. Now we had our sample of people who had died.

The details of the death and the person who dies and the person who registered the death are all shown on the **death certificate**. So, our interviewers were able to approach the person who registered the death and, after a brief interview, they determined if they were the person most involved in the care of the deceased in the year before they died. If

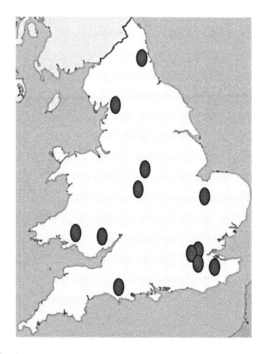

FIGURE 8.4 A solution!

they were, they sought their consent; and, if that was given, they carried on to interview them. If they were not the most appropriate person, they tried to determine who was, and they then contacted *that* person. And so on, until they had an interviewee or determined that there was no appropriate person willing to be interviewed.

Our interviewers were trained. We had developed a very highly structured questionnaire. This was not a pre-existing, *validated* questionnaire. Remember that this survey was a 'first' in the UK. So, along with our steering committee of senior researchers and academics, we worked with what was available to develop the questionnaire. What were the issues? These were outlined from what people imagined might be important issues; from what previous research on had shown (Cartwright 1964, 1967; Glaser and Strauss 1965, 1968; Hinton 1967; Hockey 1966, 1968; Marris 1958); and from what personal experiences and anecdotal evidence had suggested. These were used to develop a draft questionnaire.

This was tried out in a **pilot study** – a test run of the questionnaire to check on the **acceptability** and **feasibility** of its use on our eventual participants. This eventually led to the development of the final *23-page questionnaire*. Some researchers may only do a couple of 'pilot interviews' – often with friends and/or colleagues. I cannot stress enough just how important this stage is. *You must try to field-test your methodology on real, live people who are drawn from the type of people you will be enlisting as participants in your main study!* Of course, I realise that there may be constraints, such as time and resources which might limit this. But always ask yourself this question: 'When I come to submit a copy of the report for publication in a decent academic journal, what questions and objections might the reviewers have of my methodology?' I remember that, when we were analysing the data and writing our report on the LBD study, Michael Young and Peter Wilmott were working on their ground-breaking research in the 'Symmetrical Family' (Young and Wilmott 1973) study. Some of the researchers working on the project were bemoaning that they were on their 34th pilot study!

Once the final version of the questionnaire – all 23 pages of it – were agreed and it was printed, the interviewers had to be trained in its use. Please excuse my oncoming rant! Some researchers just go and interview their study participants without any prior testing or training – that is just not on! I have regularly run training workshops in **research skills** (see Appendices) and constantly meet people who are completely unskilled in interviewing, and, also, are unable to clearly explain the purpose of their research to participants. Training makes better! Practice and more practice make even better! Practice and training and more practice make perfection! I shall talk about ethical issues in a later section; the Health Research Authority (HRA) emphasise how important it is to be competent in the research methods you use.

So, the interviewers were closeted away for about a week in a training centre. There they practised using the questionnaire until they knew it inside out. They knew which questions there were. They knew which questions merely required a tick in a box and which ones they were expected to add notes to about what the respondent said. And they knew when to probe for more information, etc. Now they were ready to go into the field for the main study.

Whilst doing the main study interviews, all of the completed questionnaires were handed in and one of the research team would check to make sure that the questionnaire had been fully completed. Sometimes, interviewers were sent back to ask questions they had omitted. This formed part of the **quality control** within the study.

The fact that interviews were being held in 12 districts meant that there could be a maximum *team* effort to do the interviews. So, for example, if one target participant was not available on the first call, another could be approached and then the first one could be returned to later. This proved to be a relatively efficient way of maximising the effectiveness of the interviewers' time.

The results of this study proved to be ground-breaking. We were able to provide a great deal of information – much of it gloomy – about the circumstances in which people in England and Wales died. We highlighted the increasing severity of physical restrictions and symptoms which people experienced. For example: 87% of people who died of cancer were reported to have experienced pain in the year before they died – most had it for a long time and they found it very distressing. Although most people, 54%, died in a hospital, and only 35% died in their own home, most had been in and out of hospital in the last year. Home care was a vital component of the care of people who died. We found that the persons who bore the brunt of caring at home were likely to be *female relatives*, and families who might have lived quite separate lives, often adjusted to team together to provide care. We highlighted the gaps in communications about what was wrong and what was likely to happen. The person who died from cancer was less likely to be informed about what was wrong than their relatives. And relatives were more likely to be told that the person was dying than they were themselves. There was a 'conspiracy of silence' when it came to communicating about cancer and dying. How things have changed now! The book provided a cornucopia of data about people's lives in the year before they died.

A part of this work included a postal survey of the General Practitioners of the people who had died. I was put in charge of it and we got a response rate of 77% – which was a very high response rate for postal surveys of GPs at that time. I think the high response rate was due to two things: (i) GPs recognised the importance of the subject of the research, and (ii) I was a naïve researcher and misinterpreted the instructions for posting reminders. The result was that GPs were sent their questionnaire initially when we got their details in our interviews. Then a month later, they would be sent another copy with a reminder letter, then once more a month after that. But, because I made a mistake, I sent out an extra three reminders! And of course, with each posting, there was a response, so the numbers kept creeping up until we reached 77%. So, if you want to get a good response, send reminders!

Example 2: Health and Sickness: The Choice of Treatment: Perception of Illness and Use of Services in an Urban Community

Wadsworth, Butterfield, and Blaney (1973) were interested in lay people's experiences of illnesses and how they dealt with them. Up to this point in time, most research done on what illnesses people experienced and how they dealt with them had been done – yes, you've got it! – in clinical settings, either by asking GP patients or hospital patients. What's the problem with that? In criminology, the equivalent to investigating crime and criminals would be to interview – that's right – people in prison or people who have been arrested. What is the problem with that? Well, those are the *unsuccessful criminals!* Similarly, when we chose to interview existing patients, we are focusing on those people who have been unsuccessful in dealing with their illnesses! So, how did Wadsworth et al. go about it?

They decided to do a **community survey.** They chose one London Borough, and within that Borough, they took a **random sample** of 2,500 adults from the Electoral Register – 87% agreed to participate (!). The interviewers, in structured interviews, asked people about their health in the previous two weeks. In asking for detailed, specific accounts of behaviour, we tend to be able to remember what we did last week and the week before, pretty well, but thereafter things begin to blur a bit. They enquired about any signs or symptoms of disease – defined as anything that was wrong which the respondent thought should be taken to a doctor.

They found that 5% had experienced *NO* symptoms or signs of illness in the last two weeks. That is, 95% *HAD* experienced some symptoms or signs of illness in the last two weeks. About 19% took no action – they might wait and see if it went on its own. Most, 56%, took some form of non-medical action – using proprietary medicines, special diets, etc. About 17% saw a GP; 3% attended a hospital out-patient clinic, and 0.5% ended up as hospital in-patients. There was a clear **Symptom or Illness Iceberg** – for most people, the experience of having signs and symptoms of illness are an *everyday experience* (Ed: I shy away from using the term 'normal'), whilst seeking medical attention for them is comparatively speaking a rare event. Now, isn't that an interesting finding – and quite different to what it would have been if the study had been done in hospital or GP clinics.

Interestingly, I have been teaching about 'illness behaviour' since 1973, and there are always students who object when I present these findings. I got so fed up with this that I changed my teaching to get my classes of medical students to keep **health diaries** for two weeks and each hand in a summary results sheet which I would collect and analyse. I used the results in my classes on 'illness behaviour' to show that even relatively fit and well young men and women – such as medical students – might give similar results.

One of the main – and major – changes which has taken place in society since these early studies has been the growth of technology, its availability and its use. When we did the *Life Before Death* study, most households in Britain did not have a telephone. Computers were hardly heard of and there was no such thing as a pocket calculator – yes – ALL of our statistical analysis was done by hand – hence the slide rule! Now we can use pocket calculators (or our mobile phones) and computers for all of our calculations – and do them in a fraction of the time.

Along with computers and mobile phones has come the 'new technology' and all of its spin offs – such as the internet and social media. There has also been a growth of online survey engines – such as **SurveyMonkey**™. It is now possible to complete a whole survey using e-mails, telephones, etc. without leaving the comfort of your office or home study – as the next case study demonstrates.

Example 3: Musculoskeletal Injuries in Real Tennis

Joel Humphrey was a student on our MSc in Orthopaedic Surgery. I co-supervised his dissertation with Adil Ajuied, a consultant Orthopaedic Surgeon. Joel was interested in documenting injuries that were associated with 'real tennis'. As Joel wrote:

> *Real tennis is an original racquet sport from which the modern game of lawn tennis is derived. It is played indoors involving high-skill levels and strategy, and has essentially remained unchanged over the last five centuries. Real tennis was the first sport to be described as 'the beautiful game'. Currently, there are over 10,000 officially registered players in the UK, US, Australia, and France. The International Real Tennis Professional Association (IRTPA) supports real tennis professionals and drives the development of the sport worldwide. The main governing body in the UK is the Tennis & Rackets Association (T&RA).*
>
> (Humphrey et al. 2019)

I think of it as a sort of blood sport which lies somewhere between lacrosse and squash!

We developed a questionnaire to ask about respondents' personal and demographic backgrounds – age, gender, height, weight – and their tennis-playing – dominant hand, number of years played, hours played per week, whether they usually stretched pre-game, warmed-up and warmed-down, and real tennis handicap. Plus, we asked for details of any injuries (if any) they had sustained, what they did about them, etc. The T&RA is sponsored by Pol Roger (the champagne company) who donated a bottle of champagne to the study. (No! We did not benefit from it at all!) In an attempt to provide an inducement, participants in the study could opt to be included in a confidential, random draw for the champagne, which was sent directly to the winner by Pol Roger.

Our methods, definitions, and terminology were adapted from the 'Consensus statement on epidemiological studies of medical conditions in tennis, April 2009' (Pluim et al. 2009). This allowed a certain degree of standardisation which could be adapted to the aims of our study. Injuries were defined as any 'musculoskeletal complaint directly related to playing real tennis irrespective of the severity'. Severity was gauged by the number of days required off playing the sport before return, and by respondents rating each injury from 0 (insignificant) to 10 (life threatening). The questionnaire was loaded onto the **Bristol Online Survey** engine which was freely available through the university.

The T&RA co-operated by sending e-mails to all 2,036 real tennis players (aged 18 and over) on their database requesting their participation in our study by completing the anonymous online survey. We had 485 fully completed questionnaires – 438 males and 47 females – a response rate of 23.8%. These represented all 24 RT clubs in the UK, four from the USA, and two from Australia. The participants were a representative sample of the real tennis population, with low numbers of females and younger players (<25 years old).

Although the response rate was under 25%, this was thought to have been a good result when compared to another similar study of musculoskeletal injuries in lawn tennis-teaching professionals. That one only achieved an 8.7% response rate (Colberg et al. 2017).

One of the main findings was that the main factor associated with real tennis injuries is hours played per week – the more you play, the more likely you are to have an injury! The study formed a benchmark for future studies on academy and professional real tennis players.

Questionnaires and Interviews

It really annoys me when I hear people talk about doing a 'questionnaire study' when they mean a 'survey' – just don't do that! A **questionnaire** is a piece of paper with questions on it. It can be a **self-administered questionnaire (SAQ),** which is one given to people to complete on their own, or it can be an **interviewer-administered questionnaire (IAQ)**, which is one where an interviewer asks the questions of participants in the study. Questionnaires tend to fall into one of two categories – **structured** and **semi-structured**.

Structured questionnaires: Most self-administered questionnaires are highly structured – as there is no interviewer there to guide the respondent. So, it is important that everyone receives the same set of questions. The example I have described in the *Life Before Death* study above was a highly structured questionnaire. It was designed so that all interviewers had to do was tick the correct boxes and add any relevant comments where appropriate. There was no room for manoeuvre on the interviewers' part. They asked the same questions, in the same order, and with the same wording for every participant in the study. This had a **stimulus–response** logic – if every question is presented in exactly the same way (in order and wording) to each interviewee, then we know that each interviewee is responding to the same stimulus.

Semi-structured questionnaires: These are more commonly found in interviewer-administered questionnaires. They tend to allow the interviewer to have slightly more control over the interview. For sure, it is important that all the questions are asked of all respondents. But, this time, the interviewer can exert more discretion in the order they are asked, and in the actual wording that is used. So, if a respondent, in answering one question, goes on to cover the answer to another, later question, the interviewer has the discretion to follow-up on that topic, rather than saying something like 'Yes, well, we'll come on to that later'. The logic here is a more person-centred one which allows the interviewee more control and decisions in determining the shape of an interview. (We shall come back to this later when we talk about qualitative interviews.)

Interviews are study meetings arranged between a researcher and a research participant for the purpose of the researcher gathering data for the study. There are different types of interviews, but in survey research, the majority fall into the structured and semi-structured categories. **Unstructured interviews** are very uncommon in quantitative research.

Telephone and Online Interviews

When we did the Life Before Death survey, most homes did not have a telephone. Now, most people have access to a landline and mobile phones. My preference is still to do face to face interviews, although I have been involved in many studies which have relied upon telephone contacts. I like to see the person I am interviewing – I have interviewed using Skype or Face-time, but I don't feel very comfortable with them.

However, there is a lot to be said for using telephone interviews. For a start, they reduce the cost of a survey. But, then, would you want to speak to someone about sensitive topics over the phone? I wouldn't. I have done it when interviewing women in the later stages of breast cancer, and I was not comfortable with it.

Online survey engines such as Survey Monkey, Bristol Online Survey, and the like have made it very convenient to host a survey online. And they usually have useful basic statistical packages to help with some of the data analysis. Most can also interface with the most popular software used for analysing quantitative data – the **Statistical Package for the Social Sciences, (SPSS).** I have used SPSS since 1975 and it just keeps on getting better – and more complicated! So, online surveys tend to recruit participants by e-mail. These usually have information about the study and a link which participants can click on to take them directly to the survey. There are advantages, such as timing (when to complete the survey), location (where to complete the survey), privacy, and confidentiality.

TABLE 8.1   **Stages in a survey.**

Stage	Notes
1. Setting the question and defining the issues	
2. Define the population	
3. Determine a sample size	
4. Select a sampling method	
5. Pilot study – develop instruments and test feasibility	
6. Main study	
7. Data analysis	
8. Disseminating the findings – report writing	

To Sum Up

The examples shown above have all shown the emphasis on gathering numerical data – they are **quantitative** and are concerned with questions such as: 'How many people experience . . .?' and 'How severe are the injuries that people playing real tennis experience?' They all tend to the **hypothetico-deductive** end of the spectrum – they might begin with a null hypothesis such as 'People who died of cancer are no more likely to experience pain than people who died of other causes' – then the analysis of the data showed that, in fact pain was more commonly reported for people who died of cancer than people who died of other conditions. These are **observational**, in the sense that they do *not* involve any interventions or experimentations. And they all report on things which have already happened – they are **retrospective**.

Surveys can be used as a 'scattergun' approach – by including a wide spectrum of people, you may hit it lucky and come up with some significant results. So, be careful to avoid this by clearly stating your aims and your hunches – or hypotheses – at the beginning. Table 8.1 can be used as a framework for planning – or critiquing – a survey.

Our Life before Death (1973) study and Wadsworth, Butterfield, and Blaney's (1973) study described above, are examples of **community surveys.** These are a 'dying breed' of survey in which samples are drawn from the general population and researchers knock on doors to recruit participants to the study. Increasingly, **postal surveys** – such as the GP postal survey that I described in the Life Before Death study – became the norm for large-scale survey work. And these, in turn have been superseded by the **online survey** such as that carried out by Humphrey et al. (2019) in which invitations are generally sent out by e-mails to a wide audience in the hope of getting a good response. Some are targeted at specific individuals and can get a better response. With such wide-ranging surveys, issues about participants understanding the questions arise, therefore the questions have all to be at a level of reading ease that does not put off people who have difficulty reading – or have difficulty understanding English. You can't beat a good, old-fashioned interviewer administered survey!

Research is the art of the possible!

References

Cartwright A. (1964.) *Human Relations and Hospital Care*. Routledge & Kegan Paul: London.

Cartwright A. (1967). *Patients and their Doctors – A Study of General Practice*. Routledge & Kegan Paul: London.

Cartwright A, Hockey L, Anderson JL. (1973.) *Life before Death*. Routledge & Kegan Paul: London.

Colberg R, Aune K, Propst M. (2017). Prevalence of musculoskeletal conditions in tennis-teaching professionals. *Orthop. J. Sports Med.* 4(10), 2325967116668138.

Glaser BG and Strauss AL. (1965). *Awareness of Dying*. Routledge: New York.

Glaser BG and Strauss AL. (1968). *Time for Dying*. Aldine Publishing: New York.

Hinton J. (1967). *Dying*. Penguin Books: Harmondsworth.

Hockey L. (1966). *Feeling the Pulse*. Queens Institute of District Nursing: London.

Hockey L. (1968). *Care in the Balance*. Queens Institute of District Nursing: London.

Humphrey JA, Humphrey PP, Greenwood AS, et al. (2019). Musculoskeletal injuries in real tennis. *Open Access J. Sports Med* 10, 81–86.

Marris P. (1958). *Widows and Their Families*. Routledge & Kegan Paul: London.

Pluim BM, Fuller CW, Batt ME, et al. (2009). Consensus statement on epidemiological studies of medical conditions in tennis. *Br. J. Sports Med* 43, 893–897. doi:10.1136/bjsm.2009.064915.

Wadsworth MEJ, Butterfield WJH, Blaney R. (1973). *Health and Sickness: The Choice of Treatment: Perception of Illness and Use of Services in an Urban Community*, Tavistock Publications: London.

Young M and Wilmott P. (1957). *Family and Kinship in East London*. Penguin Books: Harmondsworth.

Young M and Wilmott P. (1973) *The Symmetrical Family*. Penguin Books: Harmondsworth.

CHAPTER 9

Observational Quantitative Approaches

Cross-Sectional Studies – Other Types of Study

Introduction

Surveys are not the only cross-sectional approach. They may be the most common but there are many types of study which, although they are cross-sectional, are not surveys. One critical aspect is that the study data is usually collected on one occasion only.

So, to remind you:

- We are still in the **quantitative** domain – we are still very much with gathering numerical data.
- It is still a **hypothetico-deductive** approach and we should have hypotheses in mind when we set out on this sort of endeavour.
- This is still an **observational** type of study – there is no intervention or experimentation involved.
- Again, these are **retrospective** approaches – we are investigating things which have already taken place.

Demystifying Research for Medical & Healthcare Students: An Essential Guide, First Edition. John L. Anderson.
© 2022 John Wiley & Sons Ltd. Published 2022 by John Wiley & Sons Ltd.
Companion website: www.wiley.com/go/Anderson/DemystifyingResearch

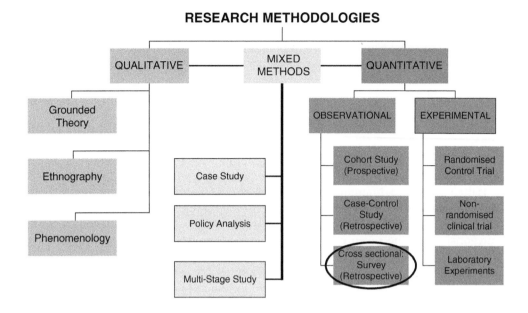

RESEARCH METHODOLOGIES

Example 1: Patients' Recall of Information In a Rheumatology Out-Patient Clinic

This study had an interesting beginning. It was at a Christmas party in the Middlesex Hospital that I first met Tony Fleming, and when Tony heard that I was a sociologist with an interest in doctor–patient communication, he replied, 'Communications, yes, that's right, patients remember about two thirds of what you tell them and they forget the rest! Any time you want to do a study of communications, you can do it in one of my clinics!'

He was partly right in thinking that 'patients remember about two thirds of what you tell them'. Philip Ley had done some research into just that (Ley and Spelman, 1964). In their study in a medical out-patient clinic, they interviewed a consecutive series of 47 new attenders. They interviewed them after they had seen the doctor and asked them to recall what they had been told. Their recall was compared to a record that the doctor had kept about the consultation. Overall, patients recalled 63% of the information given by the doctor – almost two-thirds.

So, I met with Tony and his team to discuss the possibility and the feasibility of doing a similar study within his department's out-patient clinic. The commonly held belief among the clinicians was that patients had forgotten most of what they were told within minutes of their consultation. It was agreed that this was worth investigating and the doctors all expressed their willingness to co-operate. It was agreed that we should aim for a **consecutive series** of new out-patients attending for their second visit at the rheumatology clinics. New patients – to eliminate any 'contamination' or skewing of the results as a result of their familiarity with the language of the rheumatologists; the second visit was chosen because this would be when they returned to receive the results of any tests done on the first visit. All of the doctors agreed to their consultations being audio-recorded. A vacant office was identified for the interviews to be conducted by myself and Michael Kopelman (a psychologist) with the patients. It was obvious from the discussion that the rheumatologists had a certain pattern of providing information to the patients and this helped later in categorising the information into different categories – diagnosis, prognosis, treatment, medication, effects of medication, advice, and 'other'. A start-date was agreed.

So, as the patients arrived their **informed consent** was sought. One hundred and thirty-nine (139) agreed to take part. The consultations were recorded. In the interviews, the interviewer asked some demographic (background) questions, and then asked the patients to say what they remembered about what they had been told. This was then coded into different categories and the data were transferred on to 80-column punched cards prior to being fed into the university computer system for analysis.

The information given by the doctors and reported by the patients was counted and categorised into the seven categories – diagnosis, prognosis, treatment, medication, effects of medication, advice, and 'other'. So, if a doctor said 'you have arthritis', that was counted as *one* bit of information. But if s/he said 'you probably have arthritis', that would count as *two* bits of information. Anything such as 'probably' or 'early signs of', i.e., which changed or added to the statement 'you have arthritis' (or whatever), would change that statement from being a single bit of information to two bits of information. When there was any doubt, those cases were resolved by a discussion of the researchers. In addition, a sample of the earlier consultations (about 10%) were double-checked for accuracy and consistency.

Once the interviews had been completed, the next thing we did was to check how similar our sample of new patients was to all of the new patients attending the clinic. There was a close fit in terms of age, sex, social class, and diagnostic category – *phew*!

Our results showed that, on average, patients in our sample were given 12.1 bits of information and correctly recalled 4.9 – or 40% (see Table 9.1). Interestingly, this group of patients, unlike those in Ley and Spelman's study, were more likely to remember information about treatment, medication, effects of medication, and advice – rather than about diagnosis and prognosis.

The main thing which seemed to influence the percentage recall of information was the amount of information given – the more they were given, the lower the percentage they correctly recalled. When we compared our results with those of two earlier, similar studies, these was a clear trend for the percentage of information correctly recalled to decrease with the amount of information given (see Table 9.2).

So, Tony was quite correct when, at that party, he said patients remembered about two-thirds of what they were told – when they are only given four or five bits of information! But when they are given more information – e.g. 10 (Joyce et al.) or 12 (our study), they are likely to correctly recall less than half of what they are told.

The other difference between Philip's study and ours was in the *nature of the information* that was likely to be best remembered correctly. This is shown in Table 9.3. In Philip's early study, the category of information most likely to be correctly recalled were statements about diagnosis. However, our 1978 study did not find this effect – 61% of statements about treatment were correctly recalled, compared to 56% of statements about diagnosis. The differences were not that great in our study, but the differences between our study and Philip's study are greater. This may be understood when we consider the type of clinics our studies are drawn from. Philip and Martin did their study

TABLE 9.1   Statements recorded, reported and correctly recalled.

Category	Mean number of statements recorded in consultation	Mean number of statements reported at interview	Mean number of statements recalled correctly
Diagnosis	4.2	3.0	1.7
Prognosis	1.1	0.8	0.3
Treatment	2.1	1.7	1.0
Medication	1.5	1.5	0.8
Effects of medication	0.9	0.7	0.3
Advice	0.6	0.5	0.2
Other	1.7	1.2	0.6
Total	12.1	9.4	4.9

Source: Anderson et al. (1978), with permission from Oxford University Press.

TABLE 9.2   Comparison of three studies.

Study:	Mean number of statements given to patients	Percentage of information correctly recalled
Ley and Spelman (1964)	4.6	63
Joyce et al. (1969)	10.2	47
Anderson et al (1979)	12.2	40

in a General Medicine out-patient clinic. Here one of the great concerns patients were likely to have had was 'Have I had a heart attack?' Whereas the patients in our study – rheumatology patients – were more likely to be concerned with issues like 'What can you give me to ease the pain/stiffness in my back/hip/knee/etc.?'

Using Cross-Sectional Approaches Instead of Cohort Studies

Some of my postgraduate students have opted – for reasons of time constraints – to adopt a multiple cross-sectional approach rather than to try to recruit a cohort of participants and follow them up over a period of years. This approach is, sadly, common in studies

TABLE 9.3	Category of information and percentage of statements correctly recalled.		
		Percentage of statements correctly recalled	
Category of information:		**Ley and Spelman (1964)**	**Anderson et al. (1978)**
Diagnosis		87	40
Treatment, prognosis and explanations of symptom		56	43
Instructions and advice		44	40
Other statements		67	47
All statements		63	40

of medical education where researchers wish to make comparisons of new students to medical schools and compare them to final year students. The obvious approach might be a cohort study where you recruit new entrants to medical school(s) and then you follow them up over the five years of their undergraduate course. But what if you don't have five years to wait? Then you choose the cheap, quick way of doing it – by selecting a group of students in their first year, and another group of students in their fifth year. You measure both groups in some way and – hey presto! – you interpret your results (any difference between years 1 and 5) as showing the effects of being at medical school for five years! Of course, there are huge limits to this approach . . . But it does save time until someone with more time (and better funding) comes along and does the proper study!

Example 2: An Exploration of Listening Concepts in UK Medical Students

Krishna was one of my postgraduate students whose dissertation I supervised. He is very much into studying healthcare professionals' **listening styles** and the ways in which they conceptualise 'listening'. As we all have our unique way of 'listening' and our own sets of beliefs about the roles and functions of listening, scholars in the 'listening field' argue that the way we conceptualise listening has implications for our perceptions about listening and listening behaviours. So far, research on listening in healthcare contexts has mainly focused on the behavioural listening components, he felt that there is generally a lack of focus on understanding listening conceptualisations. Thus, he wanted to investigate these conceptualisations in medical students *early* in their training and compare them with those nearing the *end* of their training.

So, now the approach is a straightforward one – to conduct two surveys. One of first-year medical students and the other of fifth-year medical students. Fortunately, he had access to a previously used and tested questionnaire – a validated questionnaire – the **Listening Concepts Inventory-Revised** measure (LCI-R) (Bodie 2010).

So, he got ethics approval from the medical school, and consent from the school office, who agreed to send out an announcement about the study to all first- and fifth-year medical students, inviting them to participate in the study and, by clicking on a link in the e-mail, to access and complete the study questionnaire. This is a very common approach which is taken to investigate aspects of students' attitudes and behaviour. We are now, at the time I am writing this, at the stage of analysing the data (Nainemi and Anderson – in preparation).

Example 3: A Study of the Use of Complementary and Alternative Medicines by Breast Cancer Patients

Kavi was another of my postgraduate students whose dissertation I supervised. He was interested in the fact that there had been a gradual and steady increase in the acceptance of **Complementary and Alternative Medicines (CAM)** by patients over the years. CAMs are popular in patients suffering from life-threatening diseases like cancer – especially in women with breast cancer. Authors in Europe and North America had previously reported this prevalence rate to be as high as 80%, with a majority of participants using CAM concurrently with conventional medicine.

Considering the possibility of harmful interactions, it is important that patients and HCPs share effective communication with regard to CAM use. However, research to date suggests that up to 77% of patients do not confide about CAM use to their HCPs. This lack of communication may threaten the fabric of the patient–doctor partnership.

In this study, the prevalence of CAM use in UK breast cancer patients was explored, focusing on the Knowledge, Attitudes and Practices (KAP) of women using CAM. A **consecutive series** of participants attending two breast cancer clinics were recruited. They were interviewed by Kavi using a structured questionnaire.

In the survey, 110 women with breast cancer and participants were agreed to participate. (A sub-set of 10 women also agreed to take part in semi-structured, qualitative interviews. Additional data was gathered from a **focus group**.)

The study estimated a prevalence rate of CAM use for the preceding 12 months at 85% – higher than previously reported in the UK – with the majority of participants using multiple CAM modalities concurrently with conventional treatment. Other issues were also highlighted – including the widespread concealment from professionals of CAM use.

This was a fairly straightforward survey which showed for the first time how high the prevalence of using CAMs was in breast cancer patients in the UK. We were fortunate in doing this study to have in our co-researcher, a clinician who was interested in the topic, and who, therefore, allowed us to access his patients and invite them to take part. We are now in the process of writing this up for publication (Sharma et al. – in preparation).

Studies of Patients' Records

A common, and relatively simple form of cross-sectional study is to look through the case notes of a series of patients to investigate some aspect of their care and treatment. These are sometimes, *wrongly,* described as **retrospective cohort studies**. As you know, cohort studies are prospective – that is the whole idea of them – you recruit a group of people and then you follow them up over a period of time, making further observations and measurements. To describe a retrospective trawl through some patients' notes as a 'retrospective cohort study' is pretentious and misleading! Don't do it!

Having said that, there are situations where questions can be answered in a relatively efficient way by reviewing what has happened to, for example, all the patients who have been treated in a certain way in one hospital or centre. This is the sort of study which junior doctors or research nurses are tasked to do by their consultants – it's a job and someone has to do it!

Some key issues should be addressed in these types of studies.

1. The purpose and hypotheses should be clearly stated in advance.
2. A data extraction sheet should be used to gather the data from the patients' notes.
3. You should check the HRA website to find out what permissions and approvals are necessary before you start rummaging through patients' information. It is not good enough just to say that these are your boss's patients and he says you can access them!
4. Check the **GDPR** regulations in place as to whether or not these records can be used for the purpose you want.
5. Remember that this is a **cross-sectional** exercise!

To Sum Up

These examples given here all demonstrate the fact that statistical information (numbers) was being collected – they were **quantitative**. There were no interventions or experimentations involved – they were all **observational** studies. They were all **retrospective** – they enquired about things which had already happened. They were all **hypothetico-deductive** – they tested hypotheses in their data analysis.

Note that all of these used **purposive sampling**, in that they targeted specific groups for inclusion. In the first, Anderson et al. (1978), we took a consecutive series of patients from new patients attending a rheumatology out-patient clinic. We were then able to compare the extent to which different types of information was correctly recalled – thus emulating an experimental design within a cross-sectional approach. (NB This was done in the data analysis.) Nainemi targeted medical students in a single centre (medical school) and invited students to self-select by volunteering to complete his online survey. He was able to get some early-year students and some later year students and could therefore make comparisons between them. Sharma et al. targeted women receiving treatment for breast cancer at a single centre (hospital) to ask them about their use of complementary and alternative medicines alongside their 'standard' medical treatments.

Research is the art of the possible!

References

Anderson JL, Dodman S, Kopelman M, et al. (1978). Patient information recall in a rheumatology clinic. *Rheumatology and Rehabilitation* (XVII), 18–22.

Bodie GD. (2010). The revised Listening Concepts Inventory (LCI-R): assessing individual and situational differences in the conceptualization of listening. *Imagination, Cognition and Personality* 30(3), 301–339.

Joyce CRB, Caple G, Mason M, et al. (1969). Quantitative study of doctor-patient communications. *The Quarterly Journal of Medicine* 38, 183.

Ley P and Spelman MS. (1974). Communications in an out-patient setting. *The British Journal of Social and Clinical Psychology* 4, 114–116.

Nainemi K and Anderson J. (2021). *Listening styles of UK medical students – an exploratory survey.* (In preparation.)

Sharma K, Simcock R, Almeida J, et al. (2019). *The use of complementary and alternative medicines (CAM) by breast cancer patients – bridging the gap in communication.* Paper presented at the 14th Conference of the European Sociological Association.

CHAPTER 10

Qualitative Ethnographic Approaches

Using Participant Observation

Introduction

Ethnographic approaches form the oldest tradition of social research. These approaches have their roots in **anthropology** – the study of human societies and cultures. Anthropologists try to understand peoples throughout the World and how different aspects of their **cultures,** such as rituals, patterns of behaviour, social rules, and so on, shape their existence. A lot of early anthropologists' efforts were spent examining 'primitive societies' with a view to helping us understand evolutionary processes. They gave us some very important research approaches which have been incorporated into social research generally. In particular, the approach known as **participant observation (PO),** in which the researcher immerses her/himself in the society or social system which they are researching by becoming a member of that social group, and by **living as of one of them,** they gain insight into the lives, the rules that guide that society, and the rituals at the core of that society – thus getting access to the parts that other methods don't. By living the life of a member of the social group you are researching, you can get rich insights into not only what people really do (as opposed to what they say they do) and why they do those things, but also into what it *feels like* too.

So, participant observation:

- Is firmly in the **qualitative** domain.
- It is **hypothetico-inductive,** that is to say you do *not* usually begin with a theoretical body of knowledge and then hypothesise as to what you might find, instead, you usually have a 'blank canvas' and your theory develops as you continue to make observations and gather data.

Demystifying Research for Medical & Healthcare Students: An Essential Guide, First Edition. John L. Anderson.
© 2022 John Wiley & Sons Ltd. Published 2022 by John Wiley & Sons Ltd.
Companion website: www.wiley.com/go/Anderson/DemystifyingResearch

- It is **prospective** – you begin making observations/gathering data and continue to over the period of time you are 'in the field' (i.e. while you are collecting your data).
- And it should be **non-interventional** – but then can you really be a participant and not contribute in some way? (Let's debate that another time!)

In this chapter, I shall introduce you to some examples of research studies using PO. In the course of this, I shall continually ask the question – 'Could this subject have been researched adequately using any other method?'

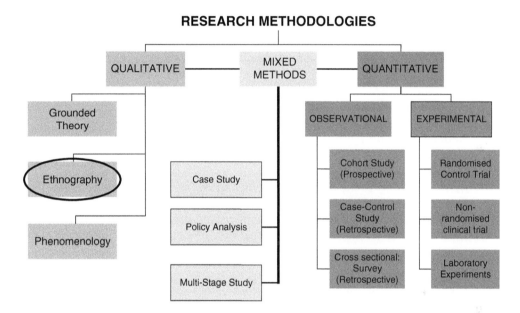

Example 1: Crime and Custom in Savage Society

One of the leading anthropologists of the twentieth century was **Bronisław Malinowski** (Figure 10.1). He is most famous for his research in the Trobriand Islands (now the Kiriwina Islands) off the southeastern coast of New Guinea in the Pacific. He spent two years doing research by participant observation, living among the people there – living in a tent, observing and questioning them to enrich his observations. He was one of the first anthropologists to leave his desk and work

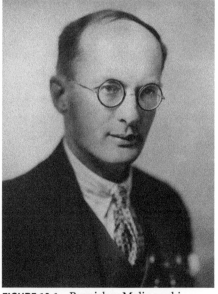

FIGURE 10.1   Bronisław Malinowski.
Source: LSE / Wikimedia Commons / Public domain.

in the field. He believed that the researcher should try to see peoples' worlds through their eyes and fully immerse themself in their lives.

> *His recommended technique implies that the investigator immerse himself in the system under analysis. For example, in discussing the obligations surrounding procurement and distribution of food, he invites the reader to join him in observing the activity of fishing: 'To enter more deeply into the nature of these binding obligations, let us follow the fishermen to the shore. Let us see what happens with the division of the catch'.*

> *(Malinowski 1926; Riley 1963)*

He emphasised the importance of observing what people actually do in real-life situations, participating in the life of the group, rather than just asking them questions about what they would or should do in those situations.

> *When the (respondent) is asked what he would do in such and such a case, he answers what he should do; he lays down the pattern of best possible conduct. When he acts as informant to a field anthropologist, it costs him nothing to retail the Ideal of the law . . . The other side, the natural impulsive code of conduct, the evasions, the compromises and non-legal usages are revealed only to the field worker who observes native life directly, registers facts, lives at such close quarters with his 'material' as to understand not only their language and their statements, but also the hidden motives of behaviour, and the hardly ever formulated spontaneous lies of conduct . . .*

> *(Malinowski 1926)*

The beauty and the art of Malinowski's work comes from the rich descriptions he provides. There is no quantification, his approach is **qualitative** and **descriptive**. In his exploratory study, he is more concerned with identifying and describing the variables – or facts – and showing how they relate to each other, than analysing them in a quantitative way using numbers.

Malinowski began from an exploratory position – 'to discover and analyse all the rules conceived and acted upon as binding obligations' in primitive societies in general, using the Trobriand Islanders as a case study. He spent a long time with these people getting to know them intimately – by observing their daily lives and by questioning **key informants** to add to the data in his observations. Thus, much of his analysis is **descriptive.** He was asking questions like 'What?' It did not come from testing hypotheses (hypothetico-deductive reasoning) but by trying to make sense of his observations and the accounts he gathered – in a **hypothetico-inductive** way. As his data collection progressed, he also became concerned with more of the detail in the data. Thus, there were global observations about society in general and more specific observations about the relationships and events he witnessed (Figure 10.2).

Read some of his work – it is classic anthropological field work at its best (e.g. Malinowski, 1922). He is rigorous – he kept a detailed set of notes in diary form (in Polish, for anonymity).

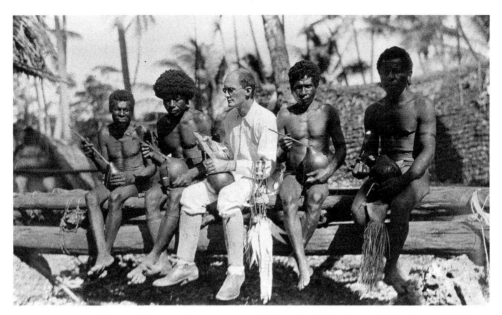

FIGURE 10.2   Malinowski comparing gourds with Trobriand Islanders, 1918. *Source:* LSE / Wikimedia Commons / Public domain.

Example 2: Street Corner Society: The Social Structure of an Italian Slum

At the time that **William Whyte** (Figure 10.3) did his research, there were a lot of concerns about life in poorer communities and the possibly 'subversive' elements in those communities – street gangs. Whyte wanted to get an 'intimate view' of life in a poor community – by living in their society and documenting his findings to present as rich and true an account of 'Street Corner Society' as was possible. He, himself, came from a well-to-do family, he thought 'Cornerville' – as the neighbourhood he was studying was referred to – was a slum, and he wanted to find out more about that 'lower class' society. Thus, he spent a total of three and a half years living in that community (Figure 10.4).

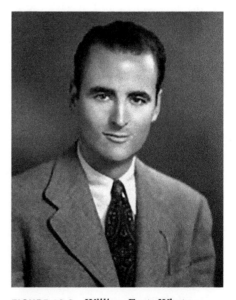

FIGURE 10.3   William Foote Whyte.

One of the aspects of Cornerville life which interested him were the 'street gangs'. There was increasing official concern in America about street gangs and the potential threat that these posed to social order. If you think about it, how else could he

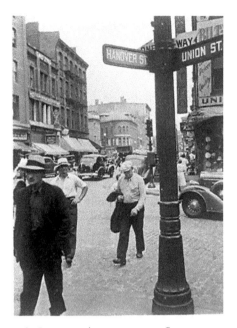

FIGURE 10.4 A street corner. *Source:* Bundesarchiv (Federal Archives) / Wikimedia commons / CC BY-SA 3.0.

reach street gang members and how might he approach them to gather information about their day-to-day life, activities, and feelings? Could he have gone to 'Google and looked up 'gangs'? This is an issue that we meet in many situations, when we are trying to identify and sample people 'on the fringe' of mainstream society. There are no directories to help us. There are problems in getting access to the data. Imagine going up to a big thug in the street and asking, 'Excuse me Mr Big, I am doing research into the activities of violent gangs and I'd like to ask you some questions . . .' Maybe not. Also, consider how honest your participants might be in answering your questions . . .

What I'm trying to say is that *PO can reach the parts of life that other methods cannot.* By living amongst the people you are researching and observing what they do – in their natural setting – you can avoid the common problem in interview research with people **'faking good'** as Malinowski also noted.

Whyte first moved to Cornerville and rented a room with an Italian family. They did not speak English, so he learnt Italian, although the younger generation – the second-generation men – spoke English. His attempt to learn Italian helped build bridges – it was appreciated and 'it gave the impression that I had a sincere and sympathetic interest in Cornerville people'. His stay with this family gave him contacts in the local community as well as insights into family life. He stayed with the family for 18 months. Then, when he got married, they went to live in their own flat.

> *This opened for me a new field of contacts. One evening I went with the son of my Italian family to a banquet on honor of the local police lieutenant. There were three groups of people present: policemen, politicians and racketeers.*

> *(Whyte 1943)*

The first challenge for him was to establish a *bona fide* genuine reason for his presence in that community. Initially he explained that he was researching Cornerville history. To this end he established support from key individuals who would vouch for him – so that he would not be taken for a 'G-Man' (one of the 'Feds'). Newcomers were suspected because of the extent of illegal activities in the community. Several of his key informants eventually formed a clear idea of his research and were able to open new doors and explain things to him. Once he was accepted within any group, he did not have to explain himself. People would ask him how his book was coming along.

A lot of his time was spent getting to know the people he was studying and getting their confidence. So, he bowled, played softball and pool, he played cards, and generally socialised with his new friends. Having things in common with them broke down barriers and made it possible for him to be accepted as an intimate member of the group. As he said:

> *I made it a rule that I would avoid influencing the actions of the group. I wanted to observe what the men did under ordinary circumstances; I did not want to lead them into different activities. I violated this rule several times . . . But on the whole I held on to it . . . I avoided making moral admonitions . . . I was there to learn about Cornerville life, not to pass judgment upon it.*

> *(Whyte 1943)*

Whyte gives a detailed account of his data collection and 'recording'. At times, he was able to take notes on the spot, but more often he had to rely upon his memory until he could write down his notes in private. He tried to make **verbatim** notes. He records that this was very difficult at first, he could only remember a few of the exact phrases used, but he became more and more skilled at doing this. Eventually, he felt confident in the accuracy of his quotations and recall of events.

Whyte observed that the street gangs he saw in Cornerville emerged from childhood friendships. He noted the relative constancy and stability of people in Cornerville.

> *The gangs grew up on the corner and remained there with remarkable persistence from early boyhood until the members reached their late twenties or early thirties. In the course of years some groups were broken up by the movement of families away from Cornerville . . . but frequently movement out of the district does not take the corner boy away from his corner. On any evening on almost any corner one finds corner boys who have come in from other parts of the city or from suburbs to be with their old friends. The residence of the corner boy may also change within the district, but nearly always he retains his allegiance to his original corner.*

> *(Whyte 1943)*

His research showed that, rather than being a completely disorganised part of society, Cornerville had 'a complex and well-established organisation of its own', It was not a seething slum of anarchists, but a community of people who lived by the laws of the land (to a greater or a lesser extent) alongside local rules and principles guiding local people's lives. He observed the sorts of social problems faced by people in this community. As a poor Italian community within an American city, things were hard for men who wanted to get on in life.

> *He is an Italian, and the Italians are looked upon by upper-class people as amongst the least desirable of the immigrant peoples . . . To get ahead, the Cornerville man must move either in the world of business and Republican politics or in the world of Democratic politics and the rackets.*

> *(Whyte, 1943)*

Whyte began with a mainly exploratory objective – 'to gain an intimate view on Cornerville life'. He wanted to get and report on life in a street corner society and Cornerville was the case he studied in depth.

In this sort of work there is always a danger of picking on extreme examples and sensationalising. Whyte was strongly criticised by some Cornerville residents for portraying the community as a slum, and a largely criminal one at that. A former Boston city councillor Frederick C. Langone who lived in Cornerville and knew Whyte said of Whyte's book:

> *What his book did to the North End was to make it look like everybody was in some kind of racket. . . In fact, the exact opposite was true. . . William Whyte's book Street Corner Society was required reading in every college. Consequently, students got the wrong perception of the North End and the Italian-American inhabitants.*

> *(Langone 1994)*

Example 3: Boys in White: Student Culture in Medical School

Howard Becker (Figure 10.5) is one of my sociological heroes! I have long admired his work and shall cite briefly another piece of his research later.

At the time this research was done, medicine was very much a male-dominated profession. That was fairly universal at the time.

> Rumour has it that a Dean of the Middlesex Hospital Medical School in London, where I started my teaching career, was in the habit of greeting prospective candidates who were attending admission interviewees at the medical school, by throwing a rugby ball at them. It they dropped it, they were out.

In the introductory section of 'Boys in White', Becker et al., talking about interviews for admission to medical school, write: 'The teachers of medicine who interview them look at them seriously and anxiously. They ask themselves and one another, "Will this bright boy really make a medical man?" For medicine is man's work. It is also woman's work . . . Although an increasing proportion of the people who have a part in the medical system are women, the medical profession itself remains overwhelmingly male.' As Brenda Beagan (2001) pointed out, 'they really were "boys" in white – in fact they were "white" boys in white'.

There were also concerns about the **mechanistic** nature of medical practice at that time. As one intern in another study put it, 'You're interested in patients; I'm interested in the disease in the body in the bed' (Duff and Hollingshead 1968).

> *But our purpose is not criticism, but observation and analysis. When we report what we have learned, it is important that we do so faithfully. We have a double duty – to our own profession of social observation and analysis and to those who have allowed us to observe their conduct. We do not report everything we observe, for to do so would violate confidences and otherwise do harm. On the*

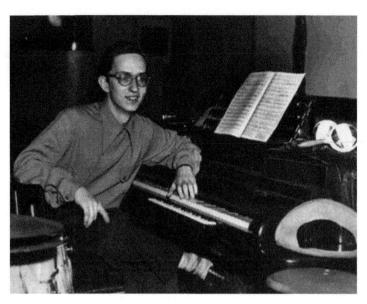

FIGURE 10.5   Howard Becker.

other hand, we must take care not to bias our analyses and conclusions. Finding a proper balance between our obligations to our informants and the organisation, on the one hand, and our scientific duty, on the other, is not easy. We have been at some pains to find such a balance.

Our aim is to bring to view and so to analyse the experiences of medical students in interaction with their teachers and their tasks that the reader may compare them with other situations of the same order.

(Becker et al. 1961)

They had no hypotheses to test. They did not use validated questionnaires to gather their data. They had no pre-determined set of data analysis methods. The 'research problem' they began with was 'to discover what medical school did to medical students other than giving them a technical education'. They did not have any assumptions about what knowledge, attitudes, and perspectives medical students *should* have. Thus, their focus was on what students learned and how they learned it. They worked with an open theoretical scheme where the variables would be discovered by doing the research, rather than by beginning with variables they could look for to test hypotheses. That is, they began with a **hypothetico-inductive** approach rather than a hypothetico-deductive approach. So, rather than proposing hypotheses and attempting to prove or disprove them, they made provisional generalisations about aspects of the medical school and medical students' experiences in it – and they revised these generalisations constantly as '**negative cases**' showed the need to revise them.

This set of concerns led to them adopting **participant observation** as their main method. This, they believed, allowed the greatest degree of flexibility to acquire information relevant to their goal. They had to decide at this point about whether to take on group (or cohort) of students and follow them up in a prospective study throughout their educational journey, or to select different year-groups of students to study. They opted for the latter because they decided it was the most time-efficient means to get their results. They started with the later years of students, in case they gained insights which might influence what they enquired about later. (They were not sure that this did not in fact have any effect.) They then planned their time to ensure that they spent time with the students in each department where they would be taught, and so that they saw each of the main teaching situations in the school. Their view was that covering as many groups of students in as many situations as possible would increase their chances of uncovering negative cases which would help in the reformulation of their generalisations – their **emerging theory**. They stressed the importance of these 'negative cases' in helping with the **refinements of their theory**.

The task they set themselves was a daunting one. In working with students in their first two years, they endeavoured to talk to every student in the class. The researchers attended school with the students, 'Following them from class to laboratory to hospital ward'. They did not pose as students – they were up front about their roles of **participant observers**, in what they referred to as a **'pseudo role' of students**. When they were engaged with a group of students, their involvement was both **continuous** and **total.** They observed different groups continuously for periods of one week to two months. And they observed the whole day's activities – according to the students' schedules.

As you might imagine, **recording their data** – their observations and their feelings – was challenging. They made it a rule to dictate their accounts of each day's observations and notes as soon as possible and to make their recordings as complete as possible – aiming for verbatim transcripts where possible. This process shines through in their accounts which were as transparent and complete as possible.

Their observations were enhanced by **informal and formal interviews.** Where possible, during each day, they questioned the students they were working with – in the form of **detailed conversations.** In addition, **formal interviews** were conducted in the medical school offices. They took a **random sample of students to interview.** These **semi-structured interviews**, using an interview guide, were audio-recorded and transcribed verbatim. This allowed them to make **quantitative analyses** of some points to augment their observational data.

As you can imagine, these methods generated huge amounts of data – about 5000 single-spaced typed pages! Their analysis was not a separate, end-stage of the research. Data gathering and the analysis went on at the same time. (You can see strong similarities in these approaches to those I describe later in **Grounded Theory– Chapter 14**). They point out that:

> We find it useful to follow the tradition of presenting illustrative quotations from our field notes . . . In presenting quotations, we present certain facts about the situation and participants in summary form so that the reader will be able to make his own assessment of the representativeness of the sample of quotations given.

> *(Becker et al. 1961)*

They confirm the fact that statements or observations are 'representative' of that case by noting the frequency it is made and the frequency that statements or observations to the contrary are made.

Because the final statement of the perspective was formulated after a great deal
of field work. . . there are usually relatively few negative cases. . . If there should
be a large number of negative cases, this would certainly require revision of any
proposition. . .

(Becker et al. 1961)

This rich source of information allowed them to present a written account of what it was like to be a medical student – from entering medical school, to going on the wards, to graduating. They describe the challenges faced by the work – from managing the sheer quantity of the work to dealing with the physical and emotional demands of the work. They describe the different cultures which influence the medical students' culture and how they influence the ways medical students think about their work and the world around them. They talk about how the predominantly white, upper-middle-class, male culture, which made up the majority of students then, influenced the ways they thought about and responded to patients.

This study had a huge impact at the time on medical education – around the world. I knew four deans of medical schools, who, after reading Becker et al.'s book, went back into the classrooms of their own medical school to find out what was going on in them.

Example 4: Being Sane in Insane Places

David Rosenhan was a psychologist at Stanford University in America (Figure 10.6). He was inspired by a lecture given by R. D. Laing – a controversial psychiatrist who challenged the orthodoxy of current psychiatric thinking – into conceiving this study. This turned out to be a study which changed the nature of modern psychiatry. I think it is a very brave study, and, although some writers describe it as an 'experiment', it adopted participant observation as its main method.

He got eight healthy people – three women and five men (including himself) – to be **pseudopatients.** They came from different backgrounds: three were psychologists, one a paediatrician, one a psychiatrist, one a painter, and one a housewife. Twelve hospitals were chosen in five states in USA. They all phoned a hospital for an appointment. There, they complained about hearing voices. These were reported as being often unclear, 'but as far as he could tell they said "empty" "hollow" and "thud"'. They also gave false names and occupations, but otherwise they played themselves. They strongly emphasised their sanity. All were admitted to the psychiatric ward. All but one were admitted with a diagnosis of **schizophrenia.**

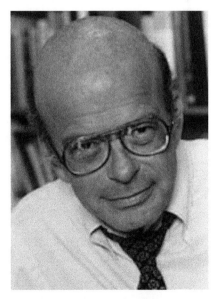

FIGURE 10.6   David Rosenhan.

They were naturally quite nervous once on the ward, but apart from that, they behaved as they would normally behave. They spoke to patients and staff as they would ordinarily. They did not report *any* more symptoms. When staff asked them how they were, they all said they were fine – they had not had any more symptoms. They complied with instructions from staff. They took their medications, but did not swallow them. Instead, they spat them out in the lavatory. Their challenge was **to get out as soon as possible by convincing staff of their sanity**.

I don't know if you, dear reader, have any idea about what life on a psychiatric ward was like in the early 1970s. I have visited many, and I found them all to be horrid places. I would not have wanted to spend even a night in any one of them. (You can get a good idea of what they were like by watching the film **One Flew Over the Cuckoo's Nest** starring Jack Nicholson, directed by Milos Forman and based upon Ken Kesey's 1962 book.) All but one of the pseudopatients wanted to be discharged as soon as they were admitted. It was a very stressful experience being on a psychiatric ward with no idea of how long they would have to stay there. (They did have a lawyer on call in case they were desperate to get out.)

So, they were left to their own devices. One of the dominant characteristics of psychiatric wards then was that they were very boring places to be in. There was very little to do. They talked to other patients. They wrote their notes about life on the ward, about the patients and the staff. Initially these notes were written secretly, but after a while, it was obvious that no one cared, so they wrote them openly.

They were essentially 'model' patients. They did what was asked of them. They were co-operative and polite. The staff reports confirmed that they were 'friendly', 'cooperative', and 'exhibited no abnormal indications'. When they were given medications and they spat them down the toilet, they noticed that some other patients had done the same, but the staff seemed to be unaware of this. (Those of you who have seen *One Flew Over the Cuckoo's Nest* may recognise that scene where Jack Nicholson, thinking he was being smart, took his medications in his mouth, then went to the lavatory to spit them out – only to find lots of other pills in the loo!) None of the pseudopatients were ever detected by the staff. Their **note-writing** was seen as part of their 'illness'. Although the staff did not detect their sanity, many of the other patients did.

> (many) patients on the admissions ward voiced their suspicions, some vigorously. 'You're not crazy. You're a journalist, or a professor [referring to the continual note-taking]. You're checking up on the hospital.' While most of the patients were reassured by the pseudopatient's insistence that he had been sick before he came in but was fine now, some continued to believe that the pseudopatient was sane throughout his hospitalization.

> (Rosenhan 1973)

All were eventually discharged – with a diagnosis of **schizophrenia 'in remission'**. They were in hospital for 7–52 days. Their average length of stay was *19 days*.

In addition to their notes, the pseudopatients collected some quantitative data – for example, on the time that staff spent 'mingling' with patients, and contacts between the pseudopatients and the staff.

> It proved impossible to obtain a 'percent mingling time' for nurses, since the amount of time they spent out of the cage was too brief. Rather, we counted

instances of emergence from the cage. On the average, daytime nurses emerged from the cage 11.5 times per shift, including instances when they left the ward entirely (range, 4 to 39 times). Late afternoon and night nurses were even less available, emerging on the average 9.4 times per shift (range, 4 to 41 times).

(Rosenhan 1973)

This made it possible to *blend the qualitative data and the quantitative data* to get a more comprehensive picture of life on the wards.

I highly recommend that you read Rosenhan's paper. In it he calls into question whether staff in psychiatric hospitals really see the patient or whether they are reacting to the **label** *that is given to them,* 'the evidence is strong that, once labeled schizophrenic, the pseudopatient was stuck with that label' (Rosenhan 1973). Deviant labels stick! (Howard Becker, 1963, is given credit for developing **Labelling Theory.**) All of the behaviours exhibited by the pseudopatients were framed by the staff within the diagnostic label of 'schizophrenia' and their stereotypes of the behaviours that 'schizophrenics' exhibit. The pseudopatients also reported a strong sense of **dehumanisation.** They were **objectified** by the staff who would often talk about them in their presence as though they didn't exist.

This study had a stunning impact, worldwide, on psychiatry. Psychiatrists began to question the dangers of giving diagnoses of schizophrenia in case those patients were labelled and treated according to that label. I remember one of the first case conferences I attended when I worked in the Academic Department of Psychiatry at the Middlesex Hospital Medical School. John Hinton, the professor of psychiatry (and a man who I had the utmost respect for) led the discussion. The case being presented was a 16-year-old boy who sometimes presented delusional experiences and the obvious temptation in the room was to treat him for schizophrenia. However, John resisted suggestions that the boy be prescribed anti-psychotic medication, on the grounds that, even though a formal diagnosis of schizophrenia had not been given, he might be labelled 'schizophrenic' by others and treated as such – without being afforded opportunities to display evidence of sanity.

Postscript: Rosenhan conducted another brief experiment. He used a prestigious teaching hospital where the staff knew about his study but claimed that such a thing could not happen with them. Famous last words! Rosenhan arranged for pseudopatients to try to be admitted to their hospital over the coming months. The staff agreed to rate every new patient in regard to their likelihood of being an imposter. They 'detected' 41 definite imposters and another 42 who they thought were 'suspect'. What do you think? That's right – in reality Rosenhan had sent no pseudopatients. *People see what they expect to see.*

Discussion

One of the greatest advantages of PO is that you can access information and participants to observe and ask questions which might not otherwise be available to you by other methods. Observing what people do filters out the responses you may get when people want to make themselves look better than they actually are. It is also a means of accessing sensitive aspects of people's lives without the embarrassment of asking formally about things.

Malinowsky, Whyte, and Becker et al. tried to access all areas of the communities they were studying. I hope you got some idea of the lengths they went to in order to be as fully inclusive as possible. Rosenhan did this also – but in a relatively smaller environment.

Becker et al. and Rosenhan were also able to blend qualitative data with quantitative data to give a fuller answer to questions like 'How often did this happen?' Even qualitative researchers can be in awe of statistics!

Note the total nature of the PO experience. Malinowski was essentially marooned on a Pacific Island for the duration of his fieldwork. Whyte spent three and a half years living in Cornerville – with his family. Note that if you embark on this sort of task, you can't usually sign off at 5.00 p.m. and leave the office. Your research becomes your life. You may not be able to escape from it for weeks, months, or even years. I'm sure that that was in Rosenhan's mind when he and his associates were first admitted to psychiatric wards. However, the longest any of them had to stay in was just over 7 weeks – 52 days.

That reminds me of one of my friends' experiences of doing PO. 'Derek' was one of my tutors at university. He was a lovely chap and became a good friend over the years. He was a very good teacher and was doing what he thought was a very good job. However, when a new Professor of Sociology was appointed, he began to shake things up and put more emphasis on research – asking people to set goals so that their research activity was visible. (You know the sort of thing.) Anyway, 'Derek' had not actually done any research for some years and found himself put on the spot by this edict. So, he came up with the idea of doing PO to study the *behaviours of people in casinos* (one of the industries that has blossomed in our society).

So, 'Derek' got a job as a croupier in a local casino. This gave him opportunities to observe the gambling behaviours of the 'punters'. Then, during his breaks, he was able to mingle and chat to people to gather more detail. Well, this went on, and 'Derek' was very happy doing his research until one day, about 18 months later. He told me that he got a letter from his Prof which more or less said, *'Dear Derek, It has been a long time since we have seen you in the department . . . I wonder if the time has come for you to make a choice and consider whether you wish to continue working as a university lecturer, of if you would rather pursue a career as a croupier?'* This shook 'Derek', because he did not want to give up his role in the casino, but at the same time still wanted to be a university lecturer. Eventually he joined Gamblers Anonymous because he realised that he had a vicarious gambling addiction. The last I heard of 'Derek' was that he was making a mint as a psychoanalyst in Harley Street. He had given up being a university teacher and re-trained as a psychoanalyst. I could imagine him being very good at it.

Problems of approach

There is a phenomenon that used to be referred to as '**going native**' – a reference to the time when anthropologists used to concentrate on doing PO in 'primitive' societies. It refers to a common event in which POs became so involved in, and sympathetic to, the group they were researching, that **they lost their objectivity.** Another old friend of mine was doing PO in a therapeutic community, and when summoned to a university departmental meeting, told his boss, 'Sorry, I can't come to the meeting tomorrow. There's an important meeting at the community and one group are trying to get power, so I have to be there to make sure they don't succeed.' His boss took him aside and gave him thorough de-briefing, and pulled him out of there soon after. He had become so overwhelmed by the events that he was meant to be observing that he had lost his objectivity. Remember what Whyte said about not interfering, and what Becker et al. nicely put:

> But our purpose is not criticism, but observation and analysis. When we report what we have learned, it is important that we do so faithfully. We have a double duty – to our own profession of social observation and analysis and to those who have allowed us to observe their conduct. We do not report everything we observe, for to do so would violate confidences and otherwise do harm. On the other hand, we must take care not to bias our analyses and conclusions. Finding a proper balance between our obligations to our informants and the organisation, on the one hand, and our scientific duty, on the other, is not easy. We have been at some pains to find such a balance.

> (Becker et al. 1961)

This phenomenon has also been observed in another sphere – that of the **undercover cop.** Policemen and journalists have often gone 'undercover' as part of their investigations. It is a way of getting at information which might otherwise have been kept secret, or only divulged to people who those being studied or investigated felt they could trust. There have been some high-profile cases where police undercover personnel have perhaps exceeded their duty and have had relationships with and had children with people in the social group they were investigating. This has led to complaints from members of the public, who felt aggrieved at being the victims of such deceit (Lewis and Evans 2011; Peachey 2013). Use Google to find other examples.

These are tricky **ethical issues.** To what extent is it a betrayal of trust as opposed to a purely academic exercise to reveal some of the 'more sinister' sides of the people you have been living with for three years?

The advice to those of you who might engage in PO is simple and clear. Use your **research supervisor** to check things out with and keep them informed of what you are doing – regularly. Remember, just because you are doing 'research' does not put you beyond the rule of the law! It can be a lonely place being a PO, so make sure that you are well-supported for that adventure.

Sampling is a big issue for those engaged in PO. The first issue to be addressed is, how do you choose your **case** to study? Will it be a useful study? What will it add to our knowledge? Then you have to consider how much of that group's life you need to involve yourself in: What events do you need to see and participate in? How will you get accepted within those settings? And so on. When you read Becker et al.'s work, you get a flavour of the almost positivist zeal with which they attempted to be all-inclusive – to be totally representative. They 'sampled' every class and clinical setting the students might experience at some point in their five years of training. But they managed to do it in one year rather than five by using all five years that were going through medical school and, because there was a whole team of researchers, they could manage it all.

Usually, the PO has to admit to her/himself that they can't be everywhere all the time. There will be events and situation they miss, but they can do their best to make up for that by gathering accounts from some of the group who were there.

Some researchers believe that **ALL ethnographic research** should involve this sort of 'immersion' in the group being studied. As my old friend Rosaline Barbour (another of the old Aberdeen group) says in her book on qualitative research:

> *most commentators are in agreement that in order to be considered as ethnography, there should be at least an element of observational fieldwork.*

> *(Barbour, 2014)*

However, as we move away from the classic sorts of anthropological studies to studies of modern, multi-cultural society, these approaches are faced with new sets of problems – particularly that of 'selection', or sampling. If you consider the analogy of someone from Mars coming to the planet Earth to study what life was like here on Earth, where would s/he land? If, for example they had, 'by chance' landed in a particular community and observed life there, who is to say that that community could 'represent' life in the country they were in – let alone the Earth as a whole? A researcher from Mars would have to immerse themselves in so many different areas as to make the research impossible, particularly when one considers the massive investment of researchers time that PO takes up. In Chapter 11, we shall look at other methods of collecting information about people's beliefs and 'cultures' using interviews and focus groups.

To Sum Up

In this chapter, I have taken you on a journey down some roads which not many students of research methods travel. We have moved from the positivist domain to the qualitative and more **interpretivist** domain – or as some of my MSc Orthopaedic Surgery students (bless them!) refer to it: the 'touchy-feely' approach. For 10 years I used to have a prize of a fine bottle of vintage wine on offer for the first MSc Orthopaedic Surgery student to do a research dissertation using qualitative methods. That prize has never been claimed.

We have moved from the quantitative world of numbers and statistics to the **qualitative** world of **themes and observations,** from the hypothetico-deductive world to the **hypothetico-inductive** world. Because PO involves studying people over a period of time, these are **prospective** studies rather than retrospective ones.

I have tried to give you a flavour of this sort of approach, so that you might understand it and be aware of some of the methodological challenges which are associated with it. I have deliberately selected four classic studies, all of which have had a major impact upon our knowledge of the world – and some which have actually had a major influence on clinical practice. In all, you can imagine that gaining access to the world they were studying was the first hurdle they had to overcome. This was usually facilitated by negotiating a socially acceptable role for them to play – Malinowski was 'the outsider who had come to study us'. Whyte was 'the new guy on the block'. Beker et al. were 'the researchers who are studying medical education'. Derek was 'the new croupier in the casino'. And Rosenhan and his colleagues had to convince doctors that they were 'insane' to get access to the world of the psychiatric hospital. Becker et al.'s study is slightly different in that the whole team were researchers and they tried to cover the whole of the undergraduate medical curriculum – and used surveys of specific groups to get more information about those specific activities they were observing. In all the other studies here, the researcher had to rely on field notes written up when they could – usually alone in the safety of their own quarters (tent, apartment, home, bed, etc.). In Rosenhan's case the very public nature of life on a psychiatric ward meant that their 'data recording' – writing their field notes – had to be done in public – sparking quite different responses from the staff and the other patients who saw them doing this.

PO is a *labour-intensive* methodology rather than a costly one. Your *time* is the main resource required to do an ethnographic study using PO.

Research is the art of the possible!

References

Barbour R. (2014). *Introducing Qualitative Research: A Student's Guide*. Sage: London.

Beagan B. (2001). Micro inequities and everyday inequalities: "race", gender, sexuality and class in medical school. *The Canadian Journal of Sociology* 2(4), 583–610.

Becker HS, Geer B, Hughes EC, et al. (1961). Boys in White: Student Culture in Medical School. Transaction Publishers.

Becker HS. (1963). *Outsiders: Studies in the Sociology of Deviance*. The Free Press: New York.

Duff R and Hollingshead A. (1968). *Sickness and Society*. Harper & Row: New York.

Kesey K. (1962). *One Flew Over the Cuckoo's Nest*. Viking Books: New York.

Langone F. (1994). *The North End: Where It All Began*. Post-Gazette, American Independence Edition: Boston, pp. 19–21.

Lewis P and Evans R. (2011). Former lovers of undercover officers sue police over deceit. *The Guardian* (16 December).

Malinowski BK. (1922). *Argonauts of the Western Pacific: An Account of Native Enterprise and Adventure in the Archipelagoes of Melanesian New Guinea*. George Routledge & Sons Ltd: London.

Malinowski BK. (1926). *Crime and Custom in Savage Society*. Harcourt Brace & World, Inc: New York.

Peachey P. (2013). Deceived lovers speak of mental 'torture' from undercover detectives. *The Independent* (1 March).

Riley MW. (1963). *Sociological Research: A Case Approach*. Harcourt Brace & World, Inc: New York.

Rosenhan DL. (1973). On Being Sane in Insane Places. *Science* 179, 250–258.

William FW. (1943). *Street Corner Society: The Social Structure of an Italian Slum*. University of Chicago Press: Chicago.

CHAPTER 11

Qualitative Ethnographic Approaches

Using Interviews and Focus Groups

Introduction

In this chapter, we shall continue to consider **ethnographic** approaches, but we have moved away from **participant observation** and shall consider other forms of ethnographic research which essentially cross-sectional approaches using **focus groups, interviews,** and **autoethnographies.**

- So, we are still in the **qualitative** domain (no numbers).
- We are looking at methods which are usually (but not always) **hypothetico-inductive – they can be hypothetico-deductive.**
- And these methods are **retrospective** – they are studying things which have already happened, about beliefs and behaviours which already exist.

We are still considering approaches which are concerned with 'cultural' aspects of a group or situation. This includes research which is trying to uncover people's beliefs, the rules – both formal and informal – which guide the ways in which they behave, and the ways in which some groups of people differ from others in our society.

You will note that using interviews and focus groups is not 'immersive' in the same way that Participant Observation is, but the experiences of conducting these interviews and focus groups can lead to a different sort of **'immersive experience'** in the lives and cultures of your participants. **Autoethnographies**, as you will see are totally immersive.

Demystifying Research for Medical & Healthcare Students: An Essential Guide, First Edition. John L. Anderson.
© 2022 John Wiley & Sons Ltd. Published 2022 by John Wiley & Sons Ltd.
Companion website: www.wiley.com/go/Anderson/DemystifyingResearch

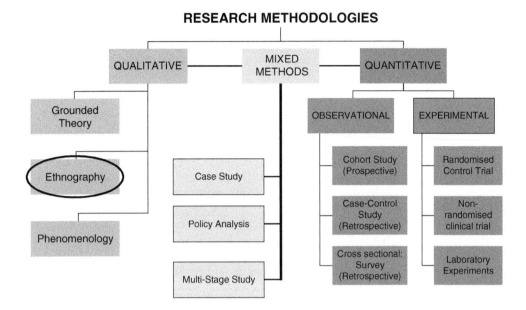

Interview methods

As you saw in the last chapter on participant observation, **interviews** – often in the form of directed conversations – are commonly used in ethnographic research. Now we shall consider some examples of ethnographic research using mainly interview methods.

Example 1: 'A comparison of HIV-related risk behaviour and risk reduction between female street working prostitutes and male rent boys in Glasgow' and 'HIV-Related Risk Practices among Glasgow Male Prostitutes: Reframing Concepts of Risk Behaviour'

(In my opinion, this is one of the most heroic programmes of study I know. Glasgow used to have a reputation as a very rough place.)

The researchers were interested in researching female and male sex workers to get some insights into their beliefs and behaviors – their 'culture' – in regard to risks of HIV infection and safer sex practices.

I have learned to be careful when I talk about their research. One time, in a lecture, I introduced their work by saying, "'Mick was interested in rent boys, and Neil was interested in street prostitutes. . .'" One wag in the class, an orthopaedic surgeon, if I remember correctly, quipped, "'Did they have any luck?!'" Well, that says a lot about some of my orthopaedic surgeon students!

This research was set in the global context of HIV transmission. At the time, it was known that in the UK, HIV infection was 'still largely associated with unprotected male homosexual sex and the shared use of unsterile needles and syringes by injecting drug users' (McKeganey et al. 1990). Research elsewhere had shown that prostitutes could play a significant part in the spread of HIV infection – as many prostitutes were known to be injecting drug users. So, they wanted to find out more about the **risk-taking** practices of male and female sex workers – 'rent boys' and 'street prostitutes' as they were known in those days – and their clients as well as their health-protecting behaviours. As they said:

While we know relatively little on each of these topics as they refer to female prostitutes, the gaps in our knowledge in relation to male prostitutes are even greater.

(McKeganey et al. 1990)

Glasgow was chosen because that is where their research units were. It was convenient.

How would you go about getting suitable participants for a study like this? Take a few minutes to think about it before going any further. Note down your ideas, then compare them with what these researchers did.

As I discussed in the last chapter about Whyte's study of Cornerville and street gangs, you cannot turn to official sources or Google for a list of street gangs, street prostitutes, or rent boys. So, I guess you probably suggested brainstorming within the unit. Perhaps you all get together and sit around and put the question 'How might we get samples of street prostitutes and rent boys?' There would probably be an embarrassed silence, maybe a few nervous laughs, and then someone might say something like, 'Well, *I've never been there myself,* but I have heard that there is a street where prostitutes hang out. . .'. Other suggestions might include STD clinics, the police, 'look at the ads in telephone boxes' and so on. (See McKeganey et al. 1990).

The researchers describe their recruitment of street prostitutes as follows:

As it is known that prostituting women make only patchy and uneven use of health services such as the clinics for sexually transmitted diseases, we sought to establish street-level contacts with the women within the areas of their working and at the times of day of their working. We time-sampled across each day of the week and across each of the time periods that the women were observed working. We report here on data collected on 208 female prostitutes contacted over 32 days fieldwork within the City's major red light district. We estimate that these figures represent approximately half of the total streetworking population in Glasgow.

*There are three dimensions to our contact with the women. First, the
maintenance of detailed records based on each period of fieldwork, listing
the number of women seen working, the number of women spoken to directly,
whether these were new or repeat contacts and whether they were injecting
drug users. Second, we have sought to develop a service-provider role within
the context of our research activities by offering the women assorted condoms,
sterile injecting equipment (if they need it), and a leaflet outlining advice on
risk reduction, sterilisation of injecting equipment and telephone numbers of
local helping agencies. It is in large part through the offering of sterile injecting
equipment to these women that we have been able to distinguish between drug-
injecting and non-drug injecting prostitutes. Thirdly, we have sought continuity
in our contact with the women as a means of establishing the rapport and trust
necessary for conducting informal street interviews with them.*

(McKeganey et al. 1990)

Note the rigour in their observations and record-keeping. By offering condoms and
clean needles, they fulfilled what they described as a 'service-provider role within the
context of our research activities'. By gaining the acquaintance of the women on a regular basis, they were able to establish their trust and help in recruiting others. Thus, I
can imagine, when Neil approached a woman to ask her if she was selling sex, and if
she would be willing to participate in their study, a rather large, threatening man might
appear out of a doorway saying, 'What dae ye want wi ma wuman?' ('What do you want
with my woman?'). Mick, who was acting as Neil's 'Minder' (bodyguard), would run up
and say 'It's OK he is a real researcher, we are from the University.'

Note also the need for a 'minder'. It is a difficult and a very brave thing to do in this
sort of research. The irony of Mick and Neil being each other's minders is that they are
two of the nicest, mildest men you could ever meet, and the thought of them having
to defend themselves against some Glasgow hard-men is a frightening one. I am filled
with admiration for their pluck and determination.

In their study of rent boys, the same issues confronted them in identifying and
recruiting participants to the study. In their pilot study they described how they
employed a former rent boy who was also an experienced interviewer to interview clients, he also helped elicit the cooperation of rent boys he knew to recruit clients for
interview. These boys were mostly bar workers (Bloor et al., 1990).

As they described the issues in recruiting male sex workers:

*Over a 16-month period, we conducted 240 hours of fieldwork, including
pilot work, and contacted 32 male prostitutes, of whom only four were not
streetworkers. In addition, we gathered information from service agencies in
contact with male prostitutes (social workers, a venereologist, and a retired
minister) and from those whom Goffman (1963) terms 'the wise' – street
vendors, toilet and bath attendants, barmen, 'punters' (clients), and cruising
gays . . . Elsewhere (Bloor et al. 1991), we have attempted to estimate the size of
the Glasgow male prostitute population during the study period, and we believe
that our 32 subjects represent more than half of that prostitute population.*

*The main methodological problem facing any study of a covert and stigmatized
activity such as male prostitution is that of establishing an adequate and
unbiased sample of research subjects. This is a problem that most previous*

studies have failed to surmount (see Allen 1980). Many have recruited samples from clinics or from agency lists of clients, or have drawn snowball samples from such lists, thus underrepresenting the range of prostitution behavior.

In this study, the problem of ensuring representation of a range of prostitution practice was tackled in three ways. First, all public places in Glasgow that were reported or rumored to be sites where male prostitutes worked (eight toilets, six pubs, four parks, two discotheques, one amusement arcade, one sauna, and one Turkish bath) were investigated, and those worthy of further investigation (two toilets, two pubs, and two parks) were subjected to systematic time sampling. Second, we did not rely exclusively on 'snowball sampling' from initial contacts; in addition, we 'cold contacted' all those at the sites in question whom we suspected from their behavior of being male prostitutes. As a result, some men in our sample were unknown not only to service agencies, but also to other prostitutes; in fact, sometimes we were the first people, apart from clients, with whom they had discussed their prostitution. And third, we supplemented these data on street-working prostitutes by contacting and interviewing nonstreetworkers – that is, Glasgow escorts, masseurs, and 'call men' (a free-lance prostitute operating in his own flat with a 'book' of regular clients). The nonstreetworkers either responded to our appeal for information in the gay press or were contacted through their own or their agencies' advertisements.

(Bloor et al. 1993)

Again, they worked in pairs for safety. You can perhaps imagine what it must be like approaching someone in a men's public lavatory in a park in Glasgow at night and asking a stranger if they sell sex . . . I remember once, when I was on a visit to Glasgow to do some interviews on a cancer study I was working on at the time, and Mick and I met to catch-up with each other. So, we met in a hotel lounge in central Glasgow. Shortly after we had sat down, Mick looked uncomfortable and said to me, 'Do you mind if we go somewhere else? There are a couple of people in here that I interviewed in our study'. So we moved on. That brought home to me the fact that even when you do research in a large city, it can still be difficult to preserve anonymity.

It is to their credit the fact that they were persistent and rigorous and that they ended up with such a good response rate. They were trying to be as comprehensive as possible in the hope that their sample would truly represent the cultures of street prostitutes in Glasgow. In this, you might ask, 'But is this not taking a quantitative approach?' In one sense it is – they were able to present **qualitative** analyses and **quantitative** analyses in their reports, thus giving a fuller picture of that culture. Saying something like 'Some people . . .' or 'The majority of people . . .' is like a red rag to a bull for a statistician! Adding 'real data' (numbers) helped make the study more acceptable to those who did not understand qualitative approaches.

They ended up with 183 typewritten pages of fieldnotes for their analysis in the study of male prostitutes from this part of the study. They used the **'Ethnograph'** software package (software which helps with the coding, searching through transcripts, and indexing of qualitative data) to help them analyse their data:

The analytic method was that known as 'deviant case analysis 'or 'analytic induction' (see Bloor 1978). The method seeks to establish both the necessary and the sufficient conditions for distinguishing, absolutely rather than probabilistically, between different analytical categories of cases. In this analysis, the task was to establish the conditions that distinguish between those male prostitutes who always practice safer sex with clients and those who currently report at least occasional unsafe commercial sex.

(Bloor et al. 1993)

This method of analysing the data is interesting. **Analytic induction** aims to develop causal explanations about social events. It involves analysing an individual case or a small number of cases and looking for similarities. This allows you to begin the formulation of a theoretical explanation of what is going on in the events you have observed (collected data about). As new cases are analysed, you look out for any that are different from your emerging theory – so-called **'deviant cases'**. These are really useful, because they help you in refining your theory and developing it further (see Chapter 14 on Grounded Theory). So, the sequence looks something like this:

a. You analyse a case (or a small number of cases).

b. You note what is going on in that case/cases, and you use this to state your preliminary theory or hypothesis.

c. You analyse another case (or small number of cases) and you check to see whether is fits your preliminary theory or hypothesis.

d. If it does not fit, then you look at them all again and you re-formulate your theory or hypothesis.

e. You repeat a) to d), revising or elaborating your theory or hypothesis, until there are no new deviant cases. That is, you have accounted for all the cases in your study and your theory becomes finalised. This is a point at which you have reached **data saturation** or **theoretical saturation**. At this point, you can stop collecting data and write up your report.

This **cyclical iteration** of your theory or hypothesis is intensive, it is thorough, and it is hard work. It is something which you should work with another person, or in a team, to allow this iterative process to take place.

Note, that this method is generally accepted as being useful for helping to define what are the **necessary conditions** for a phenomenon being studied, but it is criticised for not being able to define the **sufficient conditions**. A necessary condition has to be there for an event to happen, but that does not explain why the event happens – there has to be a sufficient condition in place for it to actually happen. (An example might be the common cold. 'Contact with the virus which causes the common cold' is a necessary condition for you to become ill with the cold. But we know that not everyone who is exposed to contact with the cold virus actually becomes ill with the cold. In order to explain why some people become ill with the cold, we need to identify what other conditions (or factors) are required for you to become ill (sufficient factors) with the cold – e.g. vulnerability or susceptibility or genetic predisposition or stress, etc.)

The researchers were able in their reports to describe the nature of the relationships which street prostitutes and rent boys had with their clients – the negotiations over payments, the conditions under which the sex workers were prepared to engage in non-safe sex, the relative power between the sex workers and their clients, and the hazards of the work.

'Mark said he only did hand jobs. I offered him condoms but he said he didn't need them. I asked if he had customers who wanted him to do other things. 'Oh yeah'. Was it sometimes difficult to refuse, 'Yeah, sometimes you get threatened'. He told me a story about a customer who had taken him to a deserted golf club. 'He was a really big guy. He was threatening, but I carry (a blade) – you have to. I slashed him across the face'.

(McKeganey et al. 1990)

Example 2: Traditional Beliefs about Respiratory Infections in Children in a Rural Area in Southeast Nigeria

I supervised Princewill's dissertation research work for his MSc in Public Health. Princewill is from Nigeria. He was born in a poor, rural part of the country in Obike, Ngor-Okpala, a small village of 10 family units. It is a subsistence farming and fishing community in South Eastern Nigeria. 'Uju' is his family name. It means 'plenty'. (For over three generations there was a fear that the family lineage was going to disappear as there was only one surviving child from these generations – Princewill's grandfather. His grandfather therefore changed his name to 'Uju' in the hope that he would have plenty of children to preserve the family line. He did. Having married several wives, he had nearly 40 children . . .)

He describes his background and his motivation for this study:

Through my early years, I remember that my grandmother was the family 'expert' on health matters. When my mother's care did not meet with her approval, she would treat me with native herbs or use scarification to get rid of my body's impurities. I still bear the scars of these folk remedies. The fact that I am still here is perhaps proof that they might have worked. So for me, growing up occurred in the context of traditional life in South Eastern Nigeria where folk beliefs and practices determined all aspects of our lives. These were and still are part of what and who I am.

*I went from junior school to senior school and eventually to medical school in Nsukka. There the deeply held traditional beliefs were purged from my system to be replaced with the professional beliefs and practices of **Modern, Western Medicine (MWM)**. This was a time of deep conflict for me. The emphasis of my training was on a largely mechanistic focus on diagnosis and treatment of disease. Social and cultural aspects were ignored. Local beliefs and practices were all ridiculed and dismissed out of hand. There was no sympathy for anyone who engaged in anything other than MWM. Indeed these 'alternative' practices were often viewed as ignorance and the cause of problems. Like my classmates, I bought into this wonderful new world of 'Scientific Medicine' purported to offer solutions to all ills. The irony of it all was that that, on leaving* *medical school, I was confronted by patients' **lay beliefs** and practices but I was not equipped with the skills to deal with them. I realised that rather than ridiculing/dismissing any patient's lay beliefs, I needed to understand them more and learn how to address them in other to make what I – as a practitioner of MWM – can offer, acceptable to them. I felt that I was limited as a health practitioner.*

*Public health attracted me in that it seemed to provide avenues towards dealing with the main problems which faced the people in my country, e.g. malaria, TB, HIV/ AIDS, leprosy etc. Here there seemed to be the opportunity to afford a meeting between the cosmologies of MWM and indigenous lay beliefs and practices. I was put back in touch with the realization that that an old village grandmother for example could understand the meaning and significance of HIV/AIDS (**obere na aja ocha** – which literarily means 'will end in the grave'), even though she does not understand its underlying scientific basis.*

This study therefore was a means of re-connecting with my roots. I see the need to understand local views and explanations of illnesses and how these influence decisions about how to deal with them. I chose to study a rural community for two reasons:

That is where traditional/folk beliefs are likely to be most strongly held and freely expressed, and because I could use my insights to help in the interpretation and understanding of these.

(Uju 2010)

He chose to study mothers' knowledge, beliefs, and practices of Acute Respiratory Infection (ARI), because these constitute a leading cause of morbidity and mortality among children especially in the developing world. Globally, statistics show that ARI accounts for 12–35% of paediatric hospitalisations and 20–40% of out-patient visits by children (Ines and Olsen 2006). Estimates suggest that there are about two billion episodes of ARI worldwide annually (Muhe 1996). They place a huge burden on the healthcare systems of such countries. Around the world, attention remains more focused on malaria, diarrhoea, and malnutrition than on ARI, and most interventions are aimed at these. However, it is acknowledged that child survival efforts cannot work without paying attention to ARI-related deaths (Kumar 1987; WHO 1995). The management of disease in the community depends on *mothers* and the success of ARI-targeted programmes must include the ability of mothers to provide the 'necessary' care in a context of limited resources and competing ideologies.

Although mothers' knowledge, attitude, and perception had been documented in several studies, Princewill's aim was to describe rural, South Eastern Nigerian, mothers' perceptions and healthcare practices in relation to ARI in children, and to understand the socio-cultural context of their beliefs about children's illnesses and how these beliefs influenced healthcare decisions.

So, Princewill decided to adopt a qualitative – **ethnographic** – approach. We agreed that **focus groups** would be a suitable method of getting data on knowledge, beliefs, and practices, and that these could be followed up by a small number (four) of **individual interviews** to allow for **triangulation** of the data. He chose his site – Ngor-Okpala, a local county in Imo State, Nigeria – because of ease of access and his familiarity with the community who are mostly from the Ibo tribe. (See Figure 11.1.) Princewill reflects:

> *My background is that of a doctor working with a non-governmental organisation involved in the HIV and tuberculosis control program in the rural areas of Nigeria. It was my primary responsibility to provide support for tuberculosis (TB) and HIV-infected clients particularly HIV-affected women and children; to facilitate the reduction of HIV-related stigma and discrimination at the community and Healthcare settings and establish community-based linkages among individuals, groups, facilities, communities and others who provide continued care of TB/HIV/ AIDS clients. It was indeed challenging, as I tried to understand the underlying socio-cultural influences in this unfamiliar community that appeared to contribute to the high prevalence of the disease in the area.*

When I therefore decided to undertake a study in my area of origin, it was mainly based on the convenience, acceptability and the relative ease of access. However, this ill prepared me for the startling revelations that were come. As I listened to account upon

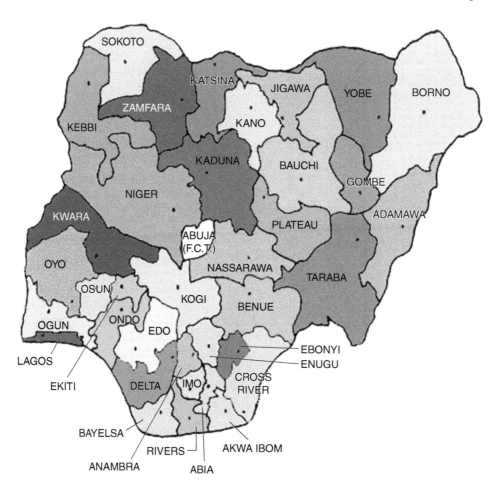

FIGURE 11.1 Map of states in Nigeria – Imo state is in the south of the country.

account, it dawned on me that contrary to my expectations, perhaps the only thing I shared in common with these lay folks was the fact that my roots can be traced to the small communities and family units aligning the creeks of rivers that made their silent course through them. I discovered that the words of Margaret Read could not be truer:

> *the scientifically trained health worker, wherever he may be, belongs to a culture, to a way of living and thinking that often has more in common with similarly trained health workers in other countries than with the illiterate population of his own country.*
>
> *(Read 1966)*

> *It was, therefore, an emotional and rude awakening for me to say the least, as I realised that I could not divorce my feelings from what I heard and was certain that it would remain a homecoming that would pervade my thoughts for years to come. As the essence of it all dawned on me and with the burst of emotions that I fought so hard to conceal I found myself stripped of every ounce of western sophistication and descended to a level where I saw it all from their simple mind's eyes. Strangely at this point, I found solace and experienced an innate joy spring forth from within me and it ceased to matter if they were right or wrong for I simply saw them for who they were, simple folks with 'simple' thoughts that seemed to define their word view.*

> *As I woke up from this seemingly trance state, I found that this journey had really been worth the while and concluded that the only change that would make sense to these folks would have to take into cognisance their world view and remain at every point, non-judgemental. . .*

> *This study, therefore, situates itself within the domain of **ethnomedicine** as it focuses on **health beliefs and practices**, cultural values, social roles and understanding the symbolic and interpersonal components of the experience of illness*
>
> *(Uju and Anderson 2014).*

Focus Groups

I shall say more about focus groups in Appendix E on research skills, but you may not have heard about this data collection method, so I shall tell you briefly about it now.

I first came across focus groups in 1980 when I worked in Hong Kong. One evening I phoned my friend Tim to ask if he fancied going out for a couple of beers. He said he could not because he was running some focus groups that evening. So, I asked him about them. Tim was a market researcher who worked for a company that had shoes manufactured in South Korea and in China. His job was to find out what sorts of styles and designs were preferred by the target client groups. He did this mainly by using focus groups. He would invite a small group of 6–10 people to meet and discuss various shoe designs. They would all sit round a table and Tim would start things off by putting a pair of shoes on the table, asking participants to have a look at them and consider what they liked about them and what they did not like about them. Then they would discuss the pros and cons of those shoes. Later, he would do the same with a different design and he would record everyone's views. In this way he was able to gauge what the prevailing thoughts and attitudes to those shoes were. *'Did people prefer the ones with the pointy toes, or the square toes, or the round toes?'* etc. By getting the group to discuss the issues amongst themselves, they could challenge others' opinions and he was able to get participants 'deeper reasoning' on topics. This discussion allowed the group to do what was difficult for him to do in a standard individual interview – challenge each other and make them explain their reasoning. Hmmm . . . interesting, I thought, and set about learning more about focus groups and practising with them.

There are two main groups of people who use focus groups – market researchers and politicians. I always imagine Prime Ministers going into their office in the morning and asking, 'Well, what are the focus groups saying today?' Businesses use them to keep a finger on the buying preferences of the general public. Politicians use them to keep a finger on the pulse of the voters in the country, so that they know which of their policies and which issues are popular. They are an excellent way of getting answers about what people *believe* – and people's beliefs are a central issue of ethnographic research. Focus groups are useful as they help to clarify arguments and they reveal diversity in views and opinions.

I remember the long hours of fun (!) I subjected Princewill to when I was coaching him on how to run a focus group. I would role play half a dozen Nigerian village women and he would play the academic researcher! I taught him how to run an **ice-breaker** – an exercise to get the group going. You choose a neutral topic and ask your participants to discuss it. This gives them a chance to warm-up, maybe even have some fun. It gives the group facilitator (the researcher) an opportunity to observe the group, to note which participants engage well in the group, which of them are reticent, and which of them might tend to hog the discussion. Then, when you bring the group back to get them to discuss the main topic or topics for discussion, you are better able to manage the group. I use the word **'manage'** deliberately, because that is what you have to do as a group facilitator. You have to be prepared to say things like: 'OK Mrs Ojimba, now let someone else say what they think . . .' or 'What about you, Mrs Adekele, you haven't said anything yet, what do you think . . .?' Sometimes, your task is to maintain order in the group and prevent any disagreements from getting out of hand. At other times you may need to be reassuring – 'It's OK to say what you think.'

I always suggest to my supervisees who use focus groups that they use a **co-facilitator.** I stress the importance of confirming beforehand what the roles are and who will lead the discussion.

Usually, the main facilitator will take the lead, and the co-facilitator will observe and make notes about what is going on in the group. S/he can, if agreed, interject to point out someone who is very quiet, or someone who is upset.

Princewill invited someone he knew from a local university to be a co-facilitator and they worked well together.

Focused Ethnographic Study (FES) of ARI

The WHO, in collaboration with several research institutes, developed the Focused Ethnographic study (FES) of ARI. This provides a framework for investigating the socio-cultural context within which families perceive and respond to ARI. It outlines the steps involved in researching lay beliefs and perceptions of ARI in children. It is a useful guide for new researchers who are new to ethnomedicine about how to conduct an ethnographic study (Hudelson 1994). Princewill found the FES useful for his study.

> *The FES design emphasizes anthropological theory and methods while limiting the scope and duration of fieldwork to a specific 'program-relevant' research problem. Findings from FES studies provide evidence of the rich vocabulary of ARI-related signs and concepts, and the interplay of structural and cultural factors that affect care-seeking for children with pneumonia.*

> *(Cove and Pelto 1993)*

He obtained his sample of mothers from those attending a weekly child welfare clinic, which is a free facility in Ngor-Okpala. Here, mothers bring children for routine immunisation and to get advice on infant feeding. About 100–200 mothers and their children attended each clinic. Because they are free – funded by government and international agencies as well as non-governmental organisations – these clinics attract people who could not otherwise pay for healthcare services.

Whilst mothers were waiting and listening to the health advice messages, the Clinic Nurses mentioned Princewill's study and invited mothers to indicate their interest. Mothers had to be over 17, have at least one child aged under 5 years, and have lived locally for at least two years. A total of 33 mothers were recruited from two clinic sessions. Two were excluded because they were health professionals. Three were school teachers and these were distributed amongst the focus groups. The mothers' recruitment to the study was preceded by a full explanation of the study. This was done in the local dialect by Princewill.

The mothers were allocated randomly into three groups of at least 10 mothers. There was some shifting around to suit the mothers' convenience. The three teachers were split between the groups – designated FG-1, FG-2, and FG-3. Travel, refreshment, and childcare costs were offered to the mothers. These were paid for by Princewill (he is a doctor and could afford it!) The focus group discussions were held in a room provided by a local district hospital. Out of the 33 recruited to the study, only 14 could make the dates and times of the groups, so only two were run. (Unfortunately, following a burst of early rains, most of the potential participants simply failed to turn up on the agreed days and time.) Six attended the first and eight the second focus group. They were a fairly homogeneous group – with the exception of the teachers.

Consent was taken before the beginning of the focus groups. Three mothers signed the form and the rest thumb-printed it. Each was given a copy of the Participant Information Sheet and the Consent form to keep. These were translated into Igbo (the local language) and back-translated to check for accuracy. They were explained in Igbo to mothers who could not read.

Ground rules were set at the start. **Confidentiality** was emphasised – both on the part of the researchers not revealing to anyone else anything that anyone was said in the focus group, and also on the part of the participants. It was also clearly explained to participants that any disclosures of potential harmful practices would be addressed and participants would be encouraged to raise such issues with their doctor or any other category of health workers accessible to them. *Researchers are not policemen.* The issue of social power was also addressed.

It was anticipated that my being of the male gender, a doctor and of a higher social status might have a potential to influence the group discussions and interviews. To counter its negative impact a few measures were taken. Firstly, I reaffirmed my position in the group as that of a student researcher and not a doctor. Secondly, my fluency in the local dialect and knowledge of the local area meant that I was more accepted and was of particular advantage in moderating the affairs of the group. Thirdly, the choice of a female assistant who contributed immensely in stimulating the group discussions and taking notes ensured that the issue of gender was neutralised. Finally, particular emphasis was placed to our dressing as we ditched our 'western looks' and appeared in conservative local attires. This is because, it has been established that the style of clothing affects people's impression about a person and their behaviour towards them.

Princewill used an icebreaker to get the groups going. He started by asking them to discuss what the best way to cook cassava was – boiled or roasted? Five mothers took part in **individual interviews** after signing/thumb-printing a consent form. A similar topic guide to that used in the focus group discussions was used.

The audio-recordings of the focus-groups and the interviews were transcribed verbatim and translated into English. He analysed his results using a **thematic analysis.** This consisted of the following steps:

1. Transcription – verbatim.
2. Immersion – reading and listening to recordings over and over again to familiarise yourself with the data.
3. Initial emergent themes – often themes or issues will jump off the page at you. You label these and keep a note of each one and where it occurs.
4. Verifying initial themes – you get a second (or even a third person) to verify your analysis. In this you would present them with your finding and they would question you about it until you both agree on the theme/issue and the best label for it.
5. Describing and reporting the themes – you then write your account of the themes which emerged from your data and give appropriate examples.

The results of this study gave a very rich account of the ways in which these mothers from southeast Nigeria perceived and responded to different aspects of ARI in their children. For example, Table 11.1 gives a description of the ways in which they perceived coughs, what they believed caused them, the steps which could be taken to deal with them, and the likely outcomes of different interventions.

In both the group discussions and interviews mothers generally agreed that family members were influential in making healthcare decisions in relation to ARIs and illnesses in children. Most of the mothers believed that the shared responsibility of illness lessens its burden. In one account a mother had this to say,

If my child is sick I tell my husband, if he is not around I will tell his brothers who will decide what to do because if I don't and something happens they will blame me (B2).

TABLE 11.1   **Type of cough; aetiology, treatment, and outcome.**

| Type of cough | Beliefs about | | |
	Origin / cause	Treatment	Outcome
Ukwara okporo (ordinary cough)	Exposure to cold Dust	Foreign medicine	Gets well after treatment
		Native herbs	Gets well after treatment
Ukwara ume oku (hot breathing)	Rainy season	Use of herbs, transpirates (foam-like discharge from plants) (Figure 11.2)	Good outcome with treatment
Ukwara oriko uwa (The cough that never dies)	Curse	Rituals can prevent	Fatal No cure
Akom (febrile illness)	Physical abuse; associated with other childhood infections.	Foreign medicine Native herbs	Good outcome with treatment.
Ukwara ooooo (whooping cough)	??	Using soup made from male lizards and insects.	Good outcome with treatment.
Ukwara uta (The slimming cough/small cough)	Poisoning, hereditary/ familial	Herbs Treatment in hospital for 6 – 12 months	Good outcome with treatment
Ukwara eburu puta uwa (the cough you are born with)	Congenital	Herbs	Good outcome with treatment.

(*Source*: adapted from Uju, 2010).

A minority thought that involving relatives might bring about confusion and cause delay.

> *Telling a lot of people will bring confusion as this person will bring one idea and the other person another idea. It is difficult to agree and the child will suffer (B3).*

Another mother had this moving tale:

> *I was once married and had one son. I was loved by my husband and his relatives but it all changed when my son was ill and I told my husband about it and he wasn't serious about it and my son died. Everybody blamed me and felt I should have done something on my own. Today I am married again with children and I will advise you, don't make the same mistakes. In this place people give you respect because of your children. If they are not there you are nothing so go to any extent for them and don't look at faces (B7).*

Many mothers complained about the state of their local hospitals and the quality of care these delivered. These were a deterrent to taking their ill children to hospital. They were specific about the lack of infrastructure and inadequate manpower. They criticised their previous experiences where they had to wait in long, seemingly endless, queues before they saw a doctor. Some mothers thought that health personnel were quite unfriendly. The staff most frequently mentioned were nurses who, they reported, were usually insensitive to their plight and talked to them rudely. Hospital clerks were accused of manipulating the order of the queues in favour of their relatives and friends irrespective of their time of arrival. Doctors were said to be absent or not in attendance as most of them were thought to engage in private practices which often conflicted with their duties in the district hospital. During interactions, there was no evidence to suggest that the hospital or clinic staff understood the mothers '*lay perceptions and beliefs*'.

All the mothers reported both **physical** and **supernatural** causes of diseases. Supernatural entities such as gods, evil forces, ghosts, malevolent spirits, and 'aggrieved' ancestors were said to be directly responsible for causing ill health. These also include beliefs in witchcraft, sorcery, magic, etc. Evil and jealous neighbours and relatives were thought to inflict illness through spells and 'poisoning' (nshi).

'Germ' concepts of disease aetiology and contagion, which are prevalent in Western medical causal models of disease, were basically non-existent in the population studied. They were more likely to attribute the causation of diseases to environmental factors. There was a general belief in the efficacy of Modern Western Medicine *in most cases*. (See Tables 11.1 and 11.2.)

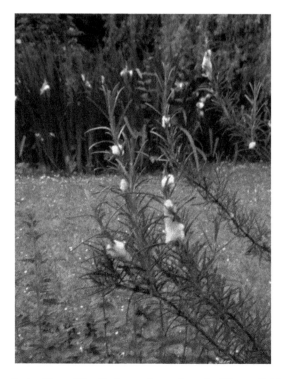

FIGURE 11.2   Transpirates (foam-like discharge from plants) – 'Cucoo Spit' – aspirates.

TABLE 11.2 Local terms and Western medical equivalents.

Local/folk terms		Western medical terms							
	Asthma	TB	Pneumonia	Whooping cough	Otitis media	Suppurative otitis media	Common cold	Uvelitis	Pharygitis/ tonsillitis
Ukwara umeoku	X		X						
Ukwara oriko									
Azuzu/oyi							X		
Ukwara eburu	X								
Ota nti					X				
Avu nti						X			
Ukwara oooo				X					
Ukwara nta	X	X							
Mgbapia								X	
Nrapa									X

(*Source*: adapted from Uju, 2010).

The interview data confirmed the same issues and themes as the focus groups' data. However, there were a couple of additional examples which were not discussed in the focus groups. During the course of the interviews, one mother reported using cow's urine and crude oil to treat convulsion in her children by rubbing it on their body or giving it to the child to drink in the bid to keep the evil spirits that were responsible at bay. When it was pointed out to her that it was a potentially dangerous practice her response replied:

> . . . if it does not cure it nothing else would. (C1)

Direct questioning of other mothers in the interviews revealed it was a common practice which they believed was effective. It was surprising that this was not mentioned during the Focus Group Discussions (FGD) – perhaps it was a practice which they felt embarrassed about discussing in the more public arena of the FGDs. He suggested that before they considered using that again, they ought to discuss it with the hospital or clinic staff first.

Princewill concluded:

> . . . mothers held firm traditional beliefs with regards to ARIs in their children. They had explanatory models of ARI causation in children which had an internal logic and consistency which helped them make sense of their child's illness and answer the questions 'how' and 'why'. Although this was not based on scientific facts, it nonetheless informed the basis of what type of action they took.

> Modifying health beliefs through health and religious messages are therefore possible. For public health messages to make sense, it should however take into cognisance the mother's explanatory model of ill health in their children. To achieve this it is imperative to note that there are other valid models of ill health apart from the western medical model. These indeed may have certain advantages over western medicine and therefore demand respect in their own right.

> It is important to note that while some folk practices may not be 'acceptable' by modern western medical standards, we must not be rash in dismissing them because it has served its users 'reliably' over time and may well be the only feasible option available to them. We should therefore resist the attempt to advise them to abolish their established traditional health values and practices without the guarantee of a viable and sustainable option, as this would only impact negatively on their natural instinct of seeking the help available to them and the psychological security this provides. When people have very little, to take that away leaves them in a powerless and helpless situation. The challenge is to learn how to integrate lay knowledge, beliefs and practices into the knowledge, beliefs and practices of Modern Western Medicine.

Now, don't you think that this is a fascinating study? It shows the power of focus groups and interviews as additional methods to get access to belief systems and patterns of behaviour. I think that Princewill's personal background and experience helped him in his understanding of and reporting of the results which he obtained.

One of the points which he made was that 'traditional beliefs' are not confined to Africa. He cites Cecil Helman's study 'Feed a cold and starve a fever' which highlights the prevalence of 'traditional beliefs' in a modern, Western society – the UK (Helman 1978). When I lived in Glastonbury, if someone was ill, it was common for friends to light a candle or say a prayer for the, Some might tie a ribbon to a sacred tree, or cast spells in the hope of helping people get better. There were more magic shops in the High Street than there were estate agents (and I know which I would trust more!) See Figures 11.3 and 11.4.

I used to invite Princewill to talk about his research in my Research Methods courses, before he moved to Glasgow to train as a GP. It was a wonderful sight – he dressed in his full Nigerian clothing and hat. At six foot four, he made a most impressive figure – and he got higher ratings in student feedback than I did.

To Sum Up

In this chapter, I have presented alternative methods to participant observation for gathering data about **cultures** – sets of beliefs about the world and appropriate ways of thinking and behaving. In the first, examples, Mick and Neil et al. demonstrated ways of getting access to a world that is usually hidden to most of us. By aiming at as large a coverage as possible, they hoped to make their findings **generalisable** to the two worlds they were studying – that of the female sex worker and that of the male sex worker. Like all good ethnographers, they went in with a sympathetic ear. Their

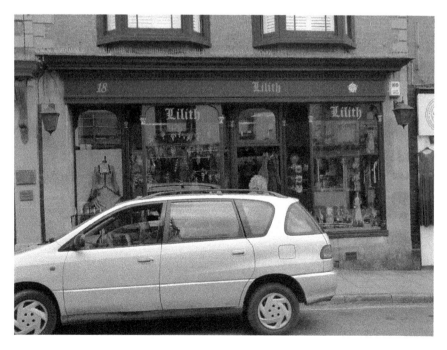

FIGURE 11.3   A magic shop in Glastonbury high street.

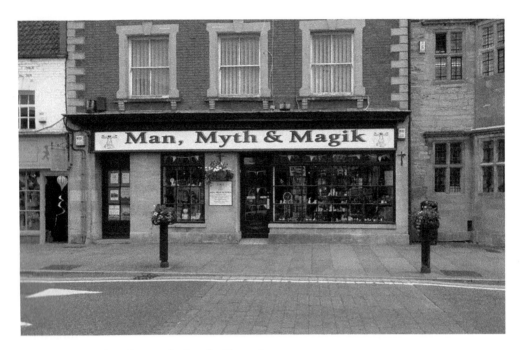

FIGURE 11.4 Another magic shop in Glastonbury.

job was to *understand not to criticise.* They used interviews as their method of data collection and. Although this was a mainly qualitative study they were able to include quantitative data as well as qualitative data. So, ethnographic research can span the quantitative/ qualitative divide.

In the same way, Princewill returned to his roots, not to convert, but to get a better insight and understanding of the world of Nigerian mothers, and to report that to others who might not appreciate or accept the views held by his participants. He did not attempt to be comprehensive in his coverage. His aim was to illustrate and to help outsiders understand their world, rather than to generalise. He used focus groups, augmented by interviews as a means of gathering his data, which was purely qualitative.

Both of these studies had the possibility of being either hypothetico-inductive or hypothetico-deductive. Neil and Mick's approach, using **analytic induction**, was hypothetico–inductive – their theory stemmed from the data they were collecting. However, Princewill, because of his own background which was immersed in the culture he was studying, meant that he had some insights and pre-conceptions already – his was more hypothetico-deductive.

Note the sampling used in each case. Neil and Mick used a 'snowballing' approach by getting the help of rent boys who worked mainly in bars to recruit others for interviews and to help spread the word that they were bona fide researchers and could be trusted. They used opportunistic approaches – whenever the opportunity arose, for example in public toilets, they would try to recruit new participants. Princewill, on the other hand, used a more conventional approach by targeting mothers who were attending an antenatal clinic. This got round the problem of recruiting from unknown rural areas – how do you know who is a mother (within two years of giving birth), etc.?

Clinics and hospitals are relatively easy targets for recruiting study participants. Both studies discussed here used *purposive sampling* – in the sense that they aimed to recruit specific groups of people to their studies.

Research is the art of the possible!

References

Bloor M, McKeganey N, and Barnard M. (1990). An ethnographic study of HIV-related risk practices among Glasgow rent boys and their clients: Report of a pilot study. *Aids Care* 2(1), 17–24.

Bloor MJ, Barnard MA, Finlay A, et al. (1993). HIV-Related Risk Practices among Glasgow Male Prostitutes: Reframing Concepts of Risk Behavior. *Medical Anthropology Quarterly*, 7(2), 152–169.

Bloor M, Neil M, and Barnard M. (2007). An ethnographic study of HIV-related risk practices among Glasgow rent boys and their clients: report of a pilot study. *Psychological and Sociomedical Aspects of AIDS/HIV* 2(1), 17–24.

Cove S and Pelto GH. (1993). Focused ethnographic studies in the WHO programme for the control of acute respiratory infections. *Medical Anthropology: Cross-Cultural Studies in Health and Illness* 15(4), 409–424.

Helman C. (1978). "Feed a cold and starve a fever": folk models of infection in an English suburban community, and their relation to medical treatment. *Culture, Medicine and Psychiatry* 2, 107–137.

Hudelson PM. (1994). The management of acute respiratory infections in Honduras: a field test of the focused ethnographic study (FES). *Medical Anthropology* 15(4), 435–446.

Ines AK and Olsen J. (2006). Determinants of acute respiratory infection in Soweto – a population based birth cohort. *South African Medical Journal* 96(7), 633–640.

Kumar V. (1987). Need for a natural control programme for acute respiratory infections. *Indian Journal of Paediatrics* 54, 145–148.

Muhe L. (1996). Mothers perception of signs and symptoms of acute respiratory infections in their children and their assessment of severity in an urban community in Ethiopia. *Annals of Tropical Paediatrics* 16(2), 129–135.

Neil M, Marina B, and Michael B. (1990). A comparison of HIV-related risk behaviour and risk reduction between female street working prostitutes and male rent boys in Glasgow. *Sociology of Health & Illness* 12(3), 274–292.

Princewill U. (2010). *Perceptions and childcare practices regarding acute respiratory infection in children: a study of mothers in a rural nigerian community.* University of Brighton, MSc dissertation.

Princewill U and Anderson JL. (2014). *Traditional beliefs about respiratory infections in children in a rural area in Southeast Nigeria.* Unpublished paper.

Read M. (1966). *Culture Health and Disease.* Tavistock Publications: London.

World Health Organisation. (1995). Division of Diarrhoeal and Acute respiratory disease control. Integrated management of the sick child. *Bulletin of World Health Organisation* 73, 735–740.

CHAPTER 12

Qualitative Ethnographic Approaches

Autoethnography

Introduction

Autoethnography is a type of ethnographic research.

- We are still in the **qualitative** domain – there are no numbers involved.
- It is **hypothetico-inductive** – we do not set out to test hypotheses, but allow the data to drive our emerging theory.
- It is **retrospective** – you study things that have already happened, rather than following people into the future.
- It is a form of **case study** – 'N = 1', but that one is you – **the researcher.**

In an autoethnography, the culture which you are studying is the **culture of you.** There is not really any sampling of participants – *you are it.* My guess is that everyone who sets out on an autoethnographic quest, wants to make a statement. So, the first thing you need to try to clarify for yourself is 'What do you want to achieve?' 'What outcomes/changes would you like to achieve?' and 'Why?' This is something that you should work through with a supervisor before you go any further – if indeed you do decide to proceed.

Autobiographical accounts can share some of the same qualities of autoethnographies. They can be very moving and leave a vivid impression on the reader. Some that I personally have found to have a profound effect on me have been (in no particular order): Adam Kaye's *This is Going to Hurt* (2018) kept me in stitches, laughing all the way through . . . and then realising the darker side of being a junior doctor and the effect that this had on him. It was funny, moving and tragic. Arthur Frank's *The Wounded Storyteller: Body, Illness and Ethics* (2013) also had a profound effect on me, as did Jane Poulson's *The Doctor Will Not See You Now* (2003), which brought home to me the juxtaposition of being a doctor and communicating, as she thought, *well,* with her patients, and then learning what it was like to be on the receiving end of

Demystifying Research for Medical & Healthcare Students: An Essential Guide, First Edition. John L. Anderson.
© 2022 John Wiley & Sons Ltd. Published 2022 by John Wiley & Sons Ltd.
Companion website: www.wiley.com/go/Anderson/DemystifyingResearch

what she had been doing for years. There are many more in the medical and nursing world. Some autobiographies blatantly set out to 're-write' history to make themselves appear in a better light. But, although these autobiographical accounts do accomplish their desired effect – they leave an imprint in our minds – they are *not* properly *auto-ethnographic*. In an **autobiography,** the psychopath can be an angel in her or his own words.

That is one of the reasons why I place such importance on forming a **research team** – even if this is just yourself and another person. Students can turn to their *supervisors*. Other researchers might consider asking a colleague (who does not appear in the autoethnography) be a co-researcher or supervisor. Some may turn to the sanctity and anonymity of a therapeutic relationship provided by a counsellor or psychotherapist. (Remember to include their fees in your research budget!) The relationships within a team also need to be spelt out.

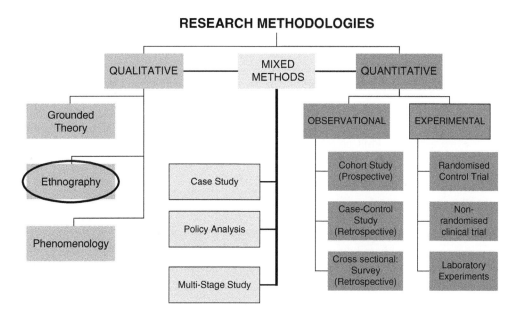

Example 1: Studying Medicine with Dyslexia: A Collaborative Autoethnography

Seb was one of my favourite postgrad students and is now a close friend as well a colleague. Seb's initial interest for his MSc in Medical Education dissertation was to document the impact that having dyslexia had on medical students. I signposted him to **interpretive phenomenology** (which we shall come to in Chapter 13) and he asked me to supervise him. I agreed. Now, at this point there is something you should know about Seb – he is a workaholic with no off switch! (We eventually agreed that he would not text or e-mail me his ideas between 10.00 p.m. and 8.00 a.m. . . .) So, Seb began with an autoethnographic account, or rather, an **assisted autoethnographic** account of his own experiences of being a medical student with dyslexia. This had five stages:

1. Seb wrote an autobiographical account.
2. I interviewed him and interrogated him about this account – this is the **assisted** element.
3. He used these two sources as the raw data to analyse thematically.
4. We wrote it up and submitted it to journals in the medical education field to publish. Here we ran into a blank wall. We got replies like:

   This paper is beautifully written, it is a compelling story, and it takes on a topic of growing interest around the world . . . They [Seb and John] acknowledge that the findings might not be generalizable and indicate that their aim is to inspire research in the area. While I am supportive of this goal, it is not clear to me that a research journal is the appropriate venue for it . . .

   (Shaw et al. 2018)

5. So, we approached Alec Grant a friend of mine from the School of Health Sciences in the University of Brighton (who is one of the leading figures in autoethnography in the UK) and invited him to join us to break through the brick wall of publishing – hence the assisted autoethnography became a **collaborative, assisted ethnography.** This collaboration worked. With Alec's greater experience, we refined the manuscript and were successful in publishing it (Shaw et al. 2018).

In our account (Shaw et al. 2016), we go into considerable detail about the roles which the three of us had in the project; and again in our account in 2018 (Shaw et al. 2018), we expand upon the roles and in particular the researcher–supervisor relationship and the need for that to be in place early on in the project. Although Seb and I had a very good working relationship, we found that involving Alec (as one of the UK's leading autoethnographers) allowed us the opportunity to have a third, more detached, researcher involved. Thus, Alec would interrogate both of us on our work, and, I believe, achieve a greater clarity and methodological purity in our work.

Here is a taste of what the final document was like.

Seb: *When you are struggling with academic requirements, your self-image and your very brain, it is easy to feel like the world is against you. Throughout my first three years at medical school, I often found myself low or even crying about this. I felt that those around me were fed up with me, thought I was inept or, even, hated me. My continuing isolation (to keep up with work) fed this situation, separating me from my peers. This remains a struggle for me to this day. My segregation from my peers has never been greater. Having focused so hard on survival and keeping up with work, I find myself able to talk to less than 10% of my cohort. For this reason, I often look at university timetables and panic when I see that I will be 'alone', with people I never took the time to get to know or maintain friendships with. Their collegiate and social groups have already formed and solidified*

(Shaw et al. 2016).

Types of Autoethnography

There are different schools of thought about autoethnographies. Some scholars prefer an approach which is an **evocative autoethnography** or an **emotional autoethnography** (Ellis 1997, 2004). The message can be conveyed in the form of texts and/ or performances to get the messages across. The account tells its own story and makes its own impact. Some would say that trying to add an analytic framework on top of it (or around it) detracts from the main points of the autoethnography, which are glaringly obvious in their own right. As Denzin (1997) puts it, evocative autoethnographies 'bypass the representational problem by invoking an epistemology of emotion, moving the reader to feel the feelings of the other' (Denzin 1997). And that is very true. A good evocative autoethnography will leave you feeling like you had read a novel or seen a play or a film and been so moved by it that you could have had the experiences yourself. The story tells its own story! Sometimes, there is an element of shocking the audience and, by so doing, making an impact and evoking their sense of guilt, or pride, or whatever.

This is in contrast to the style of autoethnographies favoured by the symbolic interactionist school of sociology – **analytical autoethnography.** This approach argues that sometimes the story itself is not enough, and to contribute to theory, autoethnographies need to adopt an analytical rather than merely emotional approach. Anderson (2006) argues that analytical autoethnography should include five key features:

1. **Complete member researcher** (**CMR**) – the autoethnographer has to be part of the world s/he is describing and studying.

2. **Analytic reflexivity** – reflexivity involves a searching of the self to enhance one's awareness of the inter-relationships between oneself and others and the situational context within which events have occurred.

3. **Narrative visibility of the researcher's self** – the researcher should be seen and heard in the accounts and the analysis and these should be included as data in the analysis.

4. **Dialogue with informants beyond the self** – although autoethnography is based upon the researcher's own experiences, s/he should also include reference to others' experiences, sometimes this will engage in the thoughts of others towards yourself.

5. **Commitment to theoretical analysis** – the researcher must go beyond the merely descriptive and engage in the analytical work, which is crucial for enhancing and advancing theory.

I would suggest that there is a third approach within autoethnography – **descriptive autoethnography.** This type lacks the emotional string-pulling of the evocative autoethnography approach, and it does not go into the analytics favoured in analytical autoethnography. Rather, descriptive autoethnography simply tells a story and leaves it to the reader to draw their own conclusions, instead of guiding the reader to the autoethnographer's conclusions by framing them within emotionally-laden accounts or within the analytic framework chosen by the analytic ethnographer.

Example 2: Ulcerative Colitis: An Autoethnographic Case Study

One of my supervisees – 'Martin' – was interested initially in doing a study to document the 'lived experiences' of young people with irritable bowel syndrome (**IBS**). When I was teaching him one to one, I asked why he was interested in this topic, he answered, 'It is an under-researched topic. There are lots of studies of adults with IBS, but almost none of younger people. And the services seem to be oriented to either children or adults . . .' I kept pressing him. 'That sounds like a good idea, but what is driving you to do this?' Eventually, he told me that he had IBS himself, and that as an adolescent he found that there were huge gaps in the services for himself and people like him. He asked me to supervise him and I agreed. I felt that his situation – as an **insider-researcher** would give him both a sensitivity in interviewing young people with IBS and a depth of insight that an 'outsider', like myself, might lack. So, we set off on our quest.

Martin identified a centre which had specialists in this area and who were interested in collaborating with us. But they insisted that one of their team must be the lead researcher in the study. We did not like the potential implications of this, and, after many months of negotiations which just went round in circles, we gave up on them. We identified another centre who might be interested, but, by then, Martin was running out of time to complete his MSc. He began to despair about succeeding in completing his work in time, so I suggested he consider an autoethnographic approach and told him more about it. He was interested, and, after giving it some consideration, he agreed to try it. His aim was clear, he wanted to use himself as a case study to illustrate the lack of sensitivity of assessments for adolescents; to show how devastating an impact IBS can have on young people; and how inadequate the services (including psychological services) can be for young people with IBS.

He mainly aimed to inform people by telling his story. He wanted to put it down in print so that others could see from it, where the gaps in understanding and treatments were. We both agreed that the messages from his narratives would paint a clear picture of what it was like to be a young man with IBS, and the lessons to take from this would be self-evident.

I was diagnosed with Ulcerative Colitis when I was 21 years old. My symptoms were classic, but severe, as I was diagnosed with Pancolitis where disease activity affected my entire large bowel. I was initially treated medically, but eventually required surgical treatment due to the severity of the disease. Over the years since I was diagnosed, I have always had a strong desire to reflect upon its impact on me and those around me. I've always had some acceptance that the condition had impacted me on more than just a physical level. This autoethnographic account explores my disease history and the impact that it has had on me individually and on others in my life. Through reflective interviewing, I have identified themes that have been present throughout my illness, many of which are shared by other sufferers. I have also explored the role for psychological interventions to help with support for such symptoms and suggest that this is an area worth further exploration.

(Anon and Anderson 2017)

The Method

The process of an autoethnography begins with *you* writing an autobiographical account of that part of your life you propose to study. But an autoethnography goes far beyond the merely *descriptive* account and the challenge for you is to provide an *analytical* account of your own lived experiences and what has happened to you in the context you are describing. In addition to the reflection, the soul-searching and the cataloguing of your experiences, the impact of them on you, and your feelings during the time you are covering and since then, your analysis might well benefit from you considering *how others saw you* and reacted to you. This might include interviews you conduct with other people who were involved or who knew you then (**witnesses**). I advocate that after you have written an autobiographical account, you get someone, perhaps your supervisor or a therapist, to interview you and challenge you on any aspects or details which might be missing, This type of 'assisted' or 'collaborative' autoethnography can be very useful in facilitating your analysis of any aspects of your narrative which you may wish to repress (Shaw et al. 2016, 2018).

> *An autobiography is a means of telling one's own story – it is DESCRIP-TIVE. An autoethnography goes beyond the mere 'telling of one's story' – it is ANALYTICAL, in an extreme depth – both in the introspection involved and in the reporting of the account.*
>
> *(Shaw, Anderson & Grant, 2016)*

Outlined below are the main steps in conducting an autoethnography:

1. Ask yourself *what you want to do* – and *why*. This last part is very important. You should be aware of your motives for this project. Why do you want to tell your story – do you want to inform the world so that people can benefit from it? Do you want to get back at people of organisations who may have harmed you? Do you want to get things off your chest? Have clear goals in mind when you set out. But beware – if your goal is revenge, remember the old Confucian saying, '*Before you set out to seek revenge, first dig two graves!*'

2. Plan what you want to do. Consider those elements of your life which you are prepared to make public and which of them you do not want to be in the public domain. At this point you might need to think about whether to publish it under your own name, or might you want to use an **alias?** Some of my MSc students whom I have supervised in the conduct of their autoethnographies have used aliases to protect their identity. Define the boundaries of your account and how you might refer to other significant people in it.

3. Get yourself someone who can supervise you or who can be there to oversee the work and who you might also use to check out any analyses that you do. Make sure that this is someone who you can trust to maintain confidences and who can be supportive – including in the way they critique your work and give you feedback. It could be a friend or colleague, but think carefully before you involve anyone who you will have an ongoing relationship with after the work is done. Let's refer to this person as your 'supervisor' for now.

4. Consider using a counsellor or a psychotherapist. (Ed: I charge 55 guineas per hour.) Seriously, two people who I have supervised have used this means of support – a therapist, but not me! Although I have undergone my training in Transactional Analysis psychotherapy, there are boundaries which supervisors should not cross. I have encouraged all my A/E supervisees to consider using the services of a counsellor or a psychotherapist. I never feel threatened by this arrangement, although I know some supervisors who would. So, if you say to your supervisor, 'This has really brought bad things back to me and I don't know how to cope with them', be prepared for her/him to say to you, 'Would you like to see someone, a counsellor, therapist or someone from student services to get support with this?' Please don't take that as a rejection. It is a good sign. It means that your supervisor is aware of **boundaries** (we are teachers, not therapists) and s/he is not going to let her/his ego come between you and the help you may need.'

5. An autoethnography can be both a challenging and incredibly rewarding piece of research. It allows a researcher to look deeply into their own experiences to infer cultural and social implications – combining autobiography and standard ethnography. In doing this, they can create a story that is both appealing and moving to others, while adding to the available literature on insufficiently scrutinized areas of research. But it has its dangers.

    The autoethnography discussed here required Seb to expose himself on a deeply vulnerable, emotional level. It was crucial that he felt 'held' emotionally throughout this process. This is where the wealth of experience from first John and later Alec formed invaluable supports. For anyone interested in conducting an autoethnographic study, we believe it is imperative to have adequate research and psychological support in place – in advance.

    (Shaw et al. 2018)

    I was crucially aware of the potential conflicts in my role as we worked very closely together through this journey. Was I teacher, mentor, therapist, colleague, father-figure, or friend? All of these, I guess. It was a very intimate process which demanded an engagement in which I believe we truly fulfilled Rogers' 'core conditions' of honesty and openness, positive regard, and empathic understanding – on both our parts (Rogers 1967). I saw Seb grow and change as a person.

    (Shaw et al. 2018)

6. Have a go. Most people want to write. *Do it!* You may find that once you have written the first sentence, e.g. 'My name is XX, and I want to tell my story . . .', you can't stop and the words just pour out on to the pages. If that happens, then go with it, but be aware of your own needs and your responsibilities. Can you take a sickie because you are writing an autoethnography? Hmmm. Interesting thought. If you find yourself sitting staring at a blank screen, then stop, pick up a pen or a pencil (a 2B pencil, so you can erase it easily!). Begin to draw a rough diagram. Put yourself – as you were – in the centre. Put yourself – as you are now – on the right-hand side. Put lines from 'you as you were' to 'bubbles' around 'you as you were' on the left, and put the events and people you want to include in your story in those bubbles.

That's right – it is a sort of spider diagram. (Believe it or not, you can download templates for these from the internet!)

7. Keep in touch with your supervisor. *When you are ready,* share your work with her/him. If you get stuck, then get support quickly.

8. Once you have got into the writing habit, carry on to write your autobiographical account – and this is where you should use 'I', 'me', 'mine', etc. This is a very **personal journey**. Take ownership of it. Be proud that you are able to write it. Describe events, people, and very importantly, your feelings. Include in your account how events and people impacted on you and your life. Also reflect during this process and write about how you were and how you contributed to events and how you affected other people around you.

9. You may find that you have already begun to be deeply reflexive and analytical in your autoethnography. Good. Now is the time when you need to go deeper. You have probably written an interesting story up to now. Next comes the job of making sense of it. This is the difficult bit. If you have been successful, your story and the points you want to make by telling it will be self-evident. However, there will always be some critic (they are called journal reviewers) who will say 'So what?' For these people, you will have to spell out the implications of your account. Say clearly how this relates to other people's lives and what can be learned from it.

10. You might wish to conduct some brief interviews with others who were involved in your life at the time you have written about. Ask them how they perceived you and how they reacted to you as you were. If possible, include some of their accounts into your own along with your reflections on them.

11. This is also the point at which you might get someone else – such as your supervisor – to *interview you*. This interview should allow them to probe more deeply into the places which you found hard to reach. It can also help in clarifying what you mean by some of the things you say. This is not obligatory, but it can be a useful event.

While broadly similar, the interview transcript did not match completely with Seb's un-assisted autobiographical recollection. The interview evoked memories of situations, thoughts, and feelings that his personal introspection had not. It was more emotional and focused less upon purely literal, experiential recollection. Therefore, the interview helped us to produce a richer pool of data to analyze and draw from. It also gave us direct quotes for use in our final case. These helped to contextualize and further humanize the dialogue. We were pleasantly surprised how successful this addition of the interview turned out to be

(Shaw et al. 2018).

12. Having written your A/E, and, if applicable, conducted your interview(s), you have your **raw data.** This can be analysed by a method of your choice. My suggestion is that a simple **thematic analysis** (see Appendix F) will be the simplest and keep you closest to the realities of your data.

13. Your next task is to write it in a report format along with a discussion section and conclusions.

As I said at the beginning, one of the first things you should consider when you are thinking about doing an autoethnography is to consider *why* you want to do it? *Who* do you want to send messages to? *What* outcomes do you want to achieve? I'd like to introduce you to a bit of Transactional Analysis theory now. I want to introduce you to the notion of the **drama triangle**. (See Figure 12.1.) At most points in our life, we tend not to be caught up in it – in the model you would be at the centre (scoring '0' – if we allocated you a score for where you were on any axis). How-

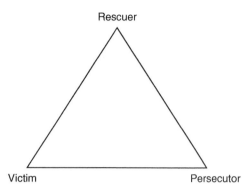

FIGURE 12.1   The drama triangle.

ever, sometimes we can gravitate out along the axis (getting nearer to a score of '10' if we allocated a score for it).

We all tend to have our own preferred place on the drama triangle, but we are not normally aware of it. The three positions on the triangle are:

- **Rescuer:** Here our inclination is to help others in difficulty.
- **Persecutor:** Here our inclination is to punish others.
- **Victim:** Here, we are in a position of needing and seeking help.

Now, take a few minutes to reflect on this – and to consider: have you found your-self in any of these positions? Which position are you most comfortable in? (We could do more, but you can read about it in depth elsewhere (Joines and Stewart 2012).)

So, let's return to your autoethnography . . . Where are you starting out on the drama triangle? Do you want to get back at someone (Persecutor)? Do you want others to know how bad things have been for you (Victim)? Do you want to help others out by telling your story (Rescuer)? Or are there parts of all three in there? How far from 0 to 10 are you along the axes? If you are very high up, please do con-sider speaking to someone about it? (If you are a student, consider going to see the student counselling service. Otherwise you might ask your GP for advice on choos-ing a counsellor.)

Example 3: Being An Echocardiographer in the UK NHS: An Autoethnographic Study

Sarah's autoethnography was another good example of an **analytical** autoethnography approach. I am so proud of the work she has done. When I first met her to discuss her MSc Cardiology dissertation, she was at a very low point. However, the prospect of doing an autoethnographic study fired her imagination and she really took off on get-ting to know the method and delving into the tasks ahead. She had worked in the NHS as an echocardiographer for 16 years and had experienced physical and psychological burnout. Her hope was that, by illustrating the situation of echocardiographers in the

NHS, she might be able to show through her own experiences some of the reasons why there is a shortage of echocardiographers.

So, she began a period of deep introspection and reflexivity along with private therapy to aid her recall and to discuss her memories and experiences. This was complemented by an in-depth interview (conducted by myself) to explore her memories in greater depth.

The results showed some important negative aspects to the role which could contribute to the national staffing problem. Issues such as musculoskeletal problems, work-related stress, working environments brimming with hazards for both the aforementioned issues, being over-stretched and under-valued, with conflicting priorities, unrealistic expectations, and a rivalry with 'non-echo' colleagues whose work is far less stressful yet somehow lines them up for faster promotion. Her account 'Broken by Tuesday' (which we are working on for publication: Merritt and Anderson, forthcoming) describes how a typical day can impact on wellbeing and lead an echocardiographer down the sorry path to exhaustion, cynicism, and professional burnout.

Thematic analysis (TA) of the results identified within the data recurring themes, grouped into four clusters as follows:

1. **Transitions**
   a. *Enthusiasm – despair*
   b. *Commitment – cynicism*
   c. *Energy – burnout*
   d. *Ambition – concern*

2. **Disappointments/juxtapositions**
   a. *Other professionals' attitudes*
   b. *Organisational issues within the NHS*
   c. *Lack of supports*
   d. *High demand – low reward*

3. **Concerns**
   a. *For self*
   b. *For the profession*

4. **Negative impacts/'costs'**
   a. *Health – physical*
   b. *Health – mental/affective/emotional*
   c. *Sapping motivation*
   d. *Relationships*

It seems that being an echocardiographer in the UK NHS can be a painful and stressful experience which may turn committed, enthusiastic individuals into exhausted cynics with a desire to leave and a reluctance to speak up. Ingrained organisational and psychosocial issues within the NHS foster chronic frustration and disappointment. Responsibility for prevention is placed largely on the individual instead of dealing with the source. Years of training and experience are wasted instead of being nurtured and valued. The costs to the NHS and to the individual are considerable.

If the current workforce is to be retained and not lost to early retirement, ill-health or career change, if undergraduates are to be enticed into the profession, and if former echocardiographers are to be persuaded back into practice, it is suggested that the issues identified here need to be carefully considered and addressed.

(Merrit 2018)

You can clearly see the application of analytic autoethnography in this study, with a clear agenda to improve the working situation of her professional group – echocardiographers.

Autoethnography vs. participant observation

Before we leave the field of autoethnography, I suspect that some of you are thinking, 'But is this not similar to the position someone finds themselves in when they do a participant observation study?' For sure, there are a lot of similarities. Both certainly tick all the boxes in the five key features of analytic autoethnography as outlined by Anderson (2006). The difference is that in PO, one is trying to map out the culture of your chosen *case* – which is a society, or social group, etc. Whereas in an autoethnography, you are studying the case that is *you,* and you are hoping to make observations which will help you, and others, understand a part of the social system that you belong to. That knowledge can be transferrable to a more general understanding of all people in that situation.

Finally, a word of warning – some qualitative methods, including autoethnography, are not at all popular with some sectors of the research community. Elaine Campbell (2017) gives an in-depth account of the 'trolling' (online abuse) which she discovered online. I cite her abstract here to give you a feel for her work.

Abstract: *Online hostility and mockery, often known as 'trolling', is a phenomenon almost as old as the internet itself. Nevertheless, the rise in trolling aimed at researchers using non-traditional, creative methodologies, such as autoethnography, remains severely under-explored. This essay seeks to fill the gap in the literature and make a contribution to the discourse on autoethnographic research. Writing autoethnographically, I share my experience of discovering vile, misogynist, and cruel trolling of autoethnographers and their work on the social media platform Twitter. I reflect on the online hatred I received when I raised the issue publically. Many of the messages I received focused on my perceived inability to cope with opinions other than my own. Therefore, I finish by offering a brief response to critiques of autoethnography; albeit criticism that comes from researchers who raise their concerns in a constructive and scholarly manner. Above all, the purpose of this essay is to bring trolling of autoethnographers to the fore and encourage others to speak about their experiences. If we do not write about trolling, then it – and our story – remains hidden.*

(Campbell 2017)

To Sum Up

The three examples I have presented above clearly show how autoethnography is a **qualitative** method with no numbers. It falls into the **ethnographic** domain – it is concerned with exploring **cultural** issues. But this time it does so not by observing or interviewing other people – it is concerned with **the 'culture' that is you.** All autoethnographies deal with events which have already happened in the researchers' lives – they are **retrospective.** It can be either **hypothetico-deductive** or **hypothetico-inductive,** in that you may have ideas or 'hypotheses' that you wish to test by embarking on this adventure, or you may not.

The three examples I have discussed here all tell different stories – they represent the realities of a new culture being explored (you), by you, the researcher – much in the same way as Malinowski when he stepped ashore in the Pacific islands for the first time and began to take in everything around him. I pointed out that there were two main approaches within autoethnographies – the **Evocative**, which tells a story and allows its impact to move the reader to their own conclusions; and the **Analytic**, which tells a story and analyses the data to make the points it wants to make to guide the reader to their conclusions. Seb's and Sarah's were firmly in the analytical branch, whilst 'Martin's' was more distinctly evocative, with leanings towards the analytic. Given that I supervised all three, the analytic propensity was probably driven by me, although all could have stood successfully on their own as pure evocative autoethnographies. The stories they tell move us and inspire us.

It is best done under some sort of **supportive supervision** in order to make sure that you get the support and help you need whilst you are doing it. You can use an **assisted** or a **collaborative** autoethnography approach – both of which (as with supervision) afford you the extra advantage of the independent observer to question, or '**interrogate**', your work. It is somewhat vilified by some hard-line quantitative researchers, but has an intrinsic value – like all autobiographical accounts of being *your* truth.

For further reading, I suggest you start with Short, Turner and Grant's book on contemporary British autoethnography (2013) and Turner et al.'s book on international perspectives on autoethnographic research and practice (2018). **Follow Alec Grant's advice – dare to publish it!** (Grant, 2019)

Research is the art of the possible!

References

Anderson L. (2006). Analytic autoethnography. *Journal of Contemporary Ethnography* 35(4), 373–395.

Anon M and Anderson J. (2017). *Ulcerative colitis: an autoethnographic case study.* University of Brighton, MSc Dissertation.

Campbell E. (2017). Apparently being a self-obsessed C**t is now academically lauded: experiencing twitter trolling of autoethnographers. *FQS Forum: Qualitative Social Research* 18(3). https://doi.org/10.17169/fqs-18.3.2819.

Denzin NK. (1997). Interpretive Ethnography: Ethnographic Practices for the Twenty-First Century. Sage: Newbury Park, CA.

Ellis C. (1997). *Evocative autoethnography: writing emotionally about our lives.* In: Representation and the Text: Re-Framing the Narrative Voice. (Tierney WG and Lincoln YS), pp. 115–142. State University of New York Press: Albany.

Ellis C. (2004). *The Ethnographic I: A Methodological Novel about Autoethnography.* AltaMira Press: Walnut Creek, CA.

Frank AW. (2013). *The Wounded Storyteller: Body, Illness and Ethics.* University of Chicago Press.

Grant A. (2019). Dare to be a wolf: Embracing autoethnography in nurse educational research. *Nurse Education Today* 82, 88–92.

Kay A. (2018). *This is Going to Hurt: Secret Diaries of a Junior Doctor.* (Main Market ed.). Picador.

Merritt S. (2018). *Being an echocardiographer in the UK NHS: an autoethnographic study.* University of Brighton, MSc Dissertation.

Merritt S and Anderson JL. (forthcoming). Broken by Tuesday.

Poulson J. (2003). *The Doctor Will Not See you Now: The Autobiography of a Blind Physician.* Novalis Press (CN).

Rogers CR. (1967). *On Becoming a Person; A Therapist's View of Psychotherapy.* Constable: London.

Shaw SCK, Anderson JL, and Grant AJ. (2016). Studying Medicine with Dyslexia: A Collaborative Autoethnography. *The Qualitative Report* 21(11, Article 2), 2036–2054. Retrieved from http://nsuworks.nova.edu/tqr/vol21/iss11/2

Shaw SCK, Grant AJ, and Anderson JL. (2018). Autoethnography in Action: A Research Methods Case Study on the Use of a Collaborative Autoethnography to Explore the Culture of Studying Medicine with Dyslexia, SAGE Research Methods Cases.

Short NP, Turner L, and Grant A. (2013). *Contemporary British Autoethnography (Studies in Professional Life and Work).* Sense Publishers.

Stewart I and Joines V. (2012). *TA Today: A New Introduction to Transactional Analysis (2).* Lifespace Publishing: Derby, UK.

Turner L, Short NP, Grant A, et al. (2018). *International Perspectives on Autoethnographic Research and Practice.* Routledge: London.

CHAPTER 13

Qualitative Approaches

Phenomenology

Introduction

In this chapter I shall turn my attention to **Phenomenology.** Why don't you practise saying it? **Phen – om – en – ology.** Now say it a few times until you get the hang of it. . . In lectures, I still sometimes stumble over it! But first, I want to tell you a story. . .

Let me transport you back in time and place, to Japan in the nineteenth century, where it was customary for Buddhist monks to wander round the country seeking out learned masters from whom they could learn and develop. One day, a wondering monk came to a small temple where two brother monks lived. He knocked on the door, and challenged them, in the customary manner to a debate for lodging – if he won the debate, he could stay and receive free food and lodging. If he lost, he would have to wander on. Anyway, the older brother, who was a very clever man, was tired from a hard day's work, so he suggested that his younger brother (who was a bit simple) join the debate in his place, but, to give his brother a chance, he instructed him to conduct the debate in silence. So, the wandering monk and the younger brother went off to the shrine for their debate.

Shortly afterwards, the wandering monk rushed out of the shrine and congratulated the older brother. 'Your brother is a fine scholar,' he said. 'He defeated me, so I must leave.'

'Please tell me about the debate,' asked the surprised older brother.

'Well, first I held up one finger to signify Buddha, the enlightened one. Then he held up two fingers to represent Buddha and his teachings. Then I held up three fingers to represent Buddha, his teachings and his followers. Then he shook his fist to indicate that all three come from the same realization. So, he won the debate and I am not worthy of staying.' The wondering monk left.

Demystifying Research for Medical & Healthcare Students: An Essential Guide, First Edition. John L. Anderson.
© 2022 John Wiley & Sons Ltd. Published 2022 by John Wiley & Sons Ltd.
Companion website: www.wiley.com/go/Anderson/DemystifyingResearch

The younger brother ran in to his older brother. 'Where is he?' he demanded.

'I hear you won the debate,' said the older brother.

'I won nothing! I'm going to give him a good beating!' Shouted the younger brother.

'Tell me what happened,' asked the confused older brother.

'He began insulting me by holding up one finger to gloat on the fact that I only have one eye! Because he was a wondering monk, I thought I had better be polite, so I held up two fingers to congratulate him for having two eyes. Then the cheeky b******** held up three fingers to rub in the fact that between us we only had three eyes! At this point, I lost my cool and began to punch him, but he ran away before I could!'

(This is adapted from a story 'Trading Dialogue For Lodging' in Paul Reps and Nyogen Senzaki's Zen Flesh, Zen Bones: a collection of Zen and pre-Zen Writings, 1957)

So, let me ask you, dear Reader. . . How many **'realities'** are there in this story? In a class, some students will answer *one* – there is only one reality. Some will answer *two* – there is the reality as experienced by the wandering monk, and the reality as experienced by the younger brother. Some will answer *three* – there is the reality as experienced by the wandering monk, the reality as experienced by the younger brother, and the reality as experienced by the older brother. Some will answer *four* – the reality as experienced by the wandering monk, the reality as experienced by the younger brother, and the reality as experienced by the older brother, and the reality as experienced by the class. Some will answer 'There is a potentially *infinite* number of realities to represent those experienced by the actors in the story and however many people hear the story'.

I love this story. It is fun. But it also makes the point of how fragile are our notions of reality – the more people who witness the event, the more likely there are to be different interpretations, or versions of that 'reality'. It very nicely encapsulates the **ontological** debate about 'What constitutes "reality"?' To me, it emphasises the need to avoid assuming that what we observe (and the sense we make of it) is the same as what everyone else observes (and the sense they make of it). To me, that is what **phenomenology** is all about – getting to know how other people experience **their** worlds and the sense(s) they make of their worlds.

- We are still in the **qualitative** domain – no numbers.
- These approaches are **retrospective** – we study people's lived experiences which have already happened.
- But this time we have a **dichotomy.** Within phenomenology, some studies are **hypothetico-inductive** (descriptive phenomenology) whilst others may also be **hypothetico-deductive** (interpretive phenomenology).

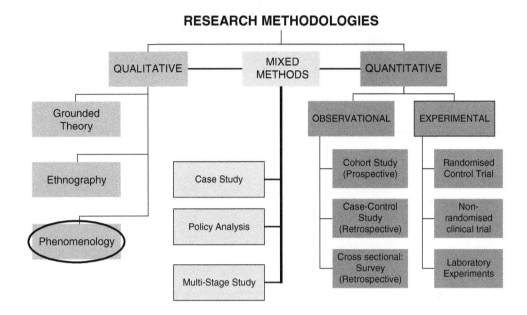

Two Main Schools of Phenomenology

There are two schools of phenomenology – **descriptive phenomenology** and **interpretive phenomenology.** Both are excellent approaches to researching what we call the 'lived experiences' of people in any situation. Both have similar goals – to discover and report on people's lived experiences, but they have different philosophical and, therefore, methodological approaches.

Descriptive Phenomenology

Once upon a time, in a country far, far away, called Germany, there was a very wise man, called Professor Husserl (Figure 13.1), who was a teacher at the big school (called a university) in Germany, He thought that human experiences could be studied by gathering data (information) about their **conscious experiences** – things that they were aware of doing or experiencing. Of course, these are very **subjective** – they are unique to each person. But, by using a scientific approach, we can identify the common features of the lived experiences shared by groups of people who we study. So Husserl insisted that, to be able to do that truthfully and honestly, we have to give up all of our **preconceptions** (what we already know and believe about the people we are studying). Some of his followers believe that we should not even read about the subject before we study it. They insist that we should not ask very specific questions other than ones like 'What is

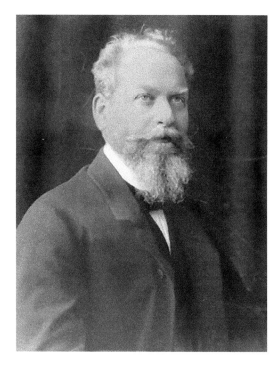

FIGURE 13.1 Edmund Husserl – looking descriptive. *Source:* Unknown author / Wikimedia Commons / Public Domain.

going on for these people?' Husserl believed that it was important to avoid any judgements or theorising about other people's lived experiences. This is called **bracketing** – the researcher shedding all preconceptions and beliefs about those people he or she is studying. This assumes that as a researcher, you can be **naïve** – innocent of prejudice because of your own thoughts and beliefs. This way of thinking, said Husserl, is free from contamination from the point of time in history and the prevailing culture withing which those experiences exist. Don't you think that Professor Husserl was a very clever man?

Interpretive Phenomenology

Now, one of Husserl's students from the big school (university) in Germany, a man called Heidegger (Figure 13.2), had a different way of thinking from Husserl. Heidegger thought that it was important to go beyond the mere *description* to search for the *meanings* in human behaviour – what is called the **hermeneutics**. He said that these meanings were not always obvious to people themselves, but they could be interpreted from the **narrative accounts** they could provide about their **lived experiences.** He thought that we could not separate human experience from time and place (history and culture), but that human experiences were firmly rooted in history and culture. For example, the experiences of the rich in a society provide them with a very different set of perspectives (ways of looking at the world) from poor people. Men and women experience life in very different ways, and so on. More than that, he insisted that it was important for us as researchers to be aware of our **location** in terms of history and

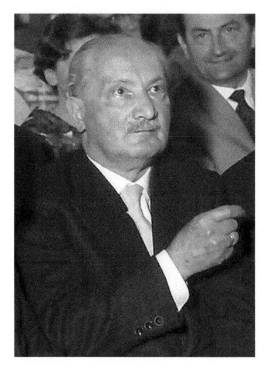

FIGURE 13.2   Martin Heidegger – looking interpretive. *Source:* Willy Pragher / Wikimedia Commons / Public Domain.

culture and to be able to recognise how these impacted upon us and the way we see the world. Heidegger also believed that prior knowledge and reading could enrich the researcher by providing insights into the world that was being studied and could lead to the development of **hypotheses** – which were compatible with his school of phenomenology. But he did think it was important for the researcher to be **open** and **honest** about his or her thinking and declare any 'biases' in advance and deal with these in their account of the research. Thus, there could be different interpretations of the meanings of the research – depending upon who was interpreting it and their locations in history and culture. My, wasn't Heidegger a very clever man too? (Lopez & Willis, 2004).

So, I have tried to make it simple for you. In Table 13.1, I have made a summary of some of the main differences between descriptive and interpretive (hermeneutic) phenomenology.

Example 1: The lived experience of postpartum depression: a phenomenological study

Cheryl Beck (Figure 13.3) carried out a **descriptive phenomenological study** of women with post-natal (post-partum) depression (PPD). Her research question, in keeping with Husserl's school of (descriptive) phenomenology was 'What is the essential

TABLE 13.1 Comparison of descriptive and interpretive phenomenology.

	Descriptive Phenomenology	Interpretive Phenomenology
Ontology	There is an 'objective' reality	Reality is subjective – it is interpreted according to the beliefs that influence us in our time in history, our place in society, and our culture.
Epistemology	'Reality' can be accessed only by an unbiased researcher who 'brackets' his or her personal beliefs, preconceptions, everyday assumptions, or prejudices. This can be accessed through the rigours of 'science'.	'Reality' can be accessed only by researchers admitting their personal beliefs and prejudices in advance and using these as a source of insight. Traditional 'science' may not adequately be able to access the phenomena being studied.
Methodology	The researcher begins with a 'blank canvas' and should not attempt to anticipate or shape the data collection in any way. This also means that hypothesising is inappropriate.	The researcher may know a lot about the topic being researched and may even be an 'insider-researcher'. She/he can use this to inform the development of the study. This includes being able to anticipate or to hypothesise.
Results	Transparency in the description allows the participants' experiences and views to be accurately reported.	Transparency in the description and analysis allows the participants' experiences and views to be accurately reported and understood.
Interpretation	Interpretation has the potential to corrupt the participants' accounts. The researcher should not go beyond describing the data.	It is the duty of the researcher to search for meaning (which may not be understood by participants themselves) and to offer her/his interpretations of the data.

structure of postpartum depression?' Many quantitative studies had been done on PPD, but the actual 'lived experiences' of women with PPD had not been researched. A *purposive sample* of seven mothers took part. They had all attended a local support group for women with PPD which Beck herself had helped to facilitate. These seven women who had experienced post-natal depression were interviewed about their subjective experiences 'prereflexively, without classifying it or categorising it into signs and symptoms'.

> *To achieve the goal of the phenomenological method, the discovery of the meaning of human experiences, researchers must reawaken their own presuppositions and make them appear by abstaining from them for a moment. This process, called bracketing, involves peeling away the layers of interpretation so the phenomena can be seen as they are, not as they are reflected through preconceptions. Bracketing does not eliminate perspective. It brings the experience into clearer focus. As the layers of meaning that give persons interpreted experiences*

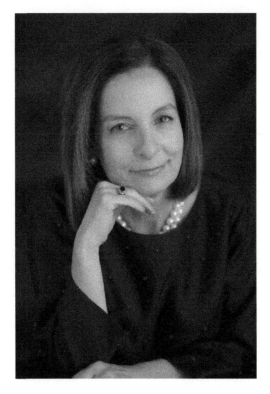

FIGURE 13.3   Cheryl T. Beck – being descriptive.

are laid aside, what is left is the perceived world prior to interpretation and explanation.

(Beck 1992)

They were invited to describe how they had experienced postpartum depression. After she obtained informed consent, Beck asked each participant to reply to this statement:

'Please describe a situation in which you experienced postpartum depression. Share all the thoughts, perceptions and feelings you can recall until you have no more to say about the situation.'

(Beck, 1992)

Her recordings were transcribed verbatim. Beck analysed the interview data using Colaizzi's (1978) method. This consists of the following seven steps:

1. Immersion – all the transcripts are read and re-read to familiarise yourself with the data.
2. Significant statements and phrases are extracted.
3. Meanings are made from these significant statements.
4. These meanings are grouped into clusters of themes.
5. The results are gathered into a comprehensive account of PPD.

6. The results are shared with participants who have the opportunity to amend or add to the data.

7. Incorporating any changes into the theoretical model.

She was able to extract 45 significant statements from the interview transcripts. These clustered into 11 themes. As Beck describes it:

> *Postpartum depression was a living nightmare filled with uncontrollable anxiety attacks, consuming guilt, and obsessive thinking. Mothers contemplated not only harming themselves but also their infants. The mothers were enveloped in loneliness and the quality of their lives was further compromised by a lack of emotions and all previous interests. Fear that their lives would never return to normal was all-encompassing.*
>
> *(Beck 1992)*

She compared these 11 theme clusters with the 21 items of the **Beck Depression Inventory (BDI)** – the then 'gold standard' instrument for measuring depression. Only three of the theme clusters identified by Cheryl were present in the BDI. These were:

a. contemplating death,

b. loss of interests, and

c. guilt.

But eight of the theme clusters which she identified were *not* represented in the BDI. These were:

d. unbearable loneliness,

e. thoughts of being a bad mother,

f. loss of self,

g. inability to concentrate,

h. feeling like a robot,

i. uncontrollable anxiety,

j. loss of control, and

k. needing to be mothered.

She concluded that further research was needed to develop a screening inventory which more accurately identified postpartum depression in women.

> *As evidenced by the findings of this study a generalised depression scale such as the BDI does not measure all of the specifics of postpartum depression, nor should it be expected to. Nurse researchers need to seriously consider whether to use a generalised depression scale in future studies on postpartum depression.*
>
> *Even one of the newest instruments designed specifically to detect postpartum depression, the Edinburgh Postnatal Depression Scale does not include some of the cluster themes of postpartum depression that emerged in this study.*
>
> *(Beck 1992)*

This was a truly descriptive phenomenological study. Beck describes in her paper how she bracketed her own perspective: 'Efforts to limit potential bias included identification of the researcher's perspective and bracketing it prior to data collection and analysis' (Beck 1992).As Polit and Beck (2010) point out,'The goal of most qualitative studies is not to generalize but rather to provide a rich, contextualized understanding of some aspect of human experience through the intensive study of particular cases.' (Polit & Beck, 2010)

Example 2: The experiences of medical students with dyslexia: an interpretive phenomenological study

You have already met Seb (Figure 13.4). Seb has dyslexia. We met on my Research Methods course when he was doing his MSc in Medical Education. He took a year out of being a medical student between years 3 and 4 of his course to do the MSc as an intercalating student. When I signposted him to **interpretive phenomenology** as a possible approach for his dissertation research, he really took off on it. It excited him as a meaningful means for accessing and reporting the 'lived experiences' of medical students with dyslexia (MSWD) and junior doctors with dyslexia (JDWD). I very

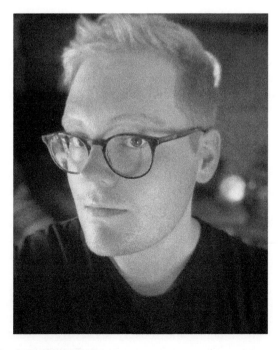

FIGURE 13.4   Seb – being interpretive.

quickly learned three things about our Seb: (i) he is very bright; (ii) he is incredibly hard working; and (iii) he has no 'OFF' switch! He bombards me with ideas ('What about a study of XXX?'), questions ('Have you read my draft about XXX yet?!'), and draughts of papers (and we all love him to bits!).

In this study, we began by reviewing the literature – or rather, bemoaning the absence of research on this topic (Shaw et al. 2017). This showed that there had been no research on the subject before. (Now, that is a double-edged sword. *Pro:* it confirms that we had a niche area for research – we were at the forefront of research into the subject. *Con:* it was difficult to convince journal editors that this was the case.) We then conducted a **collaborative autoethnography,** which you read about in the last chapter (Shaw et al. 2016, 2018). This helped us in putting together our **interview topic guide**. This is a brief outline of the topic areas to be addressed. It can act as an *aide-memoire* to check that all topic areas have been covered during the interviews – topic guides are *NOT* lists of questions to be asked!

> *Thus, before he began to access and interpret the experiences of others, he had first analysed his own thoughts, feelings, and potential biases.*
> *(Shaw and Anderson 2017)*

Our first challenge was to consider *who* we should interview. Remember, our focus was on MSWD. But if we recruited medical students, they would not have had all of their experiences as medical students. So, we agreed to focus on junior doctors with dyslexia (JDWD) – they had recently graduated, so their medical student experiences were complete, but still relatively fresh in their minds. Also, we could ask them about their experiences as junior doctors – a bonus! To recruit participants, we approached a Foundation School – a regional training school which oversees the placement and training of junior doctors in the first two years after graduation. This had the advantage of reaching out to trainees from a variety of different medical schools. If we had just tried to recruit Brighton and Sussex Medical School students (from our 'home patch') this study could have been more easily dismissed as representing the experiences of medical students from only one centre in the UK, and thus representing the experiences of that medical school's students only. As it turned out we had a good spread of participants across different medical schools.

The Foundation School agreed to publish announcements about the study in their weekly eBulletin which goes out by e-mail to all of that School's trainees. We were able to send out two reminders before closing recruitment. Trainees were invited to contact Seb directly by e-mail if they were interested in taking part in the study. We asked that only those trainees who had had a clinical diagnosis of dyslexia reply. Seb then sent them a Participant Information Sheet (**PIS**) with full details of the study and what was expected of participants. He phoned those who were still interested, checked that they understood the study, and answered any questions. Then they arranged a mutually suitable time for the interviews to take place. All interviews were conducted by telephone and were audio-recorded. This made it more convenient for accessing a population of potential participants who were all very busy, potentially wary of being interviewed, and who were from a wide geographical region. So, Seb again explained the study and answered any questions. He then obtained informed consent which was explicitly audio-recorded.

The interviews were in-depth and **loosely structured.** We described them as **unstructured,** but they did have a focus – on the participants' experiences of being a medical student with dyslexia. And there were some topic areas – as opposed to set questions – which we did wish to cover during the interviews. So, they really were very loosely structured.

> *These were unstructured to allow participants the maximum freedom and control over the content of the interviews. In this context, the term 'unstructured' refers to interviews in which topics, questions, wording and sequencing are not pre-determined. The interviewer (SS), after inviting them to tell their own story, in their own words, in the order they chose, was then able to ask probing questions as and when appropriate to get more details. This embraced SS' insider status as a medical student with dyslexia – connecting with participants through empathic understanding, enabling them to share the rawness of their experiences with someone to whom they could relate. His personal interest was declared up front. It was used to help access others' experiences and our understanding of these. His own thoughts and experiences – as a person with dyslexia – were useful in providing him with insight to ask further questions which might not have been obvious to non-dyslexic researchers, and which allowed him to check out if the participants' experiences differed from his own and each others'. This was balanced in the data analysis by JA's verification and the negotiation of agreement in the coding.*

> *(Shaw and Anderson 2017)*

Prior to conducting the interviews, Seb had attended my Research Skills Workshops on 'Obtaining Informed Consent', 'Interview Skills' and 'Analysing Qualitative Data'. In my view, all researchers should be equipped with the necessary skills to do the research – in addition to having the theoretical knowledge. I believe that this is an ethical imperative, and I encourage you to go out of your way to get training in the *skills* of research, as well as the *knowledge* of research. (I shall come back to this later in the appendices.)

Eight JDWD were interviewed. There were 13 replies to the announcements in the eBulletin. Two were discounted because they did not have a formal diagnosis of dyslexia. Three were unable to find time for the interview. Seven were female and one male. They came from five different UK medical schools.

Seb transcribed the interviews **verbatim** – word for word, without any changes, e.g. for grammatical corrections etc. These were then thematically analysed using a **framework analysis.** This is a form of **thematic analysis** in which the researcher develops a coding template that allows the main themes identified to be used to provide a structure for the rest of the analysis. Thus, there is a sort of hierarchy of the data, with main themes being identified and forming the framework or 'template' within which subsidiary or **secondary themes** fall. Then you check all of your transcriptions again to make sure you have not missed any theses in them. It may sound very structured, but in fact it allows a great deal of flexibility in the data analysis (Brooks et al. 2015). Essentially, you can identify all the themes which emerge from the data, then group them into main and sub-themes – according to what is in the data. At this point, I verified Seb's coding of the data, and any differences were resolved through discussion – in what is called an **iterative** process. You create a prototype – the initial coding. Then you test it – in the verification. Then you revise it again if necessary, until there is agreement about the final product.

These themes are shown in Table 13.2. One of the over-riding themes concerned intimidation, fear, and a lack of understanding by others. This contributed to self-deprecation and negative emotions which were reflected throughout the rest of the

TABLE 13.2 Summary of the study themes and sub-themes.

Themes	Sub-themes
Theme 1: emotional impact	Isolation; self-consciousness; hopelessness/ helplessness
Theme 2: others' reactions	Bullying and rejection; stonewalling; impact on disclosure
Theme 3: the system	Stigmatisation; competition; pride
Theme 4: supports	The good, the bad, and the wanted pastoral support; paradoxical support; others to talk to
Theme 5:	Essays, exams, and exasperation dyslexia-friendly assessments; negative assessments; lack of exam support
Theme 6: me, myself, and my dyslexia	Positive aspects; the association of dyslexia and the self

(Adapted from Shaw & Anderson 2017.)

theme clusters. One participant commented:

> *I have felt as if I am the only person in the world with dyslexia trying to get through med school – and then trying to get through training, as well . . . You feel quite isolated. Isolated because . . . I was struggling. Isolated because I would have to spend so much longer, or I would appear to spend so much longer than anyone else. (P8)*

People felt self-conscious:

> *Throughout my medical career, I constantly felt self-conscious about it. (P2)*

> *I felt like my BRAIN wasn't as good as other people's brains. (P1)*

> *I just feel embarrassed. I feel embarrassed because I struggle. Because. . . Also just the way that medics are. Medics are very highly competitive. . . So I think it's probably not as supportive an environment as you would imagine it to be. You know, even from med school when people wouldn't really share things – they wouldn't share lectures that were happening or teaching sessions that were happening. You know what I mean? It was a very highly competitive environment. So yeah – no, I've never felt comfortable admitting it. (P8)*

These sorts of experiences were made even worse by the reactions of some of their peers at medical school.

> *It didn't help me when my friends told me I was a 'fake dyslexic'. Because I am not a fake dyslexic! It's very dismissive. Which is not good! You wouldn't say to a patient who's got cancer 'oh no, you've not got cancer'. You have to help them come to terms with it, and to accept it. (P1)*

Most had to find their own ways of adapting to the high levels of demands of medical school. But there were also some positives reported.

I almost saw it (dyslexia) as a challenge. . . when I was growing up. Like, 'oh, peo-
ple think I'm dyslexic. They might think I'm stupid. I'm gonna prove them wrong
and get an A* in this exam'. Like, that would be MY attitude towards it. So. . .
When people say 'are you disabled?' – that kinda thing. . . It makes me frustrated.
Because you work very hard to overcome the problems you have. And therefore,
I don't really see it as a problem anymore. . . Because I've adapted my life, my
learning, my whatever, to be able. . . to compensate for it. So I guess. . . it's a differ-
ent way of looking at the world – a different way of seeing things. And I think you
have to compensate for those difficulties. And I think, if you can compensate for
them, then you don't have a problem – you can use it to your advantage. (P4)

One of the most disappointing findings was the lack of understanding, coupled with
the lack of psychological supports available to MSWD.

Just pastoral support. . . I think dyslexia's actually quite a big thing. (P1)

. . . It would be good to be able to talk to other people who are in the same
situation as me. (P4)

The costs, in terms of additional work which had to be done for MSWD just to keep
up with others and the consequent impact that this had on social/personal life, were
highlighted in the study.
We concluded:

His (Seb's) insider status was a strength, which was central to our interpretive
phenomenological approach, and provided contextualisation and deeper under-
standing. . . The invitation to the reader is to understand what we have reported
and to apply the knowledge where appropriate.

Further research is needed to assess the generalizability of our findings. We
therefore conducted a survey to fill this gap and shall report these results sepa-
rately. (And we did – Anderson and Shaw 2020.)

I hope that this example gives you some insights into the process and results of **inter-**
pretive phenomenology. One of the main aspects which we emphasised was the
transparency – letting our participants' accounts talk for themselves.

Example 3: Coping with Medical School: An Interpretive Phenomenological Study

This study originated from the interest inspired in Seb by my teaching about Learned
Helplessness (Seligman, 1976 and Corbin & Seligman, 1980). Seb was concerned by what
he has witnessed and experienced as a medical student – occasional periods of helplessness and hopelessness (HH) in himself and his fellow students. So, this study had a theoretical base which inspired the question: 'What are medical students' experiences of
coping with medical school – in particular, with HH?' We hypothesised that feelings of
HH might be quite commonly experienced by medical students – but we didn't know how.

We recruited participants by getting the support of a medical school to send out emails to all of its students inviting interested students to contact us, following which we sent them a participant information sheet which outlined the purpose of the study and what taking part would involve. Interviews were arranged at a mutually convenient time and place (office or telephone). Because of the potential for Seb's knowledge of the medical students, I did all the interviews using in-depth, loosely structured interviews which were audio-recorded. In the end, only three students volunteered to take part and were interviewed.

The relatively small number of participants – three – allowed us the opportunity to use a case-study approach to analyse and present the data and to abstract common-alities and differences between all three – which could then be explained using our depth of knowledge about each and relating their circumstances to Garber and Selig-man's attributional model of helplessness (Garber & Seligman, 1980). We felt that this reflected the IPA ideal of representing the 'lived experiences' of our participants as faithfully and transparently as possible.

> *Audio-recordings were transcribed verbatim. Each transcript then underwent an interpretive phenomenological analysis. This was performed by SS and verified by JA. The verification included review of the initial transcripts. The analysis was undertaken based on the steps outlined by Pietkiewicz and Smith. Firstly, SS read through the transcripts and listened to the audio recordings several times to immerse himself in the data. Whilst doing this, he made handwritten notes on a case-by-case basis. He then read back through these notes and generated initial emergent themes. These emergent themes were then reviewed in order to identify analytic themes. JA replicated this process for his verification. Any differences were discussed and resolved in an iterative manner.*
>
> *(Shaw & Anderson, 2021).*

Thus, our data analysis began with detailed descriptions of each participant's stories – or *narratives*. Here is part of **'Amy's'** account:

During her second year she had an experience with a tutor which caused her immense and lasting emotional upset and self-doubt. 'Sometimes she said harsh things to me. . . For example: "Oh, I think you should be aware of yourself, that [you're] not speaking up in the group." [And it was not about] being able to express myself. . . Just saying like I don't have enough knowledge to be in medical school. . .'.

This was devastating for her. The shame of being a failure – letting her family down. She was not good enough! How could she continue? She felt helpless and hopeless. She contemplated suicide, but thankfully did not do it. This one, 'throw-away' remark by an insensitive tutor spoilt the rest of her experience of medical school, and when I inter-viewed her, three years later, she still cried when she described the experience.

'Jess' was put into accommodation with non-medical students when she started at the university. In her naivety, she entered into the full social life that they all enjoyed – without realising that her peers in medical school were working very much harder than she was. She began to fall behind and had to repeat the first year. Her former 'friends' in medical school shunned her. She didn't fit in with the new first-year students, but had no friends or supports. She stood out as a 'deviant' rebelling against a highly-demanding system. She lost her 'home' when her old flat mate moved on without her. Even her parents shunned her when she turned to them for support. She had to move in with her new boyfriend as a desperate measure, but was not welcomed by his flatmates who wanted her out. She felt helpless and hopeless. Her 'salvation' came when the university found her a place in a hall of residence – a stable base where she could get down to the work she had to do. As she described herself: 'I was just an anonymous kind of unnamed person. . . immersed in my own kind of self-loathing and world-hating mind set'.

(Jess) 'Ryan' was a 'mature student' who had done a previous first degree. As such he was not eligible for the student loan scheme which other students got. So, to pay his medical school fees, his costs of living (accommodation and subsistence), he had managed to get five (yes – FIVE!) part-time jobs. He was getting by – but it was very hard work. Doing five part-time jobs meant that he had almost no social life and every spare moment was spent studying and revising. He was getting through, but at a cost. It got him down, but he realised that it was not personal (in the ways that Amy and Jess experienced their situations) and it would end eventually. So, although he felt helpless, he did not feel hopeless. We identified the following topics and issues which were reported:

- Isolation and a culture of silence (experienced by all three).
- Culture shock and a lack of control (experienced by Amy and Jess).
- Judgement, rejection, and interactions with others (experienced by Amy and Jess).
- Supports – personal, formal, and desired (mentioned by all three).
- Self-harm and suicidal ideation (mentioned by Amy and Jess).
- Marking and competition at medical school (mentioned by all three).

When we related the results to Helplessness theory we found that they fitted very well in to it. Amy and Jess both thought that **they** were the problem – it was **'Internal'**; whereas Ryan attributed his problems to **'External'** factors. For both Amy and Jess, the 'bad' feelings that they had about themselves were **'Global'** (they were all-encompassing) and **'Stable** (they would not change). However, Ryan saw himself and his situation as being **'Specific'** to the situation in which he found himself at that point in time. (See Table 13.3.)

We noted that 'the "culture" of medical schools is repeatedly mentioned', and we asked:

Do we need to take a closer look at what we, in medical schools, are doing to our students? Why are the experiences of medical training (at medical school and as junior doctors) so brutalising that many junior doctors either consider quitting the profession or actually do quit the profession? (Shaw & Anderson, 2021)

We concluded:

This study also highlights the importance of advertising supports to students. Whilst the ownership to take up such supports may rest with students, we can aim to maximise their knowledge of them. Heiman et al. also highlight that, 'prior to seeking therapy, students will first reach out to a tutor, faculty member, or a friend. . . It is therefore important to identify when a medical student may be on the more introjective/depressive spectrum, and to appropriately refer them to therapy'. It may therefore be prudent to ensure that all teaching staff receive some form of training in this and are aware of potential supports/are able to signpost students to appropriate individuals/services (Shaw and Anderson, 2021).

To Sum Up

Phenomenology is still in the **qualitative** domain – no numbers. As shown by all examples in this chapter, they are **retrospective.** We study people's 'lived experiences'

TABLE 13.3 Participants' experiences of helplessness, hopelessness and suicidal thoughts.

ID Nº	Gender	Pseudonym	Attributions	Feeling of Help-lessness	Feeling of Hope-lessness	Depression/ Suicidal thoughts
1	F	'Amy'	Global, Stable, Internal	Yes	Yes	Yes – did not seek help.
2	F	'Jess'	Global, Stable, Internal	Yes	Yes	Yes. Diagnosed with depression
3	M	'Ryan'	Specific, Stable, External	Yes	No	No.

of events which have already happened. But this time we have a dichotomy. Descriptive phenomenological studies are **hypothetico-inductive** – Beck's study involved her 'bracketing out' all prior knowledge and expectations to attain that 'clean slate' purity of the unbiased observer. Seb and I in the second example, on the other hand, used Seb's insider status as a MSWD to our advantage to contextualise the study and its results. Whilst we didn't go as far as to state any hypotheses, we might have done within the spirit of this approach – interpretive phenomenology may be hypothetico-deductive or hypothetico-inductive (Lopez & Willis, 2004). However, in the third example, Seb and I, in our interpretive phenomenological study – because of Seb's 'insider-researcher' status – were in a position to use our hunches and to take a **hypothetico-deductive** approach. This third example also shows how, with small numbers, you may have the luxury of greater in-depth exploration and description or the 'lived experiences' of your study participants. In a sense, the more people you include in a phenomenological study, the further your reports get from the real experiences of individuals. The **sampling** in all three cases was **purposive** – we all set out to recruit from within specified groups of people; Beck purposively sampled women who had experienced post-natal depression. In the dyslexia study, Seb and I purposively recruited junior doctors with dyslexia, and in the coping with medical school study we purposively aimed to recruit students who had experienced helplessness – although in both of these studies we invited participants to self-identify after we made the announcements about the study. Beck showed in her work, the links to **established theory** about depression and the existing 'gold standard' for measuring depression. Her subsequent work to develop a more appropriate measure for post-natal depression in women was based upon this work. In the final example, Seb and I were able to relate our findings to the established theory of human helplessness. In the dyslexia study described here, we were able to pave the way for a survey to put numbers to the issues identified in the participants in our sample. Thus, I hope you can see that all of these studies contributed to further research and the development of our knowledge of the areas we studied.

Research is the art of the possible!

References

Anderson JL and Shaw SCK. (2020). The experiences of medical students and junior doctors with dyslexia: a survey study. *International Journal of Social Sciences & Educational Studies* 7(1), 62–71.

Beck CT. (1992). The lived experience of postpartum depression: a phenomenological study. *Nursing Research* 41(3), 166–170.

Brooks J, McCluskey S, Turley E, et al. (2015). The utility of template analysis in qualitative psychology research. *Qualitative Research in Psychology* 12, 202–222.

Colaizzi P. (1978). *Psychological research as the phenomenologist's view it.* In: Existential–Phenomenological Alternatives for Psychology (Vale R and King M, eds.), pp. 48–71. Oxford University Press: New York.

Garber J and Seligman MEP. (1980). *Human Helplessness: Theory and Applications.* Academic Press: London.

Lopez KA and Willis DG (2004). Descriptive versus interpretive phenomenology: their contributions to nursing knowledge. *Qualitative Health Research* 14, 726–735.

Polit DF and Beck CT. (2010). Generalization in quantitative and qualitative research: Myths and strategies. *International Journal of Nursing Studies* 47(11), 1451–1458.

Reps P and Senzaki N. (1957). *Zen Flesh, Zen Bones: A Collection of Zen and Pre-Zen Writings.* Penguin Books Ltd: Harmondsworth.

Shaw SCK and Anderson JL. (2018). The experiences of medical students with dyslexia: an interpretive phenomenological study. *Dyslexia* 1–14. doi:10.1002/dys.1587.

Shaw SCK, Anderson JL, and Grant AJ. (2016). Studying Medicine with Dyslexia: A Collaborative Autoethnography. *The Qualitative Report* 21(11; Article 2), 2036–2054. Retrieved from http://nsuworks.nova.edu/tqr/vol21/iss11/2

Shaw SCK, Malik M, and Anderson JL. (2017). The exam performance of medical students with dyslexia: a review of the literature. *MedEdPublish* doi:10.15694/mep.2017.000116.

Shaw SCK, Grant AJ, and Anderson JL. (2018). Autoethnography in action: a research methods case study on the use of a collaborative autoethnography to explore the culture of studying medicine with dyslexia. *SAGE Research Methods Cases* doi:10.4135/9781526427229.

Shaw SCK and Anderson JL. (2021). Coping with medical school: an interpretive phenomenological study. *The Qualitative Report* 26(6).

Seligman M. (1975). *Learned Helplessness: On Depression, Development, and Death.* WH Freeman and Company: San Francisco.

CHAPTER 14

Qualitative Approaches

Grounded Theory

Introduction

Grounded theory (GT):

- Is an approach which is usually **qualitative** – no numbers.
- It is **hypothetico-inductive** – we do not begin with a theoretical background and then make hypotheses which we test – our theory is driven by what comes out of the data, rather than the other way round.
- It can be either **retrospective** (studying things which have already happened) **or prospective** (studying things as they happen).

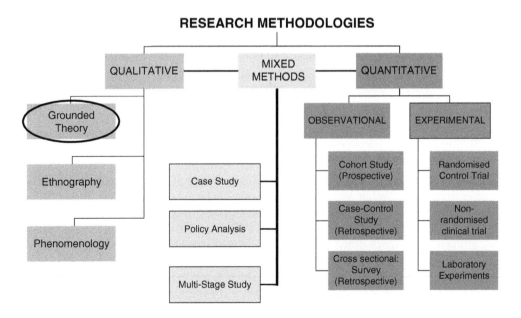

RESEARCH METHODOLOGIES

Demystifying Research for Medical & Healthcare Students: An Essential Guide, First Edition. John L. Anderson.
© 2022 John Wiley & Sons Ltd. Published 2022 by John Wiley & Sons Ltd.
Companion website: www.wiley.com/go/Anderson/DemystifyingResearch

Grounded theory: an overview

GT was developed by Barney Glaser and Anselm Strauss from the work they were doing on death and dying in America – *Awareness of Dying* (1965) and *Time for Dying* (1968). (That is why I communicated with them when I was working on the *Life Before Death* study.) You can see the embryo of their approach in Howard Becker, Blanche Geer, Everett Hughes, and Anselm Strauss's earlier work, *The Boys in White* (1961) which was a particularly thorough piece of **hypothetico-inductive** research. Andrews and Nathaniel (2015) in their 50-year anniversary homage to Glaser and Strauss's book, *The Discovery of Grounded Theory* (1967), credit the GT approach as stemming from their work on *Awareness of Dying* (1965). (Read their article for a brief explanation of their approach and the background to it.) As Glaser and Strauss state:

> *The basic theme of our book is the discovery of theory from data systematically obtained from social research.*
>
> *(Glaser and Strauss 1967)*

They point out that up until then, there was very little written on this topic, and their work aimed to fill that gap. They wanted, in particular to provide postgraduate students with a means of defending the adoption of a **hypothetico-inductive** approach. In this approach, the theory emerges from the data, rather than an existing theory driving the data collection in the traditional **hypothetico-deductive** approaches which, up until then, had dominated social research.

> *It should also help students to defend themselves against verifiers who would teach them to deny the validity of their own scientific intelligence. By making generation a legitimate enterprise, and suggesting methods for it, we hope to provide the ingredients of a defense against internalized professional mandates dictating that sociologists research and write in the verification rhetoric.*
>
> *(Glaser and Strauss 1967, p. 7)*

Anselm Strauss and Barney Glaser went their separate ways, and Anselm Strauss, with Juliet Corbin, refined the initial approach and provided more guidelines for the application of GT (Strauss & Corbin, 1997). Nowadays, GT is so firmly accepted within research tradition, particularly in nursing research (Bowen, 2006) that people, rather than saying 'What approach are you using?', are often more likely to ask: 'What school of GT are you following?'! As Bowen says, 'A grounded theory is generated by themes, and themes emerge from the data during analysis, capturing the essence of meaning or experience drawn from varied situations and contexts.' He goes on to add: 'grounded theory research, does not start with hypotheses or preconceived notions. Instead, in accordance with its inductive nature, it involves the researcher's attempts to discover, understand, and interpret what is happening in the research context' (Bowen, 2006).

One of the essential components and activities of the GT researcher is **constant comparison.** This is an ongoing activity in which you are involved in constantly reviewing your data and your emerging theory. You review each new case, or small group of cases, and compare that to what you have noted from the previous cases or groups. You will find that your observations become more meaningful as you progress.

The constant comparing of many groups draws the sociologist's attention to their many similarities and differences. Considering these leads him to generate abstract categories and their properties, which, since they emerge from the data, will clearly be important to a theory explaining the kind of behavior under observation. Lower level categories emerge rather quickly during the early phases of data collection. Higher level, overriding and integrating, conceptualizations – and the properties that elaborate them – tend to come later during the joint collection, coding and analysis of the data.

(Glaser and Strauss 1967, p. 37)

There are four stages in the **constant comparative method:**

1. *comparing incidents applicable to each category;*
2. *integrating categories and their properties;*
3. *delimiting the theory; and*
4. *writing the theory*

(Glaser and Strauss 1967, p. 105).

It really is a labour-intensive process.
Another element of GT is **theoretical sampling:**

Theoretical sampling is the process of data collection for generating theory whereby the analyst jointly collects, codes, and analyzes his data and decides what data to collect next and where to find them, in order to develop his theory as it emerges. This process of data collection is controlled by the emerging theory, whether substantive or formal. The initial decisions for theoretical collection of data are based only on a general sociological perspective and on a general subject or problem area (such as . . . what happens to students in medical school that turns them into doctors). The initial decisions are not based on a preconceived theoretical framework.

(Glaser and Strauss 1967, p. 45)

So, we set out to include groups which have features in common with your other groups – if they are dissimilar, then spurious differences would show up in meaningless parts of the data analyses. The danger is that the emerging theory will grow out of hand and deviate too much from your intended purpose in doing the research. So, if you are researching communications between doctors and people who are dying, it would be a distraction to include people who are not dying. But it would potentially enrich the development of your theory, if, in addition to including people who are dying of heart disease, you also included people who were dying of cancer. This could be a valuable piece of theoretical sampling which could add another layer of understanding to your emerging theory.

If you had found that there appeared to be open communications between doctors and patients with heart disease, and their spouses, you might extend your sampling to include cancer patients. Then (at the time Glaser and Strauss did their work on death and dying), you might observe a totally different set of communication patterns emerging in which the doctors talked openly to the wives or husband of people dying of cancer, but had a completely closed set of communications with the patients themselves. Then your task would be to understand the reasons for the differences you had observed in your data.

The third concept in GT to be aware of is that of **data saturation** or **theoretical saturation.** *Data saturation* refers to that state which you will reach when collecting new cases yields no further new information. However, that does not necessarily mean that you have reached theoretical saturation – you may need to do some more theoretical sampling to check that you have not chosen too limited a sample in the first place. Then, after broadening your sampling – within logical limits (see above) – and carrying out comparisons, if you still do not get any new results emerging, you have reached *theoretical saturation.* As Bowen (2006) put it:

> *Themes gradually emerged as a result of the combined process of my becoming intimate with the data, making logical associations with the interview questions, and considering what was learned during the initial review of the literature. At successive stages, themes moved from a low level of abstraction to become major, overarching themes rooted in the concrete evidence provided by the data. When 'theoretical saturation' occurred – that is, when additional data failed to uncover any new ideas about the developing theory – the coding process ended.*
>
> *(Bowen, 2006)*

At this point, I should emphasise the importance of **deviant cases,** and I shall. *Deviant cases can be very important in aiding the refinement of your emerging theory.* So, when you think you have come up with a nice, neat theory that accounts for all your cases, do not throw a wobbly when you suddenly find one which is markedly different from all the others and cannot be explained by the nice, neat theory that you thought you had. The challenge for you now is to explain it and reformulate your theory. So, at this point, you re-examine your data to make sure that there is not something there that you had missed. Then you might collect additional cases, perhaps broadening your initial sample base to see if you can find other deviant cases. In any event, you have to account for them as best you can. Even if it's just to say that there was one and you were unable to explain it. (There's always one, isn't there?!)

Now, I don't want to alarm you, but you should be aware that there are several **schools** of GT. Glaser came from a **positivist** background, and Strauss from an **interactionist** background. To my mind, these blended well in their initial work together. But since then, it has all become increasingly about navel-gazing and the proponents of differing approaches to GT tend to become obsessional about the detailed nature of the '39 essential steps to a perfect GT'! (I made that up.) As Tie et al. (2019) say:

> *However, philosophical perspectives have changed since Glaser's positivist version and Strauss and Corbin's postpositivism stance. Grounded theory has since seen the emergence of additional philosophical perspectives that have influenced a change in methodological development over time.*
>
> *Subsequent generations of grounded theorists have positioned themselves along a philosophical continuum, from Strauss and Corbin's theoretical perspective of symbolic interactionism, through to Charmaz's constructivist perspective. However, understanding how to position oneself philosophically can challenge novice researchers.*
>
> *Grounded theory has several distinct methodological genres: traditional GT associated with Glaser; evolved GT associated with Strauss, Corbin and Clarke; and constructivist GT associated with Charmaz. Each variant is an extension and development of the original GT by Glaser and Strauss.*

However, Birks and Mills refer to GT as a process by which theory is generated from the analysis of data. Theory is not discovered; rather, theory is constructed by the researcher who views the world through their own particular lens.

(Tie et al. 2019)

They suggest Birks and Mills' book *Grounded Theory: A Practical Guide* (2015) as a source which is easier to access by the novice researcher – i.e. people like me! I like that. Their approach makes sense to me. What was GREAT about Glaser and Strauss's initial work is that it was the first to legitimise properly **inductive** approaches. Since then, there have been so many different schools of GT and the guidelines for some are getting too complex. I truly admire Glaser and Strauss for bringing that original message to us – and suggesting other aspects of the approach, such as constant comparison, theoretical sampling, and theoretical and data saturation. However, I do not think that one has to follow any one approach's obsessive rituals in order to do a good piece of GT! You have to follow their guidelines if you want to do a Glaserian GT, or a Staussian GT, or a Charmazian GT, for sure. But these are not the only approaches. I believe that if you take a *sound* approach to gathering your data, you can use whatever analytical approach you want: use a simple thematic analysis if you want, and present it soundly, and you will have achieved something worthwhile. Then, if you are confident enough, by all means do venture further into some of the schools and find one which suits you. That is why I am writing this book – because a lot of my peers are writing to impress one another, rather than to help students learn. (An exception to this is Mick Bloor and Fiona Wood's book *Keywords in Qualitative Methods* (2006) which the publishers describe as 'an accessible and practical guide to qualitative techniques for students and researchers across the social and health sciences'.)

In the example below, I shall describe how I adapted GT to suit my needs in the analysis of *data which had already been collected*. This obviously placed some limitations on me and I had to work within these limitations. However, I hope that you will see the processes emerging in **the construction of theory from the data.** This is what gives GT its uniqueness. So far, only two of my postgraduate students have been brave enough to attempt to use a GT approach with quantitative data – which Glaser and Strauss acknowledge can be done. Let me know if you try it.

Example 1: Handling Hopelessness – Doctor–Patient Interactions in Phase 1 Oncology Trials

Introduction

When I first joined the Cancer Research UK Psychosocial Oncology Group in Brighton and Sussex Medical School (BSMS), my boss suggested that, as a sociologist, I might like to do a **qualitative analysis** of the pilot recordings that they had from the Phase I trials study which I had been brought in to manage. I agreed to give it a go. Now, at that time, I did not really understand the issues which surrounded Phase I trials. I do now, but then I thought to myself, 'I know almost nothing about phase I oncology trials. I have no "hunches" or hypotheses'. I was PI **naïve.** That was the ideal situation to be in to conduct a grounded theory study. So that is what I did. Rachel, a colleague in the Unit agreed to join me as a collaborator in this venture.

So, let's recap on what I knew about Phase I oncology trials. Unlike other Phase I clinical trials, Phase I *oncology* trials are conducted using people who have cancer, but for whom all known treatment options have been tried and the clinicians have now run out of options. Participants in these trials are not paid for taking part – unlike the healthy volunteers in other Phase I trials, who are usually paid for taking part. Their aim (at that time) was to measure the side effects of the substances (safety) being administered – the potential new drugs – and to find out what the **maximum tolerable dose (MTD)** was. They were NOT intended to measure **effectiveness** – that was started in Phase II trials.

Methods

In the pilot study (which had been completed before I joined the unit) a group of people attending a specialist Oncology Centre to discuss taking part in PI trials were approached. The research (not the PI trial) was explained and they had the opportunity to ask any questions. If they were happy to take part, then their written consent was obtained. An audio-recorder was placed in the consultation room just before they went in to see the trial doctor. This was used to record the consultations between the trial doctor and the potential participants. The participants were met after they had seen the trial doctor and were taken to a private room to be interviewed. The trial doctors were given a questionnaire to complete.

The audio-recordings of the consultation between the trial doctors and the participants formed the focus for this study. These were what I was given and invited to analyse. A **modified grounded theory** approach was used to analyse these consultations. Ideally, when interviewing participants, each interview, or a small number of interviews, would be analysed and the emerging themes would inform your emerging theory. This would be further tested in the next interviews and your theory would develop and be modified as new data was collected. In this case, all of the recordings had been made and that was it. So the theory emerged as I listened to the recordings over and over, and I read and re-read the transcripts. (Hence, we referred to it as a *modified* GT approach, in which we were guided by the work of Juliet Corbin & Anselm Strauss' book *Basics of Qualitative Research,* 2008.)

Everything was checked and double checked by Rachel. It was a truly **iterative** process. I created an embryo theory from the initial coding. Then this was put to the test in Rachel's **verification.** (She really did interrogate me and the data until she was convinced about my theory.) Then we'd revise it again if necessary, until there was agreement about the final product.

Results

As I was listening to the audio-recordings and reading the transcripts, the first thing that struck me about the trial doctors communications with the prospective trial participants, was **'It's all about treatment!'** I remember going into Rachel's office, feeling slightly confused. (Remember that this is naïve John we are talking about!) I said to her, 'I don't understand it. The doctors are all talking about treatment . . .' 'Yes', she said. 'What's wrong with that?' 'Well,' I replied, 'I thought that phase I trials were only meant to check the safety of the substance being tested to note the side effects, and to find the MTD?' 'Hmmm', she thought for a moment. 'That's what I understood. Let's have a look at some examples . . .' Here are some of them below:

Dr: In your situation really any **treatment** *that we offer is by way of being experimental . . . No guarantee of any benefit to you . . .we're looking at a* **drug** *that works by interfering with the process of cell division . . . (Case 2)*

Dr: . . . we are at the stage at least within the NHS system, we are thinking about more experimental **treatments** and newer **drugs** to see if we can make any impact on this tumour.
Pt: um hum
Dr: Which means that we are talking about **trial-based treatment**. (Case 10)

Dr: . . . one of the things we do is test new drugs that are coming out of the laboratory and are being used for the first time . . . the attraction obviously is to try and get hold of drugs that might be the standard chemotherapies of the future . . . So that what we can offer here is **treatment** *that isn't otherwise available, largely by the drugs not being in wide circulation . . . Erm and the possibility therefore of having the opportunity to try [and] deal with the tumour in the same way that your previous drugs . . . have done . . . (mentions caveats) . . . it's still the route if you like to get state of the art medication, and see whether it is something that might benefit you. (Case 12)*

'You're right!' admitted Rachel. 'They do seem to be focused on *clinical* aspects of the new "drug" rather than the *experimental* nature of the trial.' So, we stated our Emerging Theory as: **Trial doctors tend to use treatment language when talking about trials.** We noted the **'duality'** between the trial doctors' clinical and research roles. They used a mix of research language and terms with clinical language and terms. For example:

Trials were referred to as 'treatment'.

Trial agents were referred to as 'drugs'.

'Drugs' were referred to being 'effective'.

Participants were referred to as 'patients'.

One **deviant case** emerged, in which the doctor seemed to change his approach from emphasising treatment to emphasising the research when questioned by a potential participant:

Dr: . . . the study is actually only for you to be on the drug for 4 weeks. However, if you were tolerating it well and there was evidence of response then we would continue with it . . .

Pt: Would you expect to see a response in that 4 weeks, in the short term?

Dr: erm . . .The answer is **we don't know** because we have no idea what the effect would be of the drug and **the study is not designed for that.** The study is only designed to look at **side effects and to look at maximum dose** that we can give. [Case 5]

We referred to that as **confrontation and clarification.**

However, we then came across a consultation which seemed to be totally different from all the rest – **a really deviant case.** In this the potential participant was very light-hearted and joking and seemed to be only too willing to sign up to anything the trial doctor wanted. He avoided invitations to refer to the trial as treatment or offers of positive effects of the trial substance.

Dr: The (potential drug) has some side effects, we are not sure what all of them are because . . .

Pa: Oh no I'm not going to grow a beard!

Dr: That would be a very big surprise

Pa: Leave me out!

Hu – [laughs]

Pa: Yes, it's not testosterone!

Dr: No it's not a hormone like that.

Pa: [laughing]

Dr: **So you need to clear that this is of no benefit to you having the treatment, ok?**

Pa: [laughs]

Dr: **It's not really a treatment at all!**

And he managed to maintain that stance to the end.

Dr: Well just to recap, your standard treatment will happen whatever you decide about the trial. If you go into the trial **you need to be clear it's of no benefit to you.**

Pa: No I understand that.

Dr: **It's not a treatment.**

Pa: I understand that.

Dr: And you know you should feel free to refuse it having read it or thought about it you think 'I don't fancy that', okay?

Pa: Yeah, it'll be a bit mean in a way because I think about generations to come.

Revision of Theory

As you can see, there was evidence to reformulate our theory in the light of these new observations, and to ensure that the theory accounted for them. This led to the following **reformulation:**

Trial doctors tend to use treatment language when talking about trials

BUT

when potential participants are too light-hearted or joking about it

OR

when they appear too willing to take part,

THEN

trial doctors revert to the use of scientific language when talking about trials.

While we were doing our analyses, I was learning more and more about PI trials, the researchers who run them and the people who are recruited to them. I did this by reading more about the subject (see for example, Jenkins et al. 2010). Now that the GT analyses had been done, this would no longer compromise my 'naïve-researcher' status. I was learning about those who conduct these trials and the people who are recruited to take part in them from interviewing them in the main PI study. And I came to realise one of the main issues of concern in such clinical trials is that of the **therapeutic misconception** (TM) – the belief held by some people that PI trials are a form of treatment rather than research. This was first described by Paul Applebaum in 1982 as:

> *To maintain a therapeutic misconception is to deny the possibility that there may be major disadvantages to participating in clinical research that stem from the nature of the research process itself.*
>
> *(Appelbaum et al. 1987)*

Lidz and Appelbaum continued to refine their work on TM (Lidz and Appelbaum, 2002). Because of differences in the meanings attributed to the term TM, a consensus definition of 'therapeutic misconception' was proposed by Henderson et al. (2007).

> *Therapeutic misconception exists when individuals do not understand that the defining purpose of clinical research is to produce generalizable knowledge, regardless of whether the subjects enrolled in the trial may potentially benefit from the intervention under study or from other aspects of the clinical trial.*
>
> *(Henderson et al. 2007)*

At the time Rachel and I were doing this work, this was one of the critical debates in the oncology clinical trials world. And it seemed that trial doctors may have been contributing to this misconception in ways we described – possibly without being aware of doing so.

In our scrutiny of the consultations, we observed additional, more subtle ways in which PI trials may have been portrayed in a *positive light* which served to promote them. For example, we noted examples of trial doctors alluding to the fact that a similar trial was being conducted at another prestigious centre. Others seemed to aim for additional 'respectability' by informing potential participants that there were many others already enrolled in a trial.

Study Conclusions

So, the main points which we concluded were:

There was a **duality** *of:* **research** *language and* **clinical** *language . . .*

BUT:

When participants seem too eager or optimistic, or when they queried outcomes, **research** *language was used . . .*

AND:

When participants seem reticent or ambivalent, then **clinical** *language was used.*

What I have tried to do here is to show you our workings, and how our *thinking* about the situation we were observing – the recruitment of potential participants into PI oncology trials – developed as we went through our data analysis. We did not set out to test any hypotheses. Remember, I was Phase-I-oncology-trials naïve. So, GT was a natural choice of approach. The GT approach helped us to develop our theory and modify it as we went along. You can see how other studies and more general reading informed our **discussion** – but not our **data analysis.** Obviously, I have perhaps over-simplified this to make the account shorter, and to help you, dear Reader, understand the process. Unfortunately, both Rachel and I left the Unit whilst we were working to complete a version of the paper for publication, so we never did publish it. What I have reported here was made public in a conference presentation (Anderson and Ballinger 2008) – which seemed to us to be very well received.

To Sum Up

Grounded theory was first described by Barney Glaser and Anselm Strauss as an approach whereby, instead of existing theory and knowledge driving the development and testing of hypotheses (in a hypothetico-deductive approach), in their approach the theory emerged from the data – it is **hypothetico-inductive.** It is also known as the **constant-comparative** method because of the need to constantly review the data and theory emerging from existing cases and comparing new cases against these to ensure either the constancy of the theory that is emerging, or the need to re-appraise your theory. In this aspect, the search for, and accounting for, **deviant cases** is a central feature. The use of **theoretical sampling** allows the researcher to check for the consistency of the theory. And you know that you can put your jacket on and go home satisfied when you have achieved **data or theoretical saturation** – that is, when no new findings arise from the new cases you collect. Phew! Note that, although it is usually a **qualitative** approach, it can also be used with **quantitative** data too, although this latter aspect is uncommon. (Maybe that was Alexander Fleming's approach!) GT is usually **retrospective** but there is no reason it cannot be applied in **prospective** studies. Bear in mind the fact that it is a laborious task which requires a lot of time and effort to complete.

This approach suits research questions such as 'What is going on with . . .?' And if you think back over the history of science, I am sure that you will find examples of this sort of approach being used. When Darwin got off the boat in the Galapagos Islands, I don't think his first words would have been, 'It is my hypothesis that we shall discover species here that are similar to but different from species we have observed elsewhere!' Do you? When Oppenheimer said 'Go' to the detonation of the first atom bomb, they did not know how big a bang it would cause and the best advice was to 'stick your fingers in your ears, close your eyes, and pray'.

Research is the art of the possible!

References

Anderson JL and Ballinger RS. (2008). Handling Hopelessness –Doctor -Patient Interactions in Phase 1 Oncology Trials. Paper presented at the 2008 British Sociological Association, Medical Sociology Conference.

Andrews T and Nathaniel A. (2015). Awareness of dying remains relevant after fifty years. *The Grounded Theory Review* 14(2), 3–10.

Appelbaum PS, Roth LH, Lidz CW, et al. (1987). False hopes and best data: consent to research and the therapeutic misconception. *The Hastings Center Report* 17(2), 20–24. doi:10.2307/3562038. JSTOR 3562038. PMID 3294743.

Birks M and Mills J. (2015). *Grounded Theory: A Practical Guide*, 2nd ed. Sage: London.

Bloor M and Wood F. (2006). *Keywords in Qualitative Methods*. Sage: London.

Bowen GA. (2006). Grounded theory and sensitizing concepts. *International Journal of Quantitative Methods* 5(3), 12–23.

Corbin J and Strauss A. (2008). *Basics of Qualitative Research: Techniques and Procedures for Developing Grounded Theory (3)*. Sage: Thousand Oaks, CA.

Glaser BG and Strauss AL. (1965). *Awareness of Dying*. Aldine Publishing: Chicago, IL.

Glaser BG and Strauss AL. (1967). *The Discovery of Grounded Theory: Strategies for Qualitative Research*. Aldine Publishing: Chicago, IL.

Glaser BG and Strauss AL. (1968). *Time for Dying*. Aldine: Chicago, IL.'

Henderson DE, Churchill L, Davis A, et al. (2007). Clinical Trials and Medical Care: Defining the Therapeutic Misconception. *PLoS Medicine* 4(11), (Freely available online -Accessed at https://www.ncbi.nlm.nih.gov/pmc/articles/PMC2082641).

Howard SB, Blanche G, Everett CH, et al. (1961). *Boys in White: Student Culture in Medical School.* Transaction Publishers.

Jenkins V, Anderson J, and Fallowfield L. (2010). Communication and informed consent in phase 1 trials: a review of the literature from January 2005 to July 2009. *Supportive Care in Cancer* 18(9), 1115–1121.

Lidz CW and Appelbaum PS. (2002). The therapeutic misconception: problems and solutions. *Medical Care* 40, V55–V63.

Patton MQ. (2002). *Qualitative Research and Evaluation Methods*. Sage: Thousand Oaks, CA.

Strauss A and Corbin J. (1990). *Basics of Qualitative Research: Grounded Theory Procedures and Techniques*. Sage Publications: Newbury Park, CA.

Strauss AL and Corbin J. (1997). *Grounded Theory in Practice*. Sage.

Tie YC, Birks M, and Francis K. (2019). Grounded theory research: a design framework for novice researchers. *SAGE Open Medicine* 7, 1–8.

CHAPTER 15

Mixed Methods
Case Study Methods

Introduction

Case studies form the backbone of research. Almost everyone has a story about an individual case which they can tell. Individual cases fire the imagination because we can relate to individuals, especially if we have a name and a photograph to go with it. Then we can identify with that individual. We can probably relate to one or two or three cases, but beyond that we begin to deal with statistics – groups of nameless individuals. Iosif Vissarionovich Dzhugashvili (Joseph Stalin) is generally attributed with having said:

> *A single death is a tragedy, a million deaths is a statistic.*

He was right was our Joseph! Several times I have delivered *very* scholarly papers at *very* scholarly academic conferences in which I have cited my *very* grand, robust research findings, strongly backed up by some very fine statistics to make my point – only to be shot down in flames by someone who says something like, 'Well in my experience it isn't like that. I remember one patient. . .' And they have got the whole audience eating out of their hand! Being able to cite a real case, about a real individual, carries great weight.

What I have done in this book has been to give you **case studies** – in brief – about all the different methods I have presented. Now, these have been shortened because my aim was to give you a feel for and an understanding of each approach I presented. I thought that this would give the most effective impact and understanding of each approach, as opposed to discussing them all in the abstract with no examples.

So, case studies are:

- **Quantitative** or **qualitative** – often both.
- They can be **hypothetico-deductive or inductive.**
- They are usually **retrospective** but can be **prospective.**
- They can be **interventional or observational** in that they can be descriptions of interventions or they can be restricted to observational descriptions – depending upon the case and the aim of the case study.
- They all involve individual 'cases' – but these cases can be **individual people** or **group situations** or **decisions** made by organisations such as governments, or **events,** etc . . .

Demystifying Research for Medical & Healthcare Students: An Essential Guide, First Edition. John L. Anderson.
© 2022 John Wiley & Sons Ltd. Published 2022 by John Wiley & Sons Ltd.
Companion website: www.wiley.com/go/Anderson/DemystifyingResearch

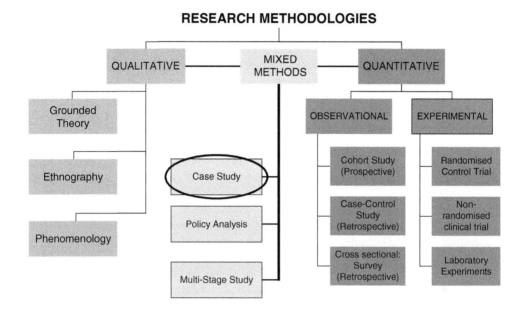

Case studies: an overview

Individual case studies are commonly found in the clinical domain, so I shall present and discuss some individual **clinical case studies** first. Then we can have a think about other types of case studies. Many major events form the focus of case studies. 'Major events' can be as 'major' as anyone thinks they are. For some NHS employees, changes which outsiders might consider as trivial may be considered world-changing to employees and others affected by them. Disasters, such as are caused by storms, floods, droughts, tsunamis, and so on, tend to attract much more general attention and examination. I wonder how many case studies will emerge from the COVID-19 pandemic. Some of these will be examples of **policy analysis** in which the different policies that were proposed and/or implemented around the world will be subject to microscopic scrutiny to determine how policies came into being, and what the results of these policies were. I shall discuss policy analysis in more depth in the next chapter, as these as important examples of case studies with particular sets of questions.

Other examples are in the methods we have encountered already – for example, in participant observation, Malinowski used the case of Polynesian island life as his case study; Whyte used 'street corner society' as his case study; Geer et al. used medical schools as their case studies; and so on. One of the issues which confronts us in researching cases is *defining the boundaries*. This can involve defining the time-period, the geographical limits, the persons involved in the group, or the event under study, and so on. NB: There are no hard and fast rules to determine this, except the notion of *relevance*, and this is largely down to the researcher's (i.e. your) judgement.

Now, have a think about what the 'case' was that was being studied in each of the research studies we have considered together so far – I bet there are different ways in which you might frame what constitutes a 'case'; for example, was the example of Doll and Hill's study of smoking and lung cancer a study of the 'case' of smoking, or of lung cancer, or of case-control studies, or. . .? It depends where you are coming from. If you are coming from a 'disease perspective' it is a case of lung cancer research. If you are coming from a 'smoking perspective' it is a case of smoking research. If you are coming from a 'research perspective' it is a case of 'research'.

And the obvious question to arise next is: 'What is the ***research question*** that is being asked in each of these cases?' That will drive the focus of the case examination (research methods) and how it is reported (data analysis).

Then you will have to consider the data that you will have to collect to present as full an account of the case as possible. Yin (2018), in his excellent and comprehensive textbook on case study research, points out some of the dangers at this stage of your journey.

> *As a caution, if you have had limited experience in conducting empirical studies, at the design stage you may not easily identify the likely analytic technique(s) or anticipate the needed data to use the techniques to their full advantage. Even more experienced researchers may find that they have either (a) collected too much data that was not later used in any analysis, or (b) collected too little data that prevented the proper use of a desired analytic technique. Sometimes, the latter situation may force researchers to return to their data collection phase (if they can), to supplement the original data. The more you can avoid either of these situations, the better off you will be.*
>
> *(Yin 2018)*

For example, one of our students wanted to examine what happened in the organisation within which she worked. Her concerns were very pertinent to her because of the emotional upheaval that was involved in the 'case' or 'instance' which she wanted to make sense of – a change within the organisation which resulted in reassignment of roles, responsibilities, and power or control. She felt very 'bruised' emotionally and wanted to make sense of what had occurred, why it had occurred (as it had), and the impact on individuals in the workplace. I guess there were two main approaches which I would have recommended – an autoethnography and a case-study approach. She chose to avoid the dangers of what she saw as 'baring her soul' in an autoethnography and opted for the case study as a more neutral approach.

This illustrates one aspect of case study approaches which is less often dealt with in the literature – the *reasons* for choosing the approach. She wanted to illustrate what went on – including what she thought of as 'bad managerial practice'. For her, the case needed to be made 'public'. I say 'public', rather than public, because for the purposes of her research she adhered to the conventions of confidentiality and anonymity within research – in concealing the names and locations involved. With this motivation, only a case study approach would really do to make the point, although, she stayed this side of the dividing line between academic research and **investigative journalism**, which could have had a greater impact but which could potentially left one open to litigation. Investigative journalism usually has the goal of making their findings known as widely as possible, as in the example below, which went 'viral' and resulted in a change in the presidency of the USA.

I have the greatest respect for high-quality investigative journalism. Some great works have been done in that field, for example, the Watergate exposures – of the

Washington Post reporters Bob Woodward and Carl Bernstein – which led to the resignation of US president Richard Nixon in 1974. (Google it or watch the movies – or better still read the case study by James M. Perry (2020), Columbia School of Journalism, Columbia University; or the book by Carl Bernstein and Bob Woodward (1974)). So, at this point you might wish to reflect upon your future career – do you want to end up an old, unknown academic researcher like me, or do you want to go on to gain fame and fortune like Carl Bernstein and Bob Woodward? In both instances, you should learn about research methods; but if you go down the investigative journalism route, skip the section on research ethics!

Ok, I guess that this will make some of our heads hurt. So, let's plunge right in and consider a couple of examples of **clinical case studies.** In clinical case studies, our goal is to share with the rest of our clinical world some example of (usually) a success, or a failure in our clinical work, so that others might learn or get ideas for further research from our work. Let's have a look.

Example 1: First clinical use of penicillin

This example of the first time that the new drug – 'penicillin' – was used on a patient was reported by Charles Fletcher (1984). (We used to meet regularly at the Royal Society of Medicine, Forum on Medical Communication. We both shared an interest in medical communication. He was a lovely unassuming, charming gentleman.) At the time he writes about (1941), he was a junior member of Professor Howard Florey's team in Oxford. Florey, who was instrumental in the clinical development of penicillin, invited Charles to join his team and help with the clinical trials of penicillin. He reports:

> *My first job was to try out various routes of administration on several volunteer patients. These just confirmed what had already been shown by animal studies, that penicillin was destroyed in the stomach, and oral administration in man also failed. Penicillin was present in blood and urine after administration with a duodenal tube but rectal administration was useless. Detectable blood concentrations were only transient after a single intravenous injection. We decided that the best route of administration would be by hourly injection into a continuous, slow running, citrate saline intravenous drip, for the high peak blood concentrations should encourage diffusion into the tissues and into collections of pus. The standard technique for such infusions then was to dissect out a superficial vein and tie in a small swan necked cannula. Simple screw caps were the only mechanism available to control the rate of flow, and they were pretty erratic. Fortunately, Marriott and Kekwick had just described a reliable flow control device using loops of capillary tubing about five inches (13 cm) long connected together by T pieces having rubber tubes with screw clips between each loop. I quickly made up two or three of these gadgets and they functioned admirably. Each penicillin injection could be flushed in by brief release of all the clips to short circuit the capillary tubes. By this means the intravenous infusions were kept to a rate of roughly 10 ml an hour.*
>
> *The time had now come to find a suitable patient for the first test of the therapeutic power of penicillin in man. Every hospital then had a 'septic' ward,*

filled with patients with chronic discharging abscesses, sinuses, septic joints, and sometimes meningitis. Patients with staphylococcal infections would be ideal because sulphonamides had no effect on them and were inactivated by pus. In the septic ward at the Radcliffe Infirmary there was then an unfortunate policeman aged 43 who had had a sore on his lips four months previously from which he had developed a combined staphylococcal and streptococcal septicaemia. He had multiple abscesses on his face and his orbits (for which one eye had been removed): he also had osteomyelitis of his right humerus with discharging sinuses, and abscesses in his lungs. He was in great pain and was desperately and pathetically ill. There was all to gain for him in a trial of penicillin and nothing to lose. Penicillin treatment was started on 12 February 1941, with 200 mg (10 000 units) intravenously initially and then 300 mg every three hours. All the patient's urine was collected, and each morning I took it over to the Dunn Laboratory on my bicycle so that the excreted penicillin could be extracted to be used again. There I was always eagerly met by Florey and Chain and other members of the team. On the first day I was able to report that for the first time throughout his illness the patient was beginning to feel a little better. Four days later there was a striking improvement, and after five days the patient was vastly better, afebrile, and eating well, and there was obvious resolution of the abscesses on his face and scalp and in his right orbit. But, alas, the supply of penicillin was exhausted: the poor man gradually deteriorated and died a month later. The total dose given over five days had been only 220,000 units, much too small a dose, as we now know, to have been able to overcome such extensive infection; but there was no doubt about the temporary clinical improvement, and, most importantly, there had been no sort of toxic effect during the five days of continuous administration of penicillin. This remarkable freedom from side effects, apart from allergy, has remained one of penicillin's most fortunate features.

(Fletcher 1984)

In this description, Sir Charles Fletcher describes clearly (well, as clearly as professional jargon will allow!) the clinical aspects of the case at the outset. He outlines the treatment in clearly understandable – and, most importantly, replicable – detail. And he clearly describes the outcomes – both short-term and final. He then accounts for those outcomes in the light of knowledge available to us today. He uses quantitative details and qualitative details to fully inform his account. I like it because it is succinct and not too wordy. It is a sad case of *'the treatment was a success, but the patient died'*. He also conveys some of his emotional responses, for example his excitement at witnessing the changes in healthcare as a result of the drug he helped test.

> *It is difficult to convey the excitement of actually witnessing the amazing power of penicillin over infections for which there had previously been no effective treatment. I could not then imagine the transformation of medicine and surgery that penicillin would produce. But I did glimpse the disappearance of the chambers of horrors, which seems the best way to describe those old septic wards, and could see that we should never again have to fear the streptococcus, whose eclipse Garrod described so vividly, or the more deadly staphylococcus.*
>
> *(Fletcher 1984)*

Example 2: First Case of 2019 Novel Coronavirus in the United States

On December 31, 2019, China reported a cluster of cases of pneumonia in people associated with the Huanan Seafood Wholesale Market in Wuhan, Hubei Province. On January 7, 2020, Chinese health authorities confirmed that this cluster was associated with a novel coronavirus, 2019-nCoV. Although cases were originally reported to be associated with exposure to the seafood market in Wuhan, current epidemiologic data indicate that person-to-person transmission of 2019-nCoV is occurring. As of January 30, 2020, a total of 9976 cases had been reported in at least 21 countries, including the first confirmed case of 2019-nCoV infection in the United States, reported on January 20, 2020. Investigations are under way worldwide to better understand transmission dynamics and the spectrum of clinical illness. This report describes the epidemiologic and clinical features of the first case of 2019-nCoV infection confirmed in the United States.

(Holshue et al. 2020)

In presenting this case, Holshue et al. describe the context of the patient.

On January 19, 2020, a 35-year-old man presented to an urgent care clinic in Snohomish County, Washington, with a 4-day history of cough and subjective fever. On checking into the clinic, the patient put on a mask in the waiting room. After waiting approximately 20 minutes, he was taken into an examination room and underwent evaluation by a provider. He disclosed that he had returned to Washington State on January 15 after traveling to visit family in Wuhan, China. The patient stated that he had seen a health alert from the U.S. Centers for Disease Control and Prevention (CDC) about the novel coronavirus outbreak in China and, because of his symptoms and recent travel, decided to see a health care provider.

They then go on to provide a detailed history of the patient's health background, and his present clinical state, along with the tests ordered for him.

Apart from a history of hypertriglyceridemia, the patient was an otherwise healthy nonsmoker. The physical examination revealed a body temperature of 37.2°C, blood pressure of 134/87 mm Hg, pulse of 110 beats per minute, respiratory rate of 16 breaths per minute, and oxygen saturation of 96% while the patient was breathing ambient air. Lung auscultation revealed rhonchi, and chest radiography was performed, which was reported as showing no abnormalities. A rapid nucleic acid amplification test (NAAT) for influenza A and B was negative. A nasopharyngeal swab specimen was obtained and sent for detection of viral respiratory pathogens by NAAT; this was reported back within 48 hours as negative for all pathogens tested, including influenza A and B, parainfluenza, respiratory syncytial virus, rhinovirus, adenovirus, and four common coronavirus strains known to cause illness in humans (HKU1, NL63, 229E, and OC43).

They notified the Centers for Disease Control and Prevention (**CDC**) and they shared their logic in determining which other tests to run on the patient.

> *Although the patient reported that he had not spent time at the Huanan seafood market and reported no known contact with ill persons during his travel to China, CDC staff concurred with the need to test the patient for 2019-nCoV on the basis of current CDC 'persons under investigation' case definitions. Specimens were collected in accordance with CDC guidance and included serum and nasopharyngeal and oropharyngeal swab specimens. After specimen collection, the patient was discharged to home isolation with active monitoring by the local health department.*

He tested positive for 2019-nCOV and was admitted to an airborne-isolation unit at the Providence Regional Medical Centre, for clinical observation. The care staff followed the CDC recommendations for appropriate protection (against contact, droplets and airborne transmission). He reported having a dry cough, nausea and vomiting, but no shortage of breath or chest pain.

They report his following days' progress. He received supportive care and appeared to stay stable, apart from some episodes of fever and tachycardia. Other symptoms he experienced included a non-productive cough and episodes of loose stools. He continued to receive supportive care along with antipyretic therapy (acetaminophen, ibuprophen), guaifenesin for his cough and normal saline for six days. On the third and fifth days in hospital, his lab tests 'reflected leukopenia, mild thrombocyte-penia, and elevated levels of creatine kinase. In addition, there were alterations in hepatic function measures.' Blood cultures showed no growth. Chest x-rays were taken on days 3 (clear), 5 (evidence of pneumonia), and 6 (suggestion of likely atypical pneumonia). These changes were accompanied by changes in his respiratory status – oxygen saturation levels dropped to 90%. His treatments altered accordingly to include supplementary oxygen and worry about a hospital acquired infection led to his being given vancomy-cin and cefepime.

His radiological changes noted on day 6 in hospital, accompanied reports from elsewhere of severe pneumonia, led to the clinicians trying out 'investigational anti-viral therapy' – intravenous remdesivir (a new 'nucleotide analogue prodrug in development'). Vancomycin was stopped on day 7 and cefepime on day 8 when his condition seemed to improve. Oxygen saturation increased from 94% to 96%, apart from an intermittent dry cough and a runny nose (rhinorrhea). On 30 January 2020, the day before the report was published in *The New England Journal of Medicine*, 'all symptoms have resolved with the exception of his cough, which is decreasing in severity'.

They give a detailed account of their specimen collection, their diagnostic testing for 2019-NCOV, and their genetic sequencing. Their report – remember that this was very early on in the spread of the pandemic – highlights some of the key elements of this case, which included how the public health warnings alerted the patient to seek help; the local healthcare workers' recognition of the significance of his recent visit to Wuhan; the following coordination of effort and information sharing between different health officials from the local hospital, state, and federal public health officials, which informed the testing and treatments which the patient received. As a result they were able quickly to determine their diagnosis of 2019-nCoV infection and treat the patient accordingly. They concluded:

> *Our report of the first confirmed case of 2019nCoV in the United States illustrates several aspects of this emerging outbreak that are not yet fully understood, including transmission dynamics and the full spectrum of clinical illness. Our case patient had travelled to Wuhan, China, but reported that he had not visited the wholesale seafood market or health care facilities or had any sick contacts during his stay in Wuhan. Although the source of his 2019-nCoV infection is unknown, evidence of person-to-person transmission has been published. Through January 30, 2020, no secondary cases of 2019-nCoV related to this case have been identified, but monitoring of close contacts continues.*

> *Finally, this report highlights the need to determine the full spectrum and natural history of clinical disease, pathogenesis, and duration of viral shedding associated with 2019-nCoV infection to inform clinical management and public health decision making.*

(Holshue et al. 2020)

Of note in this case report, like in Fletcher's, is the mix of **quantitative data;** for example, from the lab results – white cell count '6500', and **qualitative data;** for example, from the patient's reports and staff observations the patient 'appeared fatigued' – hence the term **'mixed methods'**. They have tried to be as all-inclusive as possible by including all the data that they thought was appropriate to give us a clear idea of everything of interest that was going on – and, by providing the time-line, they are able to give us a sense of what happened as a result of their interventions. Their reports are well-boundaried – they do not go into detail, for example, about the health issues faced by the cases' aunties! That is where you have to use your own discretion, following the advice of your supervisor (if you have one).

So, let me now try to pick out the main stages in case studies like this.

1. Choose your case. But in doing so, be reflexive – consider *why* you want to high-light that specific case. Consider the effects that your doing so will have, on the people in the case, on any others, and on yourself.
2. Define your research question.
3. Your research question will help clarify your aims and the data that you will need to collect to meet your goals.
4. Check whether or not you will be able to get the information you want (data) from existing data which is in the public domain (i.e. already published), or will you need to collect more data yourself. It may be a combination of both.
5. You need to do the preparatory work before you gather your data. How do you explain it to the patient who you are using as a case? How do you show that you have obtained their informed consent? If you plan to extract data from different sources, it is good practice to get a data extraction sheet (to show what information you want to extract), or to develop a questionnaire (to show what information you want to ask of them).
6. Consider what permissions you might need to access the information (data) that you need for your study. If you intend to get information from, for example, a

patient's notes, check to find out who you need to ask for permission to read them. If you want to ask other people about their experiences of the event you are studying (i.e. interview them), do you need research ethics committee approval?

7. Once you have clarified these questions about the data you want to get and the permissions you need to get, then you can start to gather your data – have fun!

8. Once you have all your data together, you need to make sense of it – to analyse it.

9. In doing the data analyses, you need to ask yourself, 'Have I got everything I want?' If the answer is 'No', then you might have to consider going back for more.

10. Then the really challenging part comes next – how to present it – to report your findings.

There, that fitted neatly into 10 steps – a nice round number. But others may say that there are 12 steps, or more, or less. It doesn't really matter; take what you will from this and I hope it helps to guide you.

Case Series

A variant of the standard case study is a **case series,** or as the name suggests a series of cases! In this approach a series of linked cases are presented and discussed – often with an analysis of the whole series. Fletcher's paper actually presented a case series – from which I selected the one that I was most interested in to make the point about a case study. I shall try to illustrate this more fully by giving an example of another of Seb and my studies.

Example 3: Coping with Medical School

This study resulted from a teaching session I had given on Martin Seligman's work on **learned helplessness** – and we have already touched on this example in Chapter 13. Seb was inspired by this topic and it resonated with his own experiences as a medical student. He wanted to document some of the experiences which medical students had of feeling helpless and hopeless. We agreed that an **interpretive phenomenological approach** would be the most suitable to adopt. So, under my supervision, he formulated the study and we got approval for the study from the medical school Ethics Committee. They insisted that Seb should not conduct any interviews with people he knew personally. That was no problem as I agreed to do these.

The medical school office agreed to send out an e-mail to all 5th year medical students to invite any interested students to contact us. Only three students responded – all of them known to Seb – so I contacted them and interviewed them (this functioned to further preserve their identity and anonymity). One was a face-to-face interview and two interviews were conducted by telephone. In these latter two, informed consent was obtained and confirmed on the audio-tape. Audio-recordings were transcribed verbatim (using a transcription service) and analysed by Seb using a **thematic analysis** which I validated. Because there were only three participants, who provided rich data, we decided to use a **case-study approach** in presenting the data. And that is why I am repeating this example here: to show how within a phenomenological approach we were able to include a case study approach – in this instance, inspired by the necessity of the fact that we only had three participants, a short series of cases. Note how we integrated the two approaches in our reporting of them. We identified each by pseudo-nyms – 'Amy', 'Jess', and 'Ryan'. Each case was presented in detail, the main issues and themes which emerged from each interview were documented, and in the discussion, these were compared and contrasted. We felt that this approach was the best to allow each of their stories to be reported for all to read, and for the overall analysis to empha-sise the common features and the individual differences.

Case 1: 'Amy'

'Amy' was a final year international student. When she began medical school she lived in halls – with other first-year 'medics'. The move from home was difficult and lonely enough, but she found the academic demands overwhelming and left her little time to get to know other students.

> *Just not being used to the environment and . . . not knowing what to expect in medical school . . . I felt the pressure.*

She began to feel increasingly 'different' from her peers – that she did not fit in, that she was not as bright or confident as they were. As a result, Amy became increasingly shy and withdrawn. In second year, an experience with a tutor left her feeling devastated, very emotionally upset and full of self-doubt.

> *Sometimes she said harsh things to me . . . For example: 'Oh, I think you should be aware of yourself, that [you're] not speaking up in the group'. [And it was not about] being able to express myself . . . Just saying like I don't have enough knowledge to be in medical school . . .*

This devastated her. Not good enough! A failure! Letting her family down! Amy began to withdraw more and more, while her tutor increasingly picked on her, telling her in class to speak up, that it reflected her lack of knowledge, and that she would not make it through medical school. When she tried to explain herself the tutor misunderstood her and told her to work on her weaknesses.

> *She said: 'well, yes I am glad that you know what your weaknesses are. I think you just have to work on it. And no one can help you with it.'*

Amy became increasingly isolated and low and started looking for a way out. In the interview, Amy was in tears. She reported that she had considered *suicide* as a strong possibility, at one stage. She was in a state of complete *hopelessness,* which haunted her throughout her time in medical school.

> *I mean apart from . . . apart from leaving medical school I also think about harming myself sometimes . . . I just kept having this thought in my mind, quite often . . . I just wanted to do something to make myself better . . . I mean I just wanted to maybe go to sleep forever.*

She began to believe that she was as bad a student as her tutor had said, and that she could not change these things – there must just be a problem with her – her *weaknesses.*

> *So that is when I thought maybe it is just me, it is just my problem.*

We found the following themes emerged from the detail of her interview:

- *Isolation* – both physically (from her family) and socially (from her classmates).
- *Judgement/failure* – That one tutor's condemnation was totally damning for her. 'What she said just kept echoing in my head. And I thought "oh, maybe I am really that kind of person and that is why I can't change for it".'
- *Guilt* – She carried a deep sense of shame – she had let her family down, and she could not discuss it with them or anyone else.
- *Lack of supports* – She was aware that there were supports in the medical school, but could not bring herself to go there. Nor could she seek help from her family or classmates. (The interview was the first time she had discussed it at all, and she took some comfort from being able to talk about it then.)
- *Academic impact* – The tutor's words became a self-fulfilling prophecy. She began to do badly in her exams and skipped all the lectures and seminars she could, until she nearly failed her attendance requirements.

We also noted a theme of *despair* running through the interview. Does this come over to you as you read this brief presentation of her experiences?

Case 2: 'Jess'

'Jess' was also a final year student. She had begun her student career positively. At university she was put into a flat with students from different courses – she did not have a medical student peer group at home. So, she followed their example of partying and socialising whilst her 'real peers' were studying hard and revising. When she began to fail exams, she realised that her classmates were really working hard – much harder than she and her flat mates – 'I guess that is when I kind of started to feel less in control'. She had to repeat her first year. Her initial classmates progressed without her and they moved on socially – they were no longer her friends.

> . . . *All of my friends were in the year above. And I didn't really talk to any of them again . . . I had a lot of friends . . . And then, you know, if I ever passed them in the corridor, I would just kind of get a sympathy nod, [with] 'how is first year?' 'It is a shame isn't it?'*

She struggled. She had no peer-reference in the first year. She felt alone – very isolated. And she wanted to change course or give up completely. Her attitude and behaviour set her apart even more.

> *I would just sit by myself and kind of turn up late in hoody and joggers and sit at the back and leave early.*

She began to sense that she was an 'outsider' who did not fit in. On top of this, she had accommodation problems. Her former flatmates did not want her back. She pleaded with them for help to be guarantors for her to rent a new flat; they refused. Now she really was excluded and had nowhere to live. She asked her family for help and they too refused her. This was in addition to the heavy demands of her course.

> *I didn't have any of my stuff with me. A few changes of clothes, and my computer I guess and a couple of books, but that was it . . .*

In the first three years, she became increasingly depressed – to the extent that she contemplated suicide.

> *I couldn't really look at anything without seeing it as a means to kill myself . . . I was having very intrusive thoughts about it that I couldn't control . . . So if I even just glanced at a balcony I would be like, 'I could jump off that, that would probably work . . . ' Or just like a curtain rail and I would be like, 'Oh I could probably just hang myself off that.'*

Out of desperation, she moved in with a boyfriend so she had a roof over her head.

Eventually she moved back into halls and had a stable 'home' at last. This was the turning point for her.

These themes and issues emerged from her story:

- *No appropriate reference group* – living with first-year students on other courses and having no friends among her classmates.
- *Rejections/being different* – being ostracised by her original classmates; by her new classmates; by her family; by almost everyone who knew her.
- *Isolation* – having no one to turn to for help or support.
- *Loss/lack of control* – she felt herself spiralling out of control.

Like 'Amy', 'Jess' had an overwhelming issue of *despair* in her life as a student – also with no one picking up on her suffering.

Case 3: 'Ryan'

'Ryan' had done a degree already and was in his second year as a medical student. He was not eligible for a student loan and began to struggle financially – far more than he had anticipated. When I interviewed him, he juggled *five* part-time jobs with his academic life – he had no time for any social life – and he felt his grades were being affected. But he had a sense that these difficulties would be time-limited.

> *I will be able to swim out of this difficulty and find myself in better waters.*

Like 'Amy' and 'Jess', he too was different to his peers. Because of his money worries, he didn't mix socially with them. He had to work in all his spare time. Although this was hard and inescapable, he didn't let it overwhelm him because he saw that his hard work would pay off in the long-term.

The themes and issues which emerged for him were:

- *Money worries* – these were constant, but he had been fortunate to make ends meet so far and believed he always could.
- *Silence culture* – he didn't ask anyone for help or complain to anyone about his situation. Like 'Amy' and 'Jess', the interview was one of the first times he had really opened up about his problems.
- *Competitive environment* – he found the constant competition within medical school a very negative aspect of being a medical student.
- *Being different* – he too was an 'outsider' who was older, did not mix socially, and had past experience of what being a student *could* be like.
- *Determination* – he felt helpless in that he *had* to work in all his free time.

Unlike Amy and Jess, there was no meta-theme of despair here. He did not drift into *hopelessness,* because he saw an end to it.

So, these three case studies (abbreviated here) describe three students' different individual situations. Despite the fact that they are all unique, you can see some common themes running through them – e.g. isolation, silence, negative aspects of medical school culture, etc. In our discussion (see Chapter 13) Seb and I elaborate upon this. However, I hope you get the feel for what it is like to record and present the results for a series of case studies which are all linked – in this instance by medical education.

To Sum Up

In case study research, a *case* can be almost anything you like to define as your 'case'. It can be an individual, a group of people, an event, an organisation, decisions (or policies) and so on. Case studies encompass both **quantitative** (with numbers) and **qualitative** (no numbers). They can be **hypothetico-deductive** or **hypothetico-inductive**. They can be **prospective** or **retrospective,** and they can be **interventional** or **observational.** In fact, they can include just about any type of research methods you can imagine!

A good case study will be clearly defined, comprehensive, and informative – they tell a story. **Clinical case studies** are often used as early descriptions of interventions with the goal of provoking further research. **Case series** are means of presenting more than one case at a time, with a view to showing how they are similar, how they are different, and what the outcomes are. The examples I have given here, are ones where I believe the authors did their best to describe in detail what they did, so that others could learn from their experience and try it out for themselves. Charles Fletcher's (1984) account is one which was essentially written for historical reasons – penicillin was well known and in wide use by then. In fact, it would have been difficult to publish such an account at the time the drug was being developed and manufactured because of official secrecy – it was the Allies 'secret weapon' against infection in World War II.

Holshue et al.'s (2020) report – 'First Case of 2019 Novel Coronavirus in the United States' – was important because it described the treatment of a new pandemic disease about which very little was known. They went into minute detail of the man's condition, his treatment, his responses to treatment, and the organisational aspects of the care he received. This account allowed others who were struggling to know how best to deal with similar cases which were appearing at an alarming rate (across America and the rest of the world), to learn from their experiences.

In the 'Coping With Medical School' study which Seb and I did, the low numbers – three participants – meant that we could adopt a case study method ***within*** an interpretive phenomenological approach. Thus, we were able to present the main details of each 'case' in order to allow the reader to understand as fully as possible what each had experienced. The similarities and differences could then be teased out within the grouped analysis of the data. This fulfilled both the case study and the phenomenological ethos of presenting the data and letting it speak for itself.

I can't end without answering the question which I know some of you will be asking: 'What about autoethnographies? Are they not case studies?' The answer is 'Yes, they are'. They are an example of a case study of information gathered and reported about 'The Self' by 'The Self'. As I discussed in Chapter 12, these carry weight because they are accounts of the realities encountered by ourselves – the researchers who dare to share.

Research is the art of the possible!

References

Carl B and Bob W. (1974). *All the President's Men*. Simon and Schuster: New York.

Fletcher C. (1984). First clinical use of penicillin. *British Medical Journal* 289, 1721–1723.

Holshue M, De Bolt C, Lindquist S, et al. (2020). First case of 2019 novel coronavirus in the United States. *The New England Journal of Medicine* 382(10), 929–936.

Leonard L. (1947). *The Washington Post, Loose-leaf notebook*. p. 9. Available at: https://www.globalsecurity.org/military/world/russia/stalin.htm (accessed on 27 August 2020).

Pakula AJ. (1976). *All the President's Men*. Warner Bros.

Perry JM. 'Watergate Case Study'. Class Syllabus for Critical Issues in Journalism. Columbia School of Journalism, Columbia University. Available at: http://www.columbia.edu/itc/journalism/j6075/edit/readings/watergate.html (accessed on 27 August 2020).

Shaw SCK and Anderson JL. (2021). Coping with medical school: an interpretive phenomenological study. *The Qualitative Report* 26(6).

Yin RK. (2018). *Case Study Research and Applications: Design and Methods*. Sage Publications: London.

CHAPTER 16

Mixed Methods

Policy Analysis

Introduction

Policy analysis (PA) is another type of **case study** approach in which the 'case' we are studying is a **policy.** There are two aspects or types of PA:

a. one which analyses an existing policy with the goal of examining in detail *what the effects of that policy have been,* these are **retrospective policy analyses** which look at things which have already taken place and help to explain why certain policies came to be; and

b. one which analyses a proposed policy with the aim of examining in detail *what the effects of the policy are likely to be,* these are **prospective policy analyses,** they try to look into the future to anticipate whether or not the policy options we identify are likely to have the effects we need from them.

c. Both of these aim to gather as much information as possible about the policy and its likely or its actual effects, from as wide a range of sources as we can, in order to provide an analysis and a report which is as comprehensive as possible.

d. In doing this, some of our data are likely to be **quantifiable** (numbers) and some of our data are likely to be **qualitative** (no numbers).

e. They can be either **hypothetico-deductive** or **hypothetico-inductive.**

But what do we mean by a 'policy'? By 'policy', we mean the sets of principles and actions which we will take to achieve any objective. Notice that I have included principles and actions. Principles are important in the sense that these can determine *how we think* about various issues, and all of our actions, which are sets of *things that have to be done,* and which will hopefully reflect the sets of guiding principles. Often policies develop as means of dealing with problems. I shall consider this as we go through this chapter.

The US CDC – Centres for Disease Control and Prevention – provide a very useful model of PA (Google it) which I shall go through later.

Demystifying Research for Medical & Healthcare Students: An Essential Guide, First Edition. John L. Anderson.
© 2022 John Wiley & Sons Ltd. Published 2022 by John Wiley & Sons Ltd.
Companion website: www.wiley.com/go/Anderson/DemystifyingResearch

There is an awful lot written on PA which is excessively detailed for our work here. For example, some writers have differentiated between Marxist PA, feminist PA, post-modern PA, etc. Try Googling PA; and when you get too confused come back here! Will you restrict yourself to existing, published work? Or, will you collect your own data as well? (Both are acceptable.) This tends to focus attention on the political standpoint of the researcher. I believe that it is important for you to examine your motives and your own driving forces for conducting a PA. Will you focus on the 'micro-approach' or the 'macro approach? Or will you, like me, take a 'middle of the road' approach and flit between the micro- and the macro- approaches? But, as with any research approach, you will be driven by your own 'biases' – or perspectives. If you feel it is important, or helpful to explain these, then by all means do so. Otherwise, you need not. How, for example, might I describe my perspective? As a 'middle of the road', 'middle-aged', 'middle class', 'male with feminist leanings', etc.? In our works on dyslexia, Seb and I have tended to declare that 'One of the authors (SS) is dyslexic'. This is often under the heading that many journals have of 'Conflicts of interest'. If you think it relevant, you should be upfront about any leanings which you might have. I do think it is important at times to look at the source of a PA. Is it from a 'Labour Party' source (or 'Democrat' in the USA) or a "Conservative Party source (or 'Republican' in the USA)? Such differences are often noted and are often cited as reasons for discounting a particular PA. Have a go, yourself, at drawing up a list of different attributes from which you might anticipate bias arising in a PA.

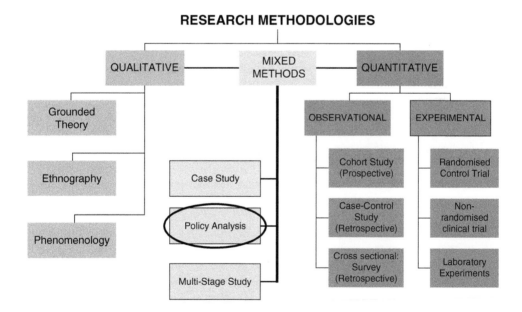

Analysis of an Existing Policy

This approach is widely used by politicians and public administrators to examine the actual outcomes of an adopted different policy. It is also very useful for identifying the factors and the 'stakeholders' who have driven the policy through. In this way we can gain some insights into the 'how' and the 'why' of the establishment of different policies.

Example 1: The Discovery of Hyperkinesis: Notes on the Medicalisation of Deviant Behaviour

This paper is one of my favourite pieces of PA – although Peter, who I met when he came to London, might prefer to refer to it as a piece of **sociological analysis.** He contextualises his work within the area of the study of **medicalisation** – the process by which medicine has increased its influence on our lives by extending its boundaries to include social, psychological, and environmental issues as areas within the scope of medicine's interest and expertise. **Ivan Illich** in his book *Limits to Medicine – Medical Nemesis: The Expropriation of Health* (1976) discusses **iatrogenesis** – physician-induced illness. He describes three types of iatrogenesis:

1. **Clinical iatrogenesis:** this refers to actual harm caused by medicine, and Illich describes: (i) Illusion of Doctors' Effectiveness, (ii) Useless Medical Treatments, and (iii) Doctor-Inflicted Injuries. Under (i) he describes the credit which the medical profession takes for the eradication, or minimalising, of the major killing diseases of the past, such as tuberculosis, measles, scarlet fever, and so on – even though most of the decline in deaths from these diseases had occurred before medical interventions had equipped doctors to do anything to combat them. Under (ii) he describes the tests and treatments performed without any validation of their effectiveness. Under (iii) he describes some of the ways by which doctors – including the research which doctors do – actually harm people. Examples of this are the problems caused by treating people with modern medicines, many of which produce side-effects which result in people being admitted to hospital for treatment for their previous treatment. He would also have mentioned diseases such as MRSA, Noro-virus, the so-called 'super-bugs', etc. which he refers to as diseases caused by medical over-treatment, and which give his argument even more weight now than it had in 1976.

2. **Social iatrogenesis:** this refers to the extent to which the medical profession is extending its scope of influence, expertise, and dominance over more and more aspects of our lives. So, it is now taken for granted that doctors can comment as experts on almost any aspect of our lives, because they influence our health. A part of this involves the exclusion of others, and other professionals, as being bona-fide contributors to people's health. This process is what he refers to as **medicalisation.** More recent commentators have referred to what Illich described as the pharmaceutical invasion ('there's a pill for every ill') as **pharmaceuticalisation** (Ahraham 2010; Williams, Gabe & Davis, 2008).

3. **Cultural iatrogenesis:** this sets in when, as Illich says 'the medical enterprise saps the will of people to suffer their reality'. It is as though 'suffering' is wrong and we have to turn to the medical specialist of life to formally endorse it and treat us for it. It refers to the fact that iatrogenesis has permeated our lives to the extent that we dare not function without the sanction of the doctor-expert.

I met Ivan when he came to visit us in Hong Kong while I was working there. He had the most powerful intellect I have ever met. He said that he wrote the book. *Limits to Medicine,* in *six months*. As he said to me, 'It was as though the medical profession was trying to commit professional suicide – the evidence was all there already, and most of it had been written by doctors themselves.' I remember when he delivered an open talk at the University of Hong Kong. It was held in the Senate chamber – a very posh semi-circular theatre, with microphones at each seat. He began by switching on his mike and saying:

My name is Ivan Illich.

Then he switched off his mike, sat back and waited. There was a stunned silence. Afterwards, when speaking to people about the event, they seemed to fall into one of two camps – half thought, 'He's a god!' and the other half thought, 'Oh God! I do not have time for this!' My friend Lawrence Goldstein was the first to break the silence after a few minutes. Lawrence switched on his mike and said in his broad Cockney accent:

Well, Dr Illich, my name's Lawrence Goldstein, but that don't get us very far does it?!

After a while, half the audience had left, and the rest of us were engaging in an interesting discussion with Ivan. At the end of his 'talk', the Dean of Education presented him with a cheque for his appearance, to which Ivan said, 'I do not have any need of this. Let us go and eat.' So, a few of us went out to dine at a nice local (Chinese) restaurant – as guests of Ivan Illich. We met a few more times before he left. It was an honour to meet him and to host an informal meeting with him at my home.

Whatever you think about it at first contact, you should read Illich's book which I believe to be one of the most prophetic and richly-referenced pieces of work I have encountered.

The theme of medicalisation was one which Peter Conrad explored in his study. He noted that **hyperkinesis** was at that time a recent diagnostic category and set out to explore how this had come to be. Hyperkinesis is characterised by hyperactivity, short attention span, restlessness and fidgeting, mood swings, clumsiness, aggressiveness, impulsivity, low frustration levels, sleeping problems, and delayed acquisition of speech. It is what many parents might have described as a typically 'naughty' child.

Conrad's question was: 'how did this very common behaviour become clinically classified as "Minimal Brain Dysfunction, Hyperactive Syndrome, Hyperkinetic Disorder Childhood, and several other diagnostic categories" for which medicine was able to provide chemical solutions to "control"'?

He noted that as far back as 1937, Bradley had described the effects of amphetamines on children with unruly behaviours – they seemed to calm the behaviours of some of these children. He tracked the history of how different labels for and responses to 'childhood behaviour disorders' were adopted (Bradley, 1937). In 1947, the term 'minimal brain injury (damage)' emerged. Then, in 1957 the term 'hyperkinetic impulse disorder' was coined. A key stage was when the US Public Health Service and the National Association for Crippled Children and Adults sponsored a task force to clarify the terminology and symptomatology for diagnosing children's behaviour. They came up with the label of **'minimal brain dysfunction' (MBD)** as the formal diagnosis for hyperkinesis.

Around the same time, a new drug was developed – Ritalin. This was approved for use in children by the US Food and Drug Administration (FDA) in 1961. Conrad notes that 'This medication became the "treatment of choice" for treating children with hyperkinesis' (1975). Publicity about the use of this new drug grew more widespread, until hyperkinesis became the most common child psychiatric problem and special clinics were set up to treat children with hyperkinesis. Knowledge of the 'new' condition and its treatment spread through the world of education and to the general public, so that it became a well-known medical disorder.

In looking at the conditions which led to the 'discovery of hyperkinesis', Conrad identified two sets of factors – what he termed the Pharmaceutical Revolution and Government Action.

1. **The Pharmaceutical Revolution:** Conrad points out that 'Until the early sixties there was little or no promotion and advertisement of any of these medications for use with childhood disorders', but that then two of the pharmaceutical 'giants' started to market these medications more aggressively in the **medical** field, and also in the **educational** sector. The growing success of psychoactive drugs for psychiatric disorders gave an increased legitimacy and confidence to pharmaceuticals.

2. **Government Action:** Conrad cites an article in the *Washington Post* in 1970 which reported that 5–10% of grammar school children in Omaha were being treated with 'behavior modification drugs to improve deportment and increase learning potential' (Grinspoon and Singer 1973) as being the catalyst for at least two government investigations.

The Congressional Subcommittee on Privacy chaired by Congressman Cornelius E. Gallagher held hearings on the issue of prescribing drugs for hyperactive school children. In general, the committee showed great concern over the facility in which the medication was prescribed; more specifically that some children at least were receiving drugs from general practitioners whose primary diagnosis was based on teachers' and parents' reports that the child was doing poorly in school. There was also a concern with the absence of follow-up studies on the long-term effects of treatment. The HEW committee was a rather hastily convened group of professionals (a majority were MDs) many of whom already had commitments to drug treatment for childrens' behavior problems. They recommended that only M.D.'s make the diagnosis and prescribe treatment, that the pharmaceutical companies promote the treatment of the disorder only through medical channels, that parents should not be coerced to accept any particular treatment and that long-term follow-up research should be done. This report served as blue ribbon approval for treating hyperkinesis with psychoactive medications

(Conrad 1975)

The pharmaceutical industry was naturally responsible for influencing the medical profession. However, he identified what Howard Becker termed **'moral entrepreneurs'** – groups or people who crusade for the creation of rules and their enforcement

(Becker 1963). These were: (i) the pharmaceutical companies and (ii) the Association for Children with Learning Disabilities.

The pharmaceutical companies spent time and money promoting their drugs for the treatment of MBD (Hyperkinesis). Conrad cites one of their ads:

MBD . . . MEDICAL MYTH OR DIAGNOSABLE DISEASE ENTITY
What medical practitioner has not, at one time or another, been called upon to examine an impulsive, excitable hyperkinetic child? A child with difficulty in concentrating. Easily frustrated. Unusually aggressive. A classroom rebel. In the absence of any organic pathology, the conduct of such children was, until a few short years ago, usually dismissed as . . . spunkiness, or evidence of youthful vitality. But it is now evident that in many of these children the hyperkinetic syndrome exists as a distinct medical entity. This syndrome is readily diagnosed through patient histories, neurologic signs, and psychometric testing-has been classified by an expert panel convened by the United States Department of Health, Education and Welfare as Minimal Brain Dysfunction, MBD.

(Conrad 1975)

These were accompanied by information packs, conferences for doctors, etc. He cites the vested interests of the pharmaceutical companies – 'CIBA had $13 million profit from Ritalin alone in 1971, which was 15% of the total gross profits'.

The Association for Children with Learning Disabilities was responsible for promoting the **medical model** of hyperkinesis by promoting conferences, sponsoring legislation, and providing support to its members. 'They have sensitized teachers and schools to the conception of hyperkinesis as a medical problem' (Conrad 1975).

Conrad locates this within the general 'medicalisation' movement (as was later described by Ivan Illich in 1976), and he describes 'another side to the medicalization of deviant behavior. The four aspects of this side of the issue include (1) the problem of expert control; (2) medical social control; (3) the individualization of social problems; and (4) the "depoliticization" of deviant behavior.'

1. **The problem of expert control:** Like Illich, Conrad notes the medical profession's monopoly over 'illness'. This is perhaps indisputable for many conditions, but other issues which are a mix of social and medical problems, like drug-taking, alcoholism, and hyperactivity, by being defined as 'medical' issues, are removed from the public domain and it becomes only doctors who are the true experts on these topics, and are, thus, dominant.

2. **Medical social control:** As Chorover (1973) termed it, **'psychotechnology'** forms a very powerful and effective method of controlling deviant behaviour – which could not be possible without the medicalisation of deviant behaviours. As Conrad put it, 'if a mechanism of medical social control seems useful, then the deviant behavior it modifies will develop a medical label or diagnosis. No overt malevolence on the part of the medical profession is implied: rather it is part of a complex process, of which the medical profession is only a part. The larger process might be called the individualization of social problems.'

3. **The individualisation of social problems:** At the time of his writing, Conrad reports the tendency for us to look for the causes and solutions to social problems

in individuals rather than within the social system. There was a culture of what Ryan (1970) called **'blaming the victim'**. As a result of 'victim-blaming' we tend to try to change the victim rather than society. By diagnosing a condition within an individual – as the medical profession does – we contribute to the individualisation of a social problem and we focus upon solutions in the individual rather than in the wider society. 'Hyperkinesis serves as a good example. Both the school and the parents are concerned with the child's behavior; the child is very difficult at home and disruptive in school. No punishments or rewards seem consistently to work in modifying the behavior; and both parents and school are at their wits' end. A medical evaluation is suggested. The diagnoses of hyperkinetic behavior leads to prescribing stimulant medications. The child's behavior seems to become more socially acceptable, reducing problems in school and at home . . . *It diverts our attention from the family or school*' (Conrad 1975).

4. **The 'depoliticisation' of deviant behaviour:** Conrad (1972) cites the example of how political dissenters (members of the political opposition) in the Soviet Union were declared mentally ill and sent to mental hospitals. 'This strategy served to neutralize the meaning of political protest and dissent, rendering it the ravings of mad persons.' By labelling the 'problem behaviour' – whatever it may be, e.g. 'Extinction Rebellion' or 'Conspiracy Theorists' – as 'madness' (i.e. a medical condition) we can sideline it and ignore its meaning in the context of society at large. 'If we focused our analysis on the school system we might see the child's behavior as symptomatic of some "dis-order" in the school or classroom situation, rather than symptomatic of an individual neurological disorder' (Conrad 1975).

Conrad concludes: 'medical social control may be the central issue, as in this role medicine becomes a de facto agent of the status quo'.

Wow! Heavy stuff! I hope I have not given you too much of a headache with this sociological analysis. Let us look at Peter Conrad's sources. He has carried out a very far-reaching literature review – going back over 50 years. And please note, those of you who have grown up not knowing a world without the interweb, that, in those days, all searches had to be done manually, there were no personal computers or internet available. What we can do now in a few minutes on our laptops or tablets, in those days took weeks or months of hard work. I think he is to be commended for his efforts and for the wide range of sources which he identified – including the political ones.

He was able to access sources from published academic papers, government reports, voluntary organisation reports, and newspaper reports. He was able to synthesise from these different sources and link that material to the sociological theory and literature of the day. He used statistics where appropriate and more general, qualitative data as well. This paper became a 'classic' example of a PA which examined *how a particular policy came to be*. This study formed his PhD work, so I guess he had the time to really get to grips with the issues.

Analysis of a Proposed Policy

This approach is widely used by politicians and public administrators (including health) to examine the likely outcomes of different policy options. A useful guide to the process involved in conducting a PA is provided in the US CDC (Centres for Disease

Control and Prevention, Office of the Associate Director for Policy and Strategy website on **www.cdc.gov/policy/polaris/policyprocess/policy_analysis.html**). You can Google it – it is intended as a guide for a prospective PA in the field of public health, but the same principles apply to any sphere. I shall use this as a 'gold standard' and go through their process in detail here. Although the CDC model is designed for a Public Health PA, it can generally be adapted and applied to *any* PA. Another approach is that presented by Beryl Radin (2019). She provides a list of 91 questions for policy analysts and a list of the necessary skills, which include:

> *Case study methods, Cost-benefit analysis, Ethical analysis, Evaluation, Futures analysis, Historical analysis, Implementation analysis, Interviewing, Legal analysis, Microeconomics, Negotiation, mediation, Operations research, Organizational analysis, Political feasibility analysis, Public speaking, Small-group facilitation, Specific program knowledge, Statistics, Survey research methods, Systems analysis*

> *(Radin 2019)*

Once you have identified the problem or the issue you need to deal with, you can then begin doing your PA. For example, in the recent COVID-19 pandemic, the overall problem was *how to minimise the spread of this disease and save lives.*

The CDC define a PA thus:

> *Policy Analysis is the process of identifying potential policy options that could address your problem and then comparing those options to choose the most effective, efficient, and feasible one.*

> *(CDC 2020)*

A thorough PA makes sure that you have *systematically* looked at different options to choose the best option for the problem being addressed. However, in the world of politics, a cynic might say that once a policy decision has been made by those in command, a PA might just be done as a justification for that policy choice – a form of 'rubber stamping' it.

As you can imagine, the sorts of options which had to be looked at in the COVID-19 pandemic included:

- Do we aim for **herd immunity** or not?
- Do we put limits or controls on people coming into or going out of the country?
- Do we put limits or controls on people mixing socially or travelling within the country?
- Do we close schools, colleges, and universities or otherwise limit contacts in them?
- Do we close workplaces – all or specific ones – or limit contacts in them?
- Do we make regulations about the wearing of protective equipment, such as masks, gowns, gloves, etc.?
- What evidence will inform any decisions about enacting controls or relaxing controls?
- Who are the 'experts' who can advise on best courses of actions?

- How do we deal with any people who are infected with the virus – or are suspected of being infected?
- How do we test for infections, immunity?
- Do we need to develop any new drugs or procedures to treat people who are infected?
- Do we need to develop any new immunisations or preventive treatments, and if so, who should be offered, or compelled, to have these?
- How do we change people's behaviour to the extent that our proposed measures work (inducements/penalties/enforcements)?

Each of these questions could require a policy decision in its own right, and all would have to be incorporated within a general policy. Thus, a series of PAs would have to take place to get the best solutions and the results coordinated by a person or group with overall powers and control of the process.

  a. The first step is to consider '*Who should be involved*?' The CDC suggest three groups of people.

    1. **Experts** who can make sense of the information gathered. These might be experts in the field/subject; economic specialists; community participants – all of whom might be able to provide the information needed and help to make sense of (interpret) that information.

    2. **People who are affected** by problems and any policies designed to deal with the problem. These might include members of the public (or their representatives) who may be affected. This could include local decision makers (e.g. from health, local authority, and voluntary services). They should be in a position to advise on how policies could affect their lives and provide social and cultural perspectives on the problem and its potential solutions. I think it is frightening to think that politicians could claim to be the representatives of the people and therefore are in a position to speak *for* the people – or as certain political viewpoints would hold, because they know better than the man and woman in the street, they are in a position to *tell them what they should think and what they should do!* Testing public opinion is one means of gathering evidence on what people think and want.

    3. **People who control resources** which may need to be engaged in helping to deal with the problem. They may be local, national, or international agencies who may have to authorise spending from their budgets or releasing other resources (including legislation). They should be able to understand the wider socio-economic context of the problem and be placed to be able to make informed decisions about allocations of resources.

  b. The next step is to conduct the PA.

    1. You have to **research and review** all available policy options.

    - **Conduct a literature review** to find out what is already known about the problem and existing alternatives which have been tried to deal with the problem. In doing this, look out for any gaps in the existing research.

    - **Conduct an 'environmental scan'** to collect information about the sort of things which might be encountered in the process.

2. Next, you need to **outline all of the different policy options** as you (and your team) see them. This involves addressing the *impact,* the *costs,* and the *feasibility* of every option. This will mean asking three types of questions.

   - **Who** will be affected by each option (the populations, groups, and sub-groups in society), and to what extent and at what points in time?
   - What are the **social, historical, cultural, and environmental contexts** within which the problem and the potential solutions are located?
   - What are the **costs and benefits** of each option? NB – make sure that appropriate specialists are involved in providing this information and making sense of it!

   In doing this, you have to constantly check on the **feasibility and acceptability** of your options. What factors might result in a failure of the proposed policy? For example, we have already seen from the chapter on Randomised Control Trials (Chapter 5) that trials of certain dietary interventions failed because the interventions were not acceptable to the groups being studied. So, will the proposed options fit the socio-cultural contexts within which they are proposed to be applied? Will they have to be adapted for various groups? And so on.

3. The third step is to put the different options into **order and choose** which one seems to you (and your advisors) to be the best. This will involve comparing the predicted benefits of each option, comparing the costs – both short-term and long term, and taking the feasibility or social acceptance into account. Then **rank them** in order on your criteria – in consultation with any 'experts' you have on hand to advise you – and see if there is one which stands out above all the rest. There usually is not, so you will have to weigh up the impact of any compromises you will have to make to ensure the greatest possible effect. Look for **feasibility, effects,** and **costs.** Hopefully this will help you to determine what you can and cannot do and what the limitations of your proposed policy will be.

   So, to check:

1. Have you done your background research to identify the best possible options, with literature reviews and environmental scans and taken examples of good practice into account?
2. Did you outline (honestly) each option's impact, costs, and feasibility?
3. Did you rank each policy option (honestly) according to their benefit, their costs, and their feasibility before choosing the best one?

If you have done all of these steps honestly and well, then you have done your job well – and you can sleep soundly in your bed at nights!

Have a look at the CDC website. Although its primary focus is on public health, which is very topical, it can be applied to any kind of PA.

A more critical view of PA is presented by Paul Cairney (2020) argues how unrealistic theoretical modelling can be when compared with the actuality of the real world (Table 16.1).

TABLE 16.1 Policy analysis in the ideal and 'real' world.

	'Rational' policy analysis	'Real world' policy analysis
Number of stakeholders	central government – few people	vague process, with many competing stakeholders and people with vested interests both within government and outside of it
Interpreting and applying lessons from 'the science'	it is straightforward to translate knowledge into practice	competing forces come in to play to shape the interpretation and use of the 'science'
Final solutions	agreement on one best solution	compromise between the different forces (pressure groups & public opinion) influencing policy makers
Ability to do the job	ideally a rational model such as a cost–benefit analysis (as discussed by Robinson et al. 2020) would be applied to shape decisions	lack of clarity in the logic and methods used to come to agree upon the final solution

Source: adapted from Paul Cairney (2020).

In truth, PA can be a very 'messy process'! For all of 1987 and 1988, I was involved in the co-ordination of joint planning between a health authority and a local authority in London. The central focus of my work was to develop appropriate strategies and policies for the implementation of community care. We did this for four main client groups: people with long-term physical disabilities; people with mental health problems; people with learning difficulties; and elderly people. The overall aim was to ensure that there was, as near as possible, seamless and comprehensive care and support from health services, local authority services, and independent (private and voluntary) services. One of the most time-consuming things was getting the working parties for all four client groups to develop and agree appropriate strategies (principles and action-plans) to meet the needs of their client groups and to get these plans approved by the relevant authorities. Then, in order to achieve the goals set out in the strategies, we had to make recommendations about future service developments. Let me tell you this – the task was like trying to herd wasps through a gate! But in the process we all learned a lot about having to develop policies which were robust – they were strong enough to face any challenges – and affordable – they had to fit within existing budgets and a small budget earmarked for joint planning projects. So, the consideration of alternatives and the future-gazing that was needed to do this work formed a formidable PA task. I wish I had known then what I know now. One of the things I learnt was that where there were existing sets of practices and allocations of resources in place, it was very difficult to develop an 'ideal' policy, because the investments in what already was were often too great to allow anything but minor tinkering with resources – both material and personnel – which are difficult to change or do away with. You need joint will for joint planning to work.

Example 2: School Closure and Management Practices during Coronavirus Outbreaks Including COVID-19: A Rapid Systematic Review

This is an example of a PA by a systematic review of the literature. As the title suggests, it was a 'rapid' one – of necessity. In March 2020, the UN Educational, Scientific, and Cultural Organization estimated that in 107 countries, school closures had been implemented as a measure to reduce the spread of COVID-19. As Viner et al. (2020) point out, 'School closures are based on evidence and assumptions from influenza outbreaks that they reduce social contacts between students and therefore interrupt the transmission.' However, there is also the possibility, as this research group suggest, that school closures can have a negative aspect in that they reduce the number of healthcare professionals (HCP) available to provide care for those who are sick (they have to stay at home to look after their own children). Previous research on school closures during influenza epidemics showed mixed results. For example, cases peaked again after schools re-opened. Also, the necessity for people to work from home could lessen the chances of exposure and transmission of the disease in the workplace. (There are also social-class differences in who can work from home – not many factory workers can take their assembly-lines home with them.) There are also some economic side-effects of closing schools.

The large-scale school closures which had taken place in so many countries by March 2020 were based upon data from influenza epidemics, but there was a lack of evidence for the effectiveness of this policy during the COVID-19 pandemic. So, the authors conducted a review of the available published evidence to answer their question: 'What is known about the use of and effectiveness and cost-effectiveness of school closure and other school social distancing practices on infection rates and transmission during coronavirus outbreaks?'

Methods

They included **quantitative** studies which evaluated the effects of school closures and other social distancing measures in schools on infection rates and transmission of coronavirus. They searched three electronic databases – PubMed, the WHO Global Research Database, and medRxiv in March 2020. All the articles were screened by three members of the team. They excluded 'opinion pieces, systematic reviews, studies addressing other viruses, university-specific settings, epidemiological studies not examining intervention effects (e.g., of prevalence of infection in schools), and studies in other languages with no English translation'. All of the full-text articles were reviewed by Viner. They searched the references and the citation-chains for additional research. Their search threw up 616 articles; 548 were rejected following the review of their titles and abstracts; 68 were assessed and 54 were excluded; and the hand search of references found another two articles. This resulted in 16 articles for review – all published articles related to the 2003 SARS outbreak; five preprints and one report related to the COVID-19 pandemic.

Results

Pre-print reports found that in Hong Kong, school closures and other *'stringent social distancing measures'* were thought to have reduced the transmission rate 'R' to below 1 – controlling the spread of the virus. No data were available in Hong Kong or in mainland China to allow for an assessment of the degree of the *impact of school closures alone* on the spread of COVID-19.

Studies of the effects of school closures in mainland China during the SARS epidemic of 2003 'added little to control of the outbreak'. In Singapore in 2003, there was no evidence of an effect of school closures.

> *A preprint study by Jackson (2020) and colleagues used routine viral surveillance to examine the effects on transmission of endemic human coronaviruses (229E, NL63, OC43, and HKU1) and other viruses of a 5-day closure of nearly all schools in the greater Seattle metropolitan area in February, 2019, due to extreme weather on transmission of these viruses. Their study estimated that the school closure resulted in a 5·6% (95% CI 4·1–6·9) reduction in coronavirus infections, similar to influenza H1N1 (7·6%; 5·2–9·7) but higher than influenza H3N2 (3·1%; 2·5–3·2), all of which were prevalent at the time.*

> *(Viner et al. 2020)*

One study looked at school closures alone – Ferguson et al. (2020), who used **modelling** to estimate the effects of social distancing measures.

> *They used UK population and schools data together with data on transmission dynamics reported from the COVID-19 outbreak in Wuhan. Using data from previous influenza outbreaks, they assumed that per-capita contacts within schools were double those in households, workplaces, or the community, and that, overall, approximately a third of transmission occurred in schools. They modelled a scenario in which all schools and 25% of universities were closed and where the effect on non-school social contacts was an increase of 50% in household contact rates for families with children and a 25% increase in community contacts during the closure. They concluded that school closure as an isolated measure was predicted to reduce total deaths by around 2–4% during a COVID-19 outbreak in the UK, whereas single measures such as case isolation would be more effective, and a combination of measures would be the most effective. The authors concluded that school closure is predicted to be insufficient to mitigate (never mind suppress) the COVID-19 pandemic in isolation, which is in contrast to seasonal influenza epidemics where children are the key drivers of transmission.*

> *(Viner et al. 2020)*

Another modelling study from Taiwan, of SARS transmission, concluded that 'a single case of SARS would infect an average of 2.6 secondary cases in a population from transmission in hospital, whereas less than 1 secondary infection would be generated per case in a school classroom' (Viner et al. 2020).

One **qualitative** study of HCPs in Canada highlighted the dilemmas faced by HCPs in balancing demands from family and work especially childcare when schools are closed. This study concluded that 'there was a need for provision of adequate resources to protect the families of health-care workers during outbreaks to maintain maximal staffing' (Viner et al. 2020).

> *Social and organizational supports are critical to help buffer the effects of stress for nurses and assist them in managing difficult role conflicts during infectious disease outbreaks. These supports are necessary to improve response capacity for bio-disasters.*
>
> *(O'Sullivan et al. 2009)*

In the results, *only the modelling studies* suggested positive impacts of school closures. The researchers concluded:

> *Currently, the evidence to support national closure of schools to combat COVID-19 is very weak and data from influenza outbreaks suggest that school closures could have relatively small effects on a virus with COVID-19's high transmissibility and apparent low clinical effect on school children. At the same time, these data also show that school closures can have profound economic and social consequences.*
>
> *More research is urgently needed on the effectiveness of school closures and other school social distancing practices to inform policies related to COVID-19.*
>
> *(Viner et al. 2020)*

So, the jury is still out as far as school closures are concerned. This analysis shows one of the problems which cause dilemmas for policy makers. 'What do you do when there is no evidence or there is very poor evidence to guide your decision?'

I know what I think of policy analyses based upon modelling – I do not think they are of any worth *unless* the assumptions upon which they are based are logical and robust; and unless they are conducted by people with no vested interests in possible outcomes.

To Sum Up

Policy analyses can analyse an existing policy with the goal of examining in detail what the effects of that policy have been. These are **retrospective policy analyses** which look at policies which have already been implemented and help to explain why these policies came to be. They are useful for helping us to answer questions such as 'How did this policy come into being?', 'Who were the interested parties (stakeholders), and what were their parts in influencing policy decisions?', and 'Who was to gain or benefit from the new policy?' Peter Conrad showed how his wide-ranging analysis of how 'difficult' behaviour in children was medicalised to become a medical entity – a

---

EXERCISE

At this point, take a break and do a bit of searching to find out how your government did in developing its policies to combat the COVID-19 pandemic. Google freely! Search for academic publications as well as other reports and policy papers. Look at:

- How well have they defined the issue or problem?
- Who has been involved in the development of the analysis and who has been left out?
- What background research have they done and how well have they analysed the results?
- What factors have been explicitly taken into account – or omitted?
- What options have been identified and are there any options which have not been considered?
- How sound is the rationale for their conclusions?
- Can you think of alternatives that have not been considered?

My guess is that you will soon identify another factor to be taken into account – **political expediency.** To what extent do the different policy options fit in with the **political will** and the **political situations** of those making the policy decisions?

---

dis-ease – which was suitable for treatment by medications. He very clearly showed the parts played by different stakeholders in that process. Policy analyses can also be used to analyse a proposed policy to predict what the likely effects of the policy – these are **prospective policy analyses.** The sort of questions these are useful for getting answers to are: 'How likely is this policy to achieve the results we want?' and 'What sorts of other consequences might there be from implementing our policy?' In doing this, some of our data are likely to be **quantifiable** (numbers) and some of our data are likely to be **qualitative** (no numbers). They can be both **hypothetico-deductive** or **hypothetico-inductive.**

References

Ahraham J. (2010). Pharmaceuticalization of society in context: theoretical, empirical and health dimensions. *Sociology* 44(4), 603–622.

Becker HS. (1963). *Outsiders: Studies in the Sociology of Deviance.* The Free Press: New York.

Bradley C. (1937). The behaviour of children receiving Benzedrine. *American Journal of Psychiatry* 94, 577–585.

Cairney P. (2020). The Coronavirus and evidence-informed policy analysis. Available at: https://paulcairney.wordpress.com/2020/03/15/the-coronavirus-and-evidence-informed-policy-analysis-long-version/ (accessed 12 March 2021).

CDC (2020). *Policy Analysis.* Available at: www.cdc.gov/policy/polaris/policyprocess/policy_analysis.html (accessed 4 September 2020).

Chorover SL. (1973). Big brother and psychotechnology. *Psychology Today* pp. 43–54.

Conrad P. (1972). Ideological deviance: An analysis of the Soviet use of mental hospitals for political dissenters. (Unpublished manuscript.).

TABLE 17.2   **Difficulties experienced as a result of dyslexia, by gender.**

	Gender		
	Males	**Females**	**All**
Difficulty	%	%	%
Inability to retain spoken information, e.g. lectures.	32	53	46
Poor spelling	68	57	61
Difficulty reading out loud	32	43	39
Slow reading speed	77	66	70
Difficulty understanding spoken information	18	17	17
Poor attention span	36	34	35
Difficulty reading from screens	23	43	36
Slow writing speed	50	40	43
Taking longer than others to grasp concepts	23	40	35
Difficulty with calculations	14	34	28
Difficulty absorbing spoken information in lectures	36	45	42
Easily distracted by noises and other people	32	51	45
Struggling with written material	32	32	32
Struggling to commit things to paper – e.g. sentences not phrased as intended	50	45	46
Struggling to articulate thoughts accurately onto paper	55	53	54
Missing out or repeating words when writing things	27	49	42
Unable to learn from lectures and any other forms of teaching – in any circumstances	5	15	12
Problems with revising or working with distractions	41	53	49
Confusion with 'left' and 'right'	9	60	43
Poor spatial awareness	0	28	19
Thinking differently to other people	45	26	32
Difficulty reading black text on a white background	9	21	17
Difficulty reading certain fonts	14	6	9
Difficulty remembering information given over the phone	18	36	30
Struggling to understand and operate computers	5	9	7
Struggling to understand written questions in exams	32	19	23
N (= 100%)*	23	52	75

* NB – these are the total numbers in the sample but the actual totals answering each question may vary.
(*Source*: Anderson & Shaw, 2020)

TABLE 17.3 Effects of dyslexia whilst at medical school by gender.

Effect of dyslexia:	At medical school:			At/since foundation school:		
	Gender			Gender		
	Male	Female	All	Male	Female	All
Shame	48	59	55	28	63	52
Inadequacy	53	89	77	50	72	66
Depression	19	47	38	6	37	28
Anxiety	38	73	62	33	70	59
Isolation	24	45	38	17	37	31
Feeling stupid	71	84	80	44	84	72
Bullying/ridicule from peers	24	23	23	11	31	25
Bullying/ridicule from Teachers	10	19	16	6	17	13
Bullying/ridicule from clinical teachers in practice	14	37	30	6	31	23
Issues of disclosure	14	57	43	6	45	33
N (=100%)[a]	23	52	75	23	52	75

[a] NB – these are the total numbers in the sample but the actual totals answering each question may vary.
(*Source*: Anderson & Shaw, 2020)

Example 2: An Experiment to Examine T2DM Decision Making

In Chapter 3, I presented this work as an example of a 'Real-Life Experiment' (McKinlay et al. 2012). Now I want to show you how the programme if research it came from was a multi-stage approach using mixed methods – a survey and an experiment.

The Survey

To investigate the size and distribution of undiagnosed Type 2 Diabetes Mellitus (T2DM) in the community, the authors designed and conducted a random sample survey in the general population in the Boston area – The Boston Area Community Health (BACH) Survey. This was an epidemiological survey of Boston residents aged between 30 and 79 years. A 'stratified two-stage cluster sample was used to recruit residents of Boston with approximately equal numbers of participants by gender, race/ethnicity (non-Hispanic black, Hispanic, non-Hispanic white), and age group (30–39, 40–49, 50–59, 60–79)'. Altogether, 5503 adults participated (1767 black, 1877 Hispanic, 1859 white, 2301 men, and 3202 women) – a response rate of 63.3% of eligible participants. Anyone who reported five of the six cardinal symptoms – fatigue; being overweight; frequent urination; thirst; not feeling well; hypertension – was considered to be highly likely to have undiagnosed T2DM' (McKinley, Marceau & Piccolo, 2012)

This part of the study showed 'no significant race/ethnic differences in the prevalence of undiagnosed signs and symptoms indicative of diabetes within any socioeconomic level. But there were significant differences between people in different socioeconomic levels - and these were consistent within each race/ethnic category.' So – *no racial/ethnic differences* in the prevalence of T2DM, but there were differences according to *socio-economic status*. This was an important finding because it was generally held, until then, that T2DM was more prevalent among people from ethnic minorities.

The Experiment

In the experimental part of the study, they used video scenarios of real clinical cases, with professional actors and actresses trained to realistically simulate a 'patient' presenting to a primary care doctor. There were 24 identical versions of the clinical scenario. These varied only with the patients' age, gender, socio-economic status, and race. The vignettes simulated an initial consultation of 5–7 minutes.

The 'subjects' were 192 primary care doctors who viewed the vignettes and were asked to give the most likely diagnosis and their degree of certainty. They were then interviewed and asked to say how they would manage the case in their practice.

Their results showed that doctors were significantly more likely to diagnose diabetes in the black and the Hispanic 'patients'. Almost three-quarters (73.4%), of the physicians' diagnosed T2DM when the 'patient' was black, two-fifths (60.9%) when Hispanic, and half (48.4%) when white ($p = 0.009$) – when fully adjusted for the 'patient's' age, gender, and SES. The percentage of physicians giving a diabetes diagnosis was not significantly different for lower SES patients than for upper SES patients. In other words, *in making an initial diagnosis, physicians focus more on the 'patient's' race/ethnicity rather than their SES*. They concluded:

> 'this paper suggests that the signs and symptoms of T2DM, when undiagnosed in the general community, are patterned by SES and not race/ethnicity and that following diagnosis by a physician they are patterned by race/ethnicity'.
>
> (McKinley, Marceau & Piccolo, 2012)

This is a good example of a research programme using one method - a **survey** to get data on the 'real' distribution of a problem – T2DM – in the community, and then the researchers followed that by using another method – an **experiment** to show how clinicians responded to that problem – and, by conforming to stereotypes, got it wrong!

To Sum Up

I hope that in this chapter I have given you some insight into the ways in which a mixed methods approach, using qualitative and quantitative methods, and different types of quantitative methods, can really complement each other and, together, provide a much fuller picture of an issue than one approach on its own. In the studies that Seb and I did, the first (qualitative) level was mainly **hypothetico-inductive** – we were not sure about what to expect. Those results provided valuable new insights into the everyday world of the medical student and junior doctor with dyslexia MSWD and JDWD), but they still left the reader with the question of 'how many experienced that?' This led on naturally to the **quantitative** enquiry of our online survey. The initial data helped us to identify the themes and the ranges of experiences of MSWD and JDWD and to incorporate these into a quantitative questionnaire which was **hypothetico-deductive**. NB there were no 'validated questionnaires' available to use, so we had to develop our own (in the same way that in the 'Life Before Death' study we used pilot studies to identify the issues and questions which were then incorporated into the final 23-page, highly-structured questionnaire. (This is an example of a **pragmatist** approach in research – you do what you need to do to get the research done!) The results were stunning – as you can see from the tables above.

John McKinley and his colleagues also developed their own measures to be used alongside previously validated measures for the survey part of this programme, and then they conducted a '**controlled factorial experiment**' to examine the influence of social class and race on the diagnostic and treatment decisions made by doctors. Both of these methodologies were quantitative, **hypothetico-deductive** approaches, but the mix of a survey approach with an experiment was an innovative mix of methods. Thus, the Boston Area Community Health Survey was able to demonstrate that Type 2 Diabetes Mellitus differs by socioeconomic status, but not by race/ethnicity, whilst the experiment showed that doctors' decision-making about diagnosis and treatment was patterned by race/ethnicity, but not by socioeconomic status. The two studies, using different approaches, formed a perfect match of methods to prove two different points within the same programme of research – this first prepared the ground for the second.

Research is the Art of the Possible!

References

Anderson JL and Shaw SCK (2020). The experiences of medical students and junior doctors with dyslexia: a survey study. *International Journal of Social Sciences & Educational Studies* 7(1), 62–71.

John BM, Lisa DM, and Rebecca JP. (2012). Do doctors contribute to the social patterning of disease? The case of race/ethnic disparities in diabetes mellitus. *Medical Care Research and Review* 69(2), 176–193.

Shaw SCK and Anderson JL. (2018). The experiences of medical students with dyslexia: an interpretive phenomenological study. *Dyslexia* 1–14.

Shaw SCK, Anderson JL, and Grant AJ. (2016). Studying medicine with dyslexia: a collaborative autoethnography. *The Qualitative Report* 21(11; Article 2), 2036–2054.

Shaw SCK, Malik M, and Anderson JL. (2017). The exam performance of medical students with dyslexia: a review of the literature. *MedEdPublish* doi:10.15694/mep.2017.000116.

CHAPTER 18

Research Ethics and Governance

The Need for Regulation

Introduction

In this section, we shall consider issues related to **research ethics** and **governance**. I shall give you examples of why we now have such strict controls over research by considering examples of past abuses and what **international regulations** there are to 'regulate' research in medicine and healthcare.

We all know what *research* is – it is about getting answers to questions. **Research ethics** are the set of **moral principles** which guide our research practices at any point in time. **Research governance** refers to the **organisational arrangements** for the scrutiny, approval, and promotion of good practice in research. So, research ethics are the *principles which guide how we do research* and research governance is about the *means by which we regulate research*.

Note that these change over time and there are variations between countries. When I first started working at the Middlesex Hospital Medical School in 1972, I asked John Hinton, my professor and boss, about getting ethical approval for the breast cancer study which Ted Chesser and I were doing. He informed me that ethical approval was usually only necessary when the body's surface was breached in some way, or when there was an intervention of some medical or surgical nature – so, as long as your study did not involve injections, taking tissue samples, or any treatments, then ethical approval was not strictly necessary. But John said he would have a word with the Chairman of the Ethics Committee the next time he saw him at lunch, just to alert him that the study was being done. We got the nod – literally. Changed days!

Demystifying Research for Medical & Healthcare Students: An Essential Guide, First Edition. John L. Anderson.
© 2022 John Wiley & Sons Ltd. Published 2022 by John Wiley & Sons Ltd.
Companion website: www.wiley.com/go/Anderson/DemystifyingResearch

Guiding Principles

According to my students, getting research ethics approvals is now seen as a long and complicated process, which is generally regarded as unhelpful rather than helpful, and which is very time-consuming. Apart from the 'S-word' (**statistics**), the two names which have inspired my students with fear and loathing over the past 10 or more years have been **ethics committees** and **research and development departments.** Let's have a look at why research and, in particular, medical research, has acquired a bad reputation over the years and why so much control is deemed necessary for its scrutiny and control.

But first, I want to give you a quick overview about some of our main guiding principles when doing research.

The Belmont Report (1979) defined three major areas of basic ethical principles. These were:

1. *'Respect for persons' – Respect for persons incorporates at least two ethical convictions: first, that individuals should be treated as* **autonomous agents***, and second, that persons with diminished autonomy are entitled to* **protection.** *The principle of respect for persons thus divides into two separate moral requirements: the requirement to acknowledge autonomy and the requirement to protect those with diminished autonomy.*

2. *'Beneficence' – Persons are treated in an ethical manner not only by respecting their decisions and protecting them from harm, but also by making efforts to secure their well-being. Such treatment falls under the principle of beneficence. The term 'beneficence is often understood to cover acts of kindness or charity that go beyond strict obligation. In this document, beneficence is understood in a stronger sense, as an obligation. Two general rules have been formulated as complementary expressions of beneficent actions in this sense: (1)* **do no harm** *and (2)* **maximize possible benefits** *and minimize possible harms'.*

3. *'Justice' – Who ought to receive the benefits of research and bear its burdens? This is a question of justice, in the sense of* **fairness in distribution** *or 'what is deserved'. An injustice occurs when some benefit to which a person is entitled is denied without good reason or when some burden is imposed unduly. Another way of conceiving the principle of justice is that equals ought to be treated equally. However, this statement requires explication. Who is equal and who is unequal? What considerations justify departure from equal distribution? Almost all commentators allow that distinctions based on experience, age, deprivation, competence, merit, and position do sometimes constitute criteria justifying differential treatment for certain purposes. It is necessary, then, to explain in what respects people should be treated equally. There are several widely accepted formulations of just ways to distribute burdens and benefits. Each formulation mentions some relevant property on the basis of which burdens and benefits should be distributed. These formulations are: (i) to each person an equal share, (ii) to each person according to individual need, (iii) to each person according to individual effort, (iv) to each person according to societal contribution, and (v) to each person according to merit.*

   (USA – The Belmont Report, 1979)

OK, first, let's consider why there is such concern over the governance of research. What has led to the situation we are in now?

Past Abuses in Research

Let's Start at World War II

In Nazi-occupied territories, a whole catalogue of atrocities were being conducted in the name of medical research. These tend to be more well-known than the Japanese abuses. It was in keeping with the Nazi's campaign to 'cleanse' Germany of 'racially impure' persons. Perhaps the most well-known are Josef Mengele's experiments on twins at Auschwitz concentration camp. He was known as the 'Angel of Death' or the 'White Angel'. He performed brutal, agonising, and lethal experiments on Jewish and Gypsy (Roma) twins. The operations he performed were without anaesthetic. He collected the eyes of his murdered victims as part of his research to find out about eye colour and how to change it. After the war, he escaped to Argentina, then to Paraguay and Brazil, where he died in 1979.

Many experiments used concentration camp prisoners in research aimed at finding ways of helping military personnel survive. At Dachau concentration camp, their **altitude research** used prisoners to find out how high you could parachute to safety from. The infamous **freezing experiments** used prisoners taken kicking and screaming to a room with a bath filled with water and ice. They were forcibly immersed in it to measure their physiological responses and their survival – or not. Prisoners were also used to test the effects of different **diseases** – like TB, typhoid, malaria, and yellow fever – and the effects of exposure to x-rays. Various **poisons**, including phosgene gas and mustard gas, were tested on prisoners.

At the **Nuremberg war crimes trials** there were also trials of some of the doctors involved – the **Doctors' Trial.** As a result of these trials the **Nuremberg Code** was established, the central feature of which was 'voluntariness'.

These are a series of examples of **'not like us'**. German, Aryan doctors exploited non-Aryans and non-Germans as their guinea pigs. Japanese doctors and military were also involved in some unspeakable experiments – see Harris (1994).

The Tuskegee and Guatemala Syphilis Studies

In the 1960s a researcher in the USA – Peter Buxton – found out about the **Tuskegee Experiment** and complained to his bosses about it. A brief investigation concluded that the study should continue until all the participants died and the data could be analysed. It was not until 1972 that a reporter broke the news and the study was shut down. It transpired that the study had begun in 1932 in Tuskegee in Alabama by the US Public Health Service. They distributed leaflets advertising 'Free Blood Test; Free Treatment, By County Health Department and Government Doctors . . . "YOU MAY FEEL WELL AND STILL HAVE BAD BLOOD. COME AND BRING ALL YOUR FAMILY"' (*Washington Post* 2017). As a result, 600 men, mostly poor sharecroppers, signed up for the study in return for promises of free meals, free healthcare, and free burial insurance. They were told that they were being treated for 'bad blood'. This term covered a variety of illnesses. Most, 399, had latent syphilis while 201 did not have the disease.

These men were followed up over the years and were informed that there was no treatment for syphilis – even when penicillin became available as a treatment for the disease in 1947. They were given placebos (aspirin and minerals) but no active treatments even when they went blind, insane, died, or had other health issues as a result of their untreated disease. By the time the study was closed down, 28 men had died of the disease and many more had died from complications of the disease.

What do you think of this 'study'? For a fuller account of it see Fred Gray's book (Gray, 1998).

I think, to use President Trump's phrase, 'It's bad, it's very bad'.

But, what makes it worse, is that the predominantly white trial doctors had recruited only **black males** to the study. So not only was it immoral, it was racist and it exploited a poor group in the community.

In 1973, the US Congress held hearings on these experiments and awarded participants or their heirs a $10 million settlement. They also issued new guidelines to protect participants in US government-funded research – the National Research Act, 1974.

On May 16, 1997, President Bill Clinton issued an apology to the eight remaining survivors of the experiment:

'The United States government did something that was wrong – deeply, profoundly, morally wrong', Clinton said. 'It was an outrage to our commitment to integrity and equality for all our citizens. To the survivors, to the wives and family members, the children and the grandchildren, I say what you know: No power on Earth can give you back the lives lost, the pain suffered, the years of internal torment and anguish. What was done cannot be undone. But we can end the silence. We can stop turning our heads away. We can look at you in the eye and finally say on behalf of the American people, what the United States government did was shameful, and I am sorry'.

(Brown, 2017)

Again, an example of 'not like us' abusive research.

Guatemala Syphilis Experiments

From 1946 to 1948, US researchers led by Dr John Cutler of the US Public Health Service, conducted a series of studies on Sexually Transmitted Diseases **STDs**) in **Guatemala**. In one study: 'Instead of conducting a long-term randomized clinical trial – which would have required more participants, time, and funding – the researchers **intentionally** exposed over 1,300 sex workers, soldiers, prisoners, and psychiatric patients to STDs to test the effectiveness of their prophylactic intervention. After exposure to STDs, only **about half** of the subjects received any form of treatment for infection. There are no records indicating that consent was obtained from the participants, and there is evidence that some were, in fact, deceived. In addition, 83 subjects died during the experiments, although the connection between the deaths and involvement in the experiments is unclear' (Spector-Bagdady and Lombardo 2019).

Another example of 'not like us' abusive research.

Drug Testing in the Third World

The Pill: "The first real large-scale trial of the pill was conducted in 1956 in Rio Pié-dras, a Puerto Rican housing project. The 200-plus women involved in the trial received little information about the safety of the product they were given, as there was none to give, and no one thought that it might be necessary to provide such information. That was the standard of the day. Women who stepped forward to describe side effects of nausea, dizziness, headaches, and blood clots were discounted as 'unreliable historians'. Despite the substantial positive effect of the pill, 'its history is marked by a lack of consent, a lack of full disclosure, a lack of true informed choice, and a lack of clinically relevant research regarding risk. These are the pill's cautionary tales' (Liao 2012).

Yet another example of 'not like us' abusive research.

Generally

There has been something of a 'tradition' of drugs testing in poorer counties – in Africa, Central America, and in Asia. In many Third World countries, there is more obvious corruption, so, it is easier to bribe the necessary officials to get permissions to conduct trials and for pharmaceutical companies to do what they please. It is also easier to convince poorer 'native' people that trials are really treatments which are for their benefit. But, crucially, it is more difficult for poor people in other countries to sue the researchers who may be based in the USA and/or Europe.

In the same way that it is cheaper to mass produce goods in poorer countries in the developing world, it is cheaper and less risky to conduct drug trials in these countries rather than in the USA and Europe where a relatively well-educated population has the knowledge and access to legal systems which can allow them to sue. Often corruption is cited as enabling such illegal trials, but the days of the hundred-dollar bill tucked into a document have been superseded both in sophistication and dimension. See Sonia Shah's award-winning book *The Body Hunters: Testing New Drugs on the World's Poorest Patients* (Shah, 2006) for more background on this. She points out that up to 80% of patients recruited to drug trials in in some developing countries are not told details of the study they are taking part in. Many don't feel able to quit the trials, in case they or their children forfeit treatment as a result (Shah, 2006).

You can imagine just how easy it is for modern Western doctors to appear in a poor part of the world and offer to treat some of the diseases that people there suffered from.

1. If people are harmed by side effects of an experimental medicine, you can imagine how easy it is for the doctor to say 'Sorry, the treatment didn't work'.
2. How can a poor, peasant farmer tell if that doctor is telling the truth or not?
3. Even if that poor person realised there was something wrong with the 'treatment', who could they turn to for help?
4. If they sought help and were told they could sue the doctor, how could they afford the legal costs?
5. If they could afford legal costs, how difficult would it be to sue someone who is in another country altogether?
6. Etc., etc.

The world is – or was – ripe for exploitation. Some of you may have read John le Carre's book *The Constant Gardner* – or seen the film based on the book. It tells the story of a young embassy official in Africa (played in the film by Ralph Fiennes), whose wife, who was involved in charity work, was found murdered. This man spends the rest of the story trying to find out what happened to his wife. In the process, he learns that she was an Amnesty International activist. He is initially assured by a Foreign Office official (played by one of my favourite actors, Bill Nighy) that he would get the full support of the FO. However, as he continues his quest and runs into the activities of a drug company using local people to test a TB drug, he is threatened and told to back off; but he persists . . . And if you want to know any more, you will have to read the book or see the film! The story is vaguely based upon a true case in Nigeria. I like le Carre's works. Like many of my favourite authors he really does his research into his topic. That is why I found le Carre's postscript so chilling. He wrote:

> But let me tell you this. As my journey through the pharmaceutical jungle progressed, I came to realise that, by comparison with the reality, my story was tame as a holiday postcard.
>
> *(Le Carre 2001, p. 490)*

There is much published about the exploitation of Developing or Third World countries by pharmaceutical multinationals and about other ways in which results of drug trials have been misrepresented and exaggerated. Read Ben Godacre's bestselling book *Bad Pharma: How Medicine is Broken, and How We Can Fix It*. He cites the source of le Carre's story as being in Kano in Nigeria (Goldacre 2013). Another awful example of 'not like us'.

Clinical Trials (Phase I Trials)

You saw earlier when I gave an example of the work I was involved in looking at Phase I trials in the UK that the issue of informed consent was the main issue. It is not only in developing countries that doctors have been accused of misleading trial participants into believing that they were receiving treatment when they were, in fact, taking part in a drug trial – a **therapeutic misconception.**

> Therapeutic misconception implies that patients are motivated to join P1 trials because they have misunderstood the primary aims of such trials and believe the novel drugs are a treatment from which they will derive benefit. This calls into question the validity of the informed consent and by default the communication skills of the clinician during P1 trial discussions.
>
> *(Jenkins et al. 2010)*

Which raises the question of the intent of the trial doctor who said:

> One of the things we do is test new drugs that are coming out of the laboratory and are being used for the first time . . . the attraction obviously is to try and get hold of drugs that might be the standard chemotherapies of the future . . . So

that what we can offer here is treatment that isn't otherwise available, largely by the drugs not being in wide circulation . . . Erm and the possibility therefore of having the opportunity to try [and] deal with the tumour in the same way that your previous drugs . . . have done . . . (mentions caveats) . . . it's still the route if you like to get state of the art medication, and see whether it is something that might benefit you.

(Anderson and Ballinger 2008)

Falsification in Research

There are constant examples of 'falsification' in the reporting of drug research. For example, the Swiss company Novartis was involved in a scandal over claims that falsified data was used to exaggerate the benefits of a blood-pressure drug.

Novartis Japan unit charged over research manipulation

Japanese prosecutors Tuesday laid charges against the local unit of Swiss pharmaceutical giant Novartis in a widening scandal over claims that falsified data were used to exaggerate the benefits of a popular blood-pressure drug.

Prosecutors also indicted former employee Nobuo Shirahashi, 63, alleging he manipulated the data in clinical studies that were later used in marketing the drug Valsartan.

The dual charges laid by the Tokyo District Public Prosecutor's Office – which allege that Novartis bore responsibility for Shirahashi's actions – came several weeks after he was first arrested and authorities raided the offices of Novartis Pharma KK in the Japanese capital.

The drug studies suggested Valsartan – sold under the brand name Diovan in Japan, and licensed for use in more than 100 countries – could help prevent strokes and angina, in addition to its acknowledged benefits in combating blood pressure.

The firm used data from those studies to market its drug, playing up its supposed additional benefits.

'We take the arrest of our former employee and the indictment of our company very seriously', the unit said in a statement on its website.

'We deeply apologise to patients, their families and medical workers as well as Japanese people for causing these concerns and trouble', it added.

The pharmaceutical giant's Japan unit has also been embroiled in another scandal over allegations it did not properly disclose the possible side effects of leukaemia treatments.

In April, Novartis replaced the top executives at its Japanese arm over those allegations.

(Medical Xpress July 1, 2014)

In a critique of another group's research, Darrel Francis of Imperial College, London writes:

> *Amongst 48 reports from the group, there appeared to be 5 actual clinical studies ('families' of reports). Duplicate or overlapping reports were common, with contradictory experimental design, recruitment and results. Readers cannot always tell whether a study is randomised versus not, open-controlled or blinded placebo-controlled, or lacking a control group. There were conflicts in recruitment dates, criteria, sample sizes, million-fold differences in cell counts, sex reclassification, fractional numbers of patients and conflation of competitors' studies with authors' own. Contradictory results were also common. These included arithmetical miscalculations, statistical errors, suppression of significant changes, exaggerated description of own findings, possible silent patient deletions, fractional numbers of coronary arteries, identical results with contradictory sample sizes, contradictory results with identical sample sizes, misrepresented survival graphs and a patient with a negative NYHA class. We tabulate over 200 discrepancies amongst the reports.*
>
> *(Francis et al. 2013)*

Corruption in research? Not in our time???

In 2012, Jefferson et al. published a *Cochrane Review* of 50 trials of **influenza vaccines.** They concluded that 'Influenza vaccines have a modest effect in reducing influenza symptoms and working days lost. There is no evidence that they affect complications, such as pneumonia, or transmission' (Jefferson et al. 2012). The authors published a 'Warning' in their publication:

> *This review includes 15 out of 36 trials funded by industry (four had no funding declaration). An earlier systematic review of 274 influenza vaccine studies published up to 2007 found industry funded studies were published in more prestigious journals and cited more than other studies independently from methodological quality and size. Studies funded from public sources were significantly less likely to report conclusions favorable to the vaccines. The review showed that reliable evidence on influenza vaccines is thin but there is evidence of widespread manipulation of conclusions and spurious notoriety of the studies. The content and conclusions of this review should be interpreted in light of this finding.*
>
> *(Jefferson et al. 2012)*

This sort of criticism of industry-funded research is not new or unique. The authors noted widespread misrepresentation of the conclusions of studies. They also brought our attention to the fact that when manufacturers' studies do *not* show favourable results, they may be discarded.

We tend to expect our watchdogs, such as the UK the National Institute of Clinical Excellence (**NICE**), or in the USA, the Food and Drug Administration (**FDA**), to be fair and impartial. On 22 October 2014, BBC News's Adam Brimelow reported that a group of doctors and researchers had urged MPs to investigate 'potential conflicts of interest' within NICE. They were concerned about the recent decision by NICE to recommend the use of Statins (cholesterol-lowering drugs) to millions of people who were at *low risk* of developing heart disease. They pointed out that most of the experts on the NICE panel who made that recommendation had links with pharmaceutical companies. Dr Aseem Malhotra (a signatory to the letter to MPs) is outspoken over what he calls 'Too Much Medicine & The Great Statin Con'. In a presentation delivered at the Public Health Collaboration Conference in 2017 (and available as a video on **YouTube** – watch it – it is both informative and fun!), Dr Malhotra points to harmful side effects of statins (Malhotra 2017). He points out the financial incentives made to doctors to prescribe statins and other treatments and questions the necessity and efficacy of these and the reluctance of researchers to share their raw data about the benefits of statins. He denounces doctors who 'collude with industry for financial gain'. A survey of statin use in the USA found that 'Nearly 75% of new users discontinue their therapy by the end of the first year . . . More than six in ten respondents (62%) said they discontinued their statin due to side effects' (The Statin Usage Survey 2017).

'In conclusion, we believe that unless access to the raw clinical trial data is released, any claims about the true efficacy and harms of statins cannot be considered to be evidence based' (Malhotra et al., 2016).

A Swine Flu Conspiracy?

Do you remember the last pandemic scare? It was in 2009–2010 when the Director-General of WHO announced: 'On the basis of available evidence, and these expert assessments of the evidence, the scientific criteria for an influenza pandemic have been met . . . The world is now at the start of the 2009 influenza pandemic' (Chan 2009).

Cohen and Carter, in a collaboration by the *BMJ* and the Bureau of Investigative Journalism, London investigated the 'pandemic' and, in particular, WHO's response to it. They highlight the fact that some of the key scientists who advised WHO on planning for the 'pandemic' had received payments from the pharmaceutical companies who stood to make fortunes out of the results of their advice. They further point out that WHO have never given details of the conflicts of interests in its advisors and dismissed any enquiries into its handling of the 'pandemic' as 'conspiracy theories'. They point out that the culmination of this is that:

> *one year on, governments that took advice from WHO are unwinding their vaccine contracts, and billions of dollars' worth of stockpiled oseltamivir (Tamiflu) and zanamivir (Relenza) – bought from health budgets already under tight constraints – lie unused in warehouses around the world.*
>
> *(Cohen and Carter 2010)*

'Cock-up or conspiracy'? Meirion R. Evans, who declares a conflict of interest in the article as a member of the UK Scientific Pandemic Influenza Advisory Committee and the UK Scientific Advisory Group on Emergencies, wrote in the *Journal of Public Health* (Evans 2010) taking a softer stance in the editorial reviewing the 'pandemic':

> *So was swine flu a scam? Did the pharmaceutical industry manipulate a fake pandemic? Were the scientific experts, consciously or unconsciously, part of a conspiracy to promote anti-viral stockpiles and boost vaccine sales? Corporate*

influences on epidemiology have a long history. The tobacco industry has undertaken elaborate campaigns to undermine WHO activities on tobacco control in the past. More recently, the alcohol beverage industry and the food industry have come under scrutiny for possible attempts to influence public opinion, regulation and the conduct of science. But the swine flu affair smells more of cock-up than conspiracy.

(Evans 2010)

It is interesting that in the current COVID-19 pandemic, WHO is coming under a great deal of accusation and criticism – you can Google it if you are interested in such things.

Corruption in research? Not in our country!

Fraud in Research

Ranstam et al. in 2000 published their results of an international survey of biostatisticians in which they asked about their knowledge of and participation in 'fraud' in research. They suggested that 'fraud' was endemic both in scientific disciplines and in different countries. So, they set out to investigate fraud in medical research by conducting a survey of members of the International Society of Clinical Biostatistics (ISCB). They sent a questionnaire to all members of the ISCB and set up an online version, inviting members to participate. They had a response rate of 37% – 163 out of a total of 442 members, which was slightly disappointing. They defined 'fraud' as 'a deliberate attempt to mislead others in the design, conduct, analysis, or reporting of a study' – as opposed to carelessness or incompetence. Thus, poor methodology was excluded. Most, 76%, thought that 'career and power' were the main reasons behind fraud; 65% believed that fraud was a major problem in the progress of science; 51% admitted to knowing of at least one project nearby which was fraudulent; 31% had been involved in a project where fraud took place, and 13% said that they had been asked to support fraud (Ranstam et al. 2000).

In the magazine *What Doctors Don't Tell You* in September 2016, there was a feature on the widespread nature of 'fraud' in medical research. The editor, in his review of different types of falsification (or 'fraud') and the widespread nature of it, concluded that:

Fraud is the cancer at the heart of medicine. It's been estimated that up to 70 per cent of all medical research has been infected. It could be that the summary – which after all is often the only part of the research paper ever read – has been massaged to tell a different story from the one actually suggested by the results, or even that inconvenient data have gone missing, so altering the results and conclusions.

He cites Karmal Mahtani, director of the Centre for Evidence-Based Medicine, who referred to it as:

'unconscious prejudice', and it happens when results jar with the researcher's world view. It then matters more to the researcher that his beliefs about how the world operates are vindicated than it is to just report the findings as reflected by the data.

I could go on, but I'm sure you get the message.

International Regulations and General Principles

Following the **Nuremberg war crimes trials** in Germany after the end of the World War II, in August 1947, the Nuremberg Code was drawn up by judges in the infamous 'Doctors' Trial'. This Code set out for the first time in international circles, 10 principles to guide medical research. Shuster (1997) outlines the 10 points in the Code:

The Nuremberg Code

1. The voluntary consent of the human subject is absolutely essential. This means that the person involved should have legal capacity to give consent; should be so situated as to be able to exercise free power of choice, without the intervention of any element of force, fraud, deceit, duress, overreaching, or other ulterior form of constraint or coercion; and should have sufficient knowledge and comprehension of the elements of the subject matter involved as to enable him to make an understanding and enlightened decision. This latter element requires that before the acceptance of an affirmative decision by the experimental subject there should be made known to him the nature, duration, and purpose of the experiment; the method and means by which it is to be conducted; all inconveniences and hazards reasonably to be expected; and the effects upon his health or person which may possibly come from his participation in the experiment. The duty and responsibility for ascertaining the quality of the consent rests upon each individual who initiates, directs or engages in the experiment. It is a personal duty and responsibility which may not be delegated to another with impunity.

2. The experiment should be such as to yield fruitful results for the good of society, unprocurable by other methods or means of study, and not random and unnecessary in nature.

3. The experiment should be so designed and based on the results of animal experimentation and a knowledge of the natural history of the disease or other problem under study that the anticipated results will justify the performance of the experiment.

4. The experiment should be so conducted as to avoid all unnecessary physical and mental suffering and injury.

5. No experiment should be conducted where there is an a priori reason to believe that death or disabling injury will occur; except, perhaps, in those experiments where the experimental physicians also serve as subjects.

6. The degree of risk to be taken should never exceed that determined by the humanitarian importance of the problem to be solved by the experiment.

7. Proper preparations should be made and adequate facilities provided to protect the experimental subject against even remote possibilities of injury, disability, or death.

8. The experiment should be conducted only by scientifically qualified persons. The highest degree of skill and care should be required through all stages of the experiment of those who conduct or engage in the experiment.

9. During the course of the experiment the human subject should be at liberty to bring the experiment to an end if he has reached the physical or mental state where continuation of the experiment seems to him to be impossible.

10. During the course of the experiment the scientist in charge must be prepared to terminate the experiment at any stage, if he has probable cause to believe, in the exercise of the good faith, superior skill, and careful judgement required of him, that a continuation of the experiment is likely to result in injury, disability, or death to the experimental subject.

Source: (Shuster 1997)

Note that the concept of **voluntary consent** is central to the whole of the code, as is the notion **do no harm.** Shuster (1997) points out that, since its creation in 1947, the Nuremberg Code has **not been adopted in its entirety by any country as law**, nor by any major medical association. The notion of **informed consent** *has* been universally accepted as law by the United Nations.

It is concerning to note, as Shuster points out, that:

The World Medical Association, established during World War II, has been accused of purposely trying to undermine Nuremberg in order to distance physicians from Nazi medical crimes. The election of a former Nazi physician and SS member, Hans Joachim Sewering, to the presidency of that organization in 1992 added credibility to that accusation. (Because of public criticism, Sewering later withdrew.)

(Shuster 1997)

The Declaration of Helsinki

In 1964 the World Medical Association (WMA) at its 18th General Assembly in Helsinki, Finland, drew up and adopted what is now referred to as the **Declaration of Helsinki.** This has been amended or clarified in 1975, 1983, 1989, 1996, 2000, 2002, 2004, 2008 and the latest (to date) in 2013 (World Medical Association 2013). You can access this from the WMA website at: **www.wma.net/policies-post/wma-declaration-of-helsinki-ethical-principles-for-medical-research-involving-human-subjects**.

Again, like the Nuremberg Code, this is *not* legally binding under international law, but carries great weight from the fact that many countries, including the UK, actually use it as the cornerstone for their own sets of ethical and legal codes which govern medical research in their country. And that is what we shall turn to in the next chapter.

To Sum Up

In this chapter, I have tried to show you some of the unethical practices which have happened in the past – all of them in the last 100 years. Some of these were so repugnant – certainly by today's standards – that it is difficult to believe that human beings could be so terrible to other human beings, and all supposedly for the sake of medical science – or for profits! No country is free of guilt in this. Atrocities carried out in the name of medical research are global and span the whole history of medicine and healthcare – up to the present day. It has been the reaction to these events which has driven the regulation of research that we experience today – starting with the Nuremberg Code and leading up to the ever-evolving Declaration of Helsinki. We truly do *live in the shadow of our past.* So, whilst we may complain about over-restrictive regulations and practices, take a moment to reflect upon the reason why they are there. They are there to help protect those innocent persons who are noble enough to take part in healthcare research. And, to a lesser extent, they are there to prevent any well-meaning, but over-exuberant researchers going beyond reasonable boundaries to get the results they need.

References

Anderson JL and Ballinger RS. (2008). *Handling hopelessness –doctor -patient interactions in phase 1 oncology trials*. Paper presented at the BSA Medical Sociology Group Conference, 2008.

Brown DL. (2017). *You've got bad blood. Washington Post (16 May)*. Available at: HYPERLINK "http://www.washingtonpost.com/news/retropolis/wp/2017/05/16/youve-got-bad-blood-the-horror-of-the-tuskegee-syphilis-experiment" www.washingtonpost.com/news/retropolis/wp/2017/05/16/youve-got-bad-blood-the-horror-of-the-tuskegee-syphilis-experiment (accessed 10 September 2020).

Chan M. (2009). Cited in Cohen D & Carter P "WHO and the pandemic flu 'conspiracies'. *British Medical Journal* 340, c2912.

Cohen D and Carter P. (2010). WHO and the pandemic flu "conspiracies". *BMJ* 340, 1274–1279.

Evans MR. (2010). The swine flu scam? *Journal of Public Health* 32(3), 296–297.

Francis DP, Mielewczik M, Zargaran D, et al. (2013). Autologous bone marrow-derived stem cell therapy in heart disease: discrepancies and contradictions. *International Journal of Cardiology* 168(4), 3381–403.

Goldacre B. (2013.) *Bad Pharma: How Medicine Is Broken, and how we Can Fix it 4*. Harper Collins: London.

Gray FD. (1998). *The Tuskegee Syphilis Study: The Real Story and Beyond*. NewSouth Books: Montgomery, Alabama.

Harris SH. (1994). *Factories of Death: Japanese Biological Warfare, 1932–45, and the American Cover Up*. Routledge: London.

Health Research Authority (2020). *UK Policy Framework for Health and Social Care Research*. Available at HYPERLINK "http://www.hra.nhs.uk/planning-and-improving-research/policies-standards-legislation/uk-policy-framework-health-social-care-research" www.hra.nhs.uk/planning-and-improving-research/policies-standards-legislation/uk-policy-framework-health-social-care-research (accessed 18 September 2020).

Jefferson T, Rivetti A, Harnden A, et al. (2012). Vaccines for preventing influenza in healthy adults. *Cochrane Database of Systematic Reviews* 8, CD004879.

Jenkins VA, Anderson JL, and Fallowfield LJ. (2010). Communication and informed consent in phase 1 trials: a review of the literature from January 2005 to July 2009. *Support Care Cancer* 18, 1115–1121.

Le Carre J. (2001). *The Constant Gardner*. Hodder: London.

Liao PV. (2012). Half a century of the oral contraceptive pill historical review and view to the future. *Canadian Family Physician* 58, 757–760.

Malhotra A. (2017). *Too much medicine and the great statin con. Presentation delivered at the Public Health Collaboration Conference*, 2017.

Malhotra A, Abramson J, De Longeril M, et al. (2016). More clarity needed on the true benefits and risks of statins. *Prescriber* 27(12), 15–17.

Medical Xpress (2014). *Novartis Japan unit charged over research manipulation*. Available at https://medicalxpress.com/news/2014-07-novartis-japan.html (accessed 15 September 2020).

Ranstam J, Buyse M, George SL, et al. (2000). Fraud in medical research: an international survey of biostatisticians. *Controlled Clinical Trials* 21, 415–427.

Shah S. (2006). *The Body Hunters: Testing New Drugs on the World's Poorest Patients*. The New Press: New York.

Shuster E. (1997). Fifty years later: the significance of the Nuremberg code. *The New England Journal of Medicine* 337, 1436–1440.

Spector-Bagdady K and Lombardo PA. (2019). U.S. Public Health Service STD experiments in Guatemala (1946–1948) and their aftermath. *Ethics & Human Research* 41(2), 29–34.

The Statin Usage Survey (2017). *Understanding statin use in America and gaps in education*. Available at HYPERLINK "http://www.statinusage.com/Pages/about-the-survey.aspx" www.statinusage.com/Pages/about-the-survey.aspx (accessed 15 September 2020).

United States. (1978). The Belmont report: ethical principles and guidelines for the protection of human subjects of research. [Bethesda, Md.], The Commission.

World Medical Association (2013). WMA Declaration of Helsinki – Ethical Principles for Medical Research Involving Human Subjects. Available at https://www.wma.net/policies-post/wma-declaration-of-helsinki-ethical-principles-for-medical-research-involving-human-subjects (accessed 16 September 2020).

CHAPTER 19

Research Ethics and Governance

Regulations, Approvals, and Permissions

Introduction

In this chapter I shall discuss the issues involved in **regulations** governing research and the sorts of **permissions** you are likely to need for different kinds of research projects. I shall introduce you to some of the different research ethics committees in the UK and some of the processes you may have to go through to get the correct approvals for your study. As a basic principle, we should bear in mind that *people have a right not to be researched*.

It is important to bear in mind that almost all research projects should be subject to at least a basic level of research ethics scrutiny before you begin your study. If you are doing your study as a student, then you must always get approval from your college or university before you start your project, and, at this point, you are likely to be signposted to additional approvals you will require. For example, when I was co-ordinating our MSc students' research dissertations in the Department of Medical Education at the Brighton & Sussex Medical school, I chaired our Dissertation Panel which provided the first level of scrutiny for all the dissertation research projects. In addition to making sure that the projects were at the correct (Master's) level, that the proposals were clearly and logically set out and the methods proposed were appropriate for the research aims, we would try to signpost students to the appropriate regulatory bodies which might be necessary for approving their projects. These might include our **Medical School Research Governance and Ethics Committee (RGEC)** (which I served on for about 10 years); a **UK National Health Service Trust Research & Development Department (R&D)**; a **Health Research Authority (HRA) Ethics Committee;** an **Overseas Research Ethics Committee** (I used to be something of an expert as far as getting approvals from Nigerian RECs was concerned – and no! That did not mean I suggested slipping a $10000 dollar bill in with the application!); and other institutional approvals where necessary. But, please don't lose heart just yet, not

Demystifying Research for Medical & Healthcare Students: An Essential Guide, First Edition. John L. Anderson.
© 2022 John Wiley & Sons Ltd. Published 2022 by John Wiley & Sons Ltd.
Companion website: www.wiley.com/go/Anderson/DemystifyingResearch

all projects have to go through all of these steps, and they are not always obstructive, painful, or time-consuming. In principle, these should all be **facilitative** – that is, they are meant to *help* the research process by safeguarding both the researcher and the research participants, they are *not* meant to be unduly critical, obstructive, or block any project without good cause (even though some are!).

So, remember that *all* student research projects will require some form of **institutional approval** and should be **supervised** by an experienced researcher.

A **HOT TIP** here – always look for a supervisor who you feel you can get on with and someone who will be able to give you the time that you will need.

If you are not a student, then consider who else might wish to approve your study (in addition to an REC). Will your employer require you to seek their permission? The answer is almost certainly 'Yes' – especially if you are conducting your study in your employer's time, or in your employer's workplace. Even then, if you are doing this independently, but can be identified as an employee of 'X', then bear in mind that your employer may be concerned with **'reputational risk'**. That is, will your employer's reputation be at risk as a result of how you conduct that study or by the results which you publish? If there is a risk, then it is important that you inform them and get written confirmation that they are happy for you to do the study.

The Health Research Authority provides the following approvals and opinions for research studies. '**What approvals and decisions do I need**' in this section will help you understand what services you require and how to navigate and manage your application.

Before you begin your application and submit your project for approval there are a number of planning and preparation activities you need to complete. Visit the '**planning and improving research**' section to ensure your application is 'right first time'.

To support you with writing and submitting your application for HRA Approval, we have created a series of top tips, which can be found within the **IRAS help section**.

(Sourced at: https://www.hra.nhs.uk/approvals-ammendments/ on 8 February 2022)

For information about research ethics and governance in the UK, visit the HRA website at **https://www.hra.nhs.uk**. It contains lots of useful information and guidance.

Research vs Practice

It is important to be aware that there is a distinction between research and practice.

Research is something which is aimed at benefitting *all* people, but not necessarily those involved in the research project. Usually in health and social care research, we tell our participants, that, although we hope that, in the future, patients or service-users may benefit from the application of the results of a study, it is unlikely that there will be any immediate benefit to them. Research is not designed to be of specific benefit to any individual *at the time of doing the study.* They may benefit, along with others *in the future* as a result of actions being taken in response to the results of your study. **Experimentation within a study requires REC approvals – as does the study of all people receiving care.**

Practice is what you do to benefit those *individuals who receive your care.* They should expect to benefit from your interventions *in the here and now* as well as in the future. Practice is and should be directly tailored to meet the needs of every individual receiving that service or care. **Experimentation, as a part of finding the best care for an individual client or patient, does not require REC approvals.** Two important aspects of care are: (i) the regulation of standards of care, which is done by **audit;** and (ii) the improvement of services wherever possible, which is done by **service evaluation.** Both of these are activities which clinicians and practitioners are expected to engage in (Table 19.1).

So, in health and social care (and other professions) you are expected as a competent **practitioner** to audit your work and the service you provide – as an *essential aspect of your work role.* You are expected to experiment to get the best possible fit between your patients/clients and the interventions you apply – as a normal part of your role. Hence, this does not usually entail REC review – it is a matter of professional discretion, although it is one which you should share with your manager. Many R&D departments like to be informed of, and keep a record of, audits and service evaluations done in their organisation, so do consult with them.

Not all Research Activities are Classed as Research by the HRA

Not many people know this, but not all research activities are classed as research by the HRA (Health Research Authority 2020). In these cases, there is no need to apply for HRA or HRA REC approvals (Figure 19.1). But you should check with your organisation (R&D Dept.) in case any local permissions or reviews are needed. In the case of audits,

TABLE 19.1   Aspects of research, audit, and service evaluation.

	Research	Audit	Service evaluation
Aims:	To generate new knowledge	To check the quality of care or a service against an agreed standard	To identify current levels of care or a service
Outcomes:	May test a new (novel) intervention	No new (novel) interventions	No new (novel) interventions
Methods:	Best application of appropriate research methods	Best application of appropriate research methods	Best application of appropriate research methods
REC review:	Necessary	Not required	Not required
Who conducts this:	Researchers	Clinicians	Clinicians

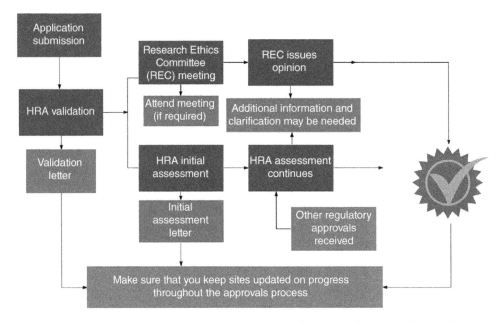

FIGURE 19.1 HRA approvals processes. (*Source*: HRA Website, March 2021), with permission from HRA.

NHS Caldicott Guardians may provide advice. A **Confidentiality Advisory Group (CAG)** will advise you on the use of patient data which is accessed without consent.

Studies which are classed as research and are managed as research require **REC scrutiny.** To tell if your project is classified as research, the HRA has a very useful 'Decision Tool' – 'Is my study research?' It is available on the HRA website at: **www. hra-decisiontools.org.uk/research**.

My project is categorised as research:

If your research project is:
- a Clinical Trial of an Investigational Medicinal Product (CTIMP) (with the exception of Phase 1 trials in healthy volunteers taking place outside the NHS)
- a Clinical Investigation or other study of a Medical Device
- a combined trial of an Investigational Medicinal Product and an Investigational Medical Device
- a Clinical Trial to study a novel intervention or randomised Clinical Trial to compare interventions in clinical practice
- a basic science study involving procedures with human participants
- a study administering questionnaires/interviews for quantitative analysis, or using mixed qualitative/quantitative methodology
- a study involving qualitative methods only
- a study limited to working with human tissue samples (or other human biological samples) and data (specific project only)
- a study limited to working with data (specific project only).

Then you *will* need to apply for **HRA Approval.**

If your project does not fall into the categories above but is:

- a Research Tissue Bank;
- a Research Database; or
- taking place in a non-NHS setting (a Phase 1 clinical trial in health volunteers, for example)

Then you will *not* need HRA Approval but *may* still need approval from a **Research Ethics Committee.**

(*Source*: HRA Website, March 2021)

The HRA has many forms of guidance and advice on its website which you can access freely on **www.hra.nhs.uk**.

If your research does not fall into the category of research as defined by the HRA, it may still require approvals by other bodies. Check!

The HRA will consider applications for student research, including PhD and MSc students.

Research Sponsorship

A research **sponsor** is 'An individual, company, institution, organisation or group of organisations that takes on responsibility for initiation, management and financing (or arranging the financing) of the research' (HRA).

All research should have a sponsor. Why? Because one of the main financial benefits of having a sponsor, is that *the sponsor underwrites the research.* In practice this means that, if any of your research participants has reason to believe that you have caused them any harm, in any way – including emotional or mental harm, for example by saying something which causes offence to them – then you are **insured** against this eventuality. 'But that's not likely to happen!' you might say. If a participant sues you for using offensive language, say, and wins the case, leaving you with a bill for legal fees and an award of £250,000 for damages, against you, could you afford to pay it? Your professional insurance may cover you. (Check!) But it could mean you losing your house and life savings! Do you see the value of a sponsor? I do!

If you are a student, approval by a university or college body (such as a faculty research committee or a REC) should, implicitly affirm their sponsorship of your project – but best check.

Guidance for sponsors of student research

The UK Policy Framework for Health and Social Care stipulates that *universities and colleges are expected to accept the role of sponsor for all educational research conducted by their own students, unless the student is employed by a health or social care provider that prefers to do this.* (My emphasis.)

Sponsors of educational research should ensure that their supervisors can and do carry out the activities involved in fulfilling this role. It is expected that the sponsor will provide any advice and support to students using this process.

(*Source*: HRA Website, March, 2021)

The sponsor for your project can be:

- your university or college if you are a student or a member of staff;
- an NHS Trust if you are employed by one;
- a funding body such as a research foundation or other funding organisation;
- a commercial source, such as a pharmaceutical company or an equipment manufacturer – if they are funding the project;
- another source of funding and support.

So, when a university acts as sponsor, it will usually have a REC or **sponsorship committee** who will scrutinise the study proposal with a particular interest in the potential risks of the project. There will probably be at least one member who is an insurer, or an underwriter, who will look at the proposal through 'cash-register eyes'. If you see them thinking, they will probably be counting on their fingers as they consider how much their block 'research' policy will cost. Clinical trials are likely to be the most risky and therefore the most costly! Whilst observational studies are likely to carry the least risks. If the university agrees to sponsor your study, you will be given the magic numbers – the **insurance policy numbers** which must be put in the correct place on the **Integrated Research Application Service (IRAS)** form (see below). *You cannot submit the form without them* – hence my reference to them as the magic numbers!

Chief/Principal Investigator (CI/PI)

The **Chief/Principal Investigator (CI/PI)** is the individual who is responsible for the whole project. S/he should have sufficient research expertise to be able to supervise all aspects of the research and communicate with other agencies such as RECs and other review bodies throughout the research process. There should be a PI at each site where the research takes place. If there is only one site, then the CI and the PI are normally the same person.

For student research projects at Undergraduate, Postgraduate, and PhD level, the CI/PI is normally expected to be the student's dissertation or thesis **supervisor.** Once you have gained enough experience of conducting research projects under the guidance of a supervisor – having proved that you can plan, execute, and publish research – you will be considered for a CI/PI role in a research project. But PLEASE – do not be disappointed or take offence because you are not allowed to be the CI/PI. That's just the way things are. I know it might seem harsh that you have thought of a project and put so much into the planning of it, and then someone else gets all the glory by being CI/PI. The project will still be yours and you should still be the **first author** on publications arising from the project. Hopefully, your supervisor will have contributed enough so that you will be proud to co-author publications with her/him. In that case, s/he will normally be the **last-named author.** That is the convention. Any other contributors may be invited by you to join the author list – and journals tend to insist, and ask for written confirmation, that all authors have made a *meaningful contribution* to the article for publication.

Chief/Principal Investigator

The **UK Policy framework** stipulates that students should not normally take the role of chief investigator at any level of study, as this function should be undertaken by supervisors or course leaders, although exceptions are made in some circumstances.

Supervisors are encouraged to develop and lead research projects that individual students can contribute to, always acknowledging their contribution.

The framework further states that sponsors can create a 'research culture' by promoting students' awareness of health and social care research, research ethics and public involvement, and enabling them to develop skills in research methods.

(*Source*: HRA website, March, 2021)

Remember that when you ask the question, 'Who bears the brunt if anything goes wrong in the study?' in this eventuality, ***the buck stops at the CI/PI's door.*** The CI/PI is responsible for ensuring that the study is carried out properly – Purposefully. Ethically. Methodologically. Honestly. And legally. S/he is the person who is responsible for ensuring **compliance** with regulations such as General Data Protection Regulation (**GDPR**), Good Clinical Practice (**GCP**), etc. So, they probably do earn their title, don't you think? (Figure 19.2)

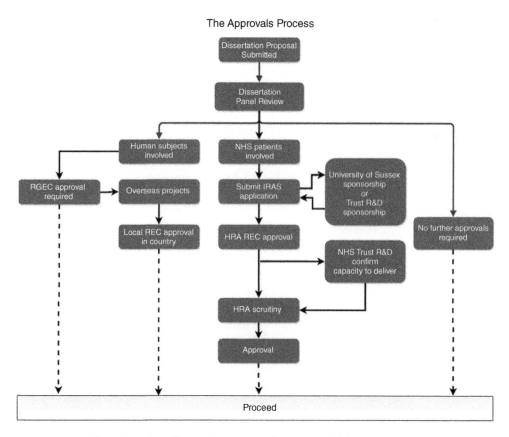

FIGURE 19.2   The PG student dissertation approvals process within DME, BSMS.

Research and Development Departments (R&D)

NHS R&D departments used to have a wide remit for the approval of and support for research. This used to be very contentious according to many of my students, some of whom referred to them as 'Review and Destroy' departments. They seemed to be the most unpopular group of people in the research field. But as with most areas of life, if I've met some right *plonkers* in R&D, I have also met some wonderful, helpful, and facilitative people in R&D.

Example 1: 'Audrey's story

'Audrey' planned to do a study of doctors' nurses' and HCP's attitudes towards influenza vaccinations in an NHS Trust. She was directed to the R&D department in her trust to discuss the project with them. The next day she phoned her supervisor. 'Help! They say I have to get NHS Ethics Committee approval via the IRAS system.' 'Don't worry' I said. 'I'll have a word with them.' So, I phoned the Director of the R&D department and pointed out, 'You are aware that, from September 2011, REC approval is not required for research involving NHS staff?' 'Oh, you're quite right' said the Director, 'I'll refer it to my deputy to deal with.' So I told 'Audrey' to contact the Deputy. She phoned back the next day. 'Help! She says I have to go through IRAS to get REC approval!' 'OK – Leave it with me' I said. I phoned the Deputy. 'You are aware that, from September 2011, REC approval is not required for research involving NHS staff?' The Deputy replied, 'You're quite right. All she has to do is to apply to us.' 'How does she do that?' I asked. The Deputy replied, 'She has to go through IRAS . . .' Snookered!

To cut a long story short, 'Audrey' applied for an NHS REC review through IRAS. Her study was approved, and eventually the R&D department were fully cooperative with her and facilitated the project. However, it did take her an extra six weeks to begin her field-work. I use this as an example of how **risk-averse,** how **do-it-by-the-book** some R&D employees can be! It was within their remit to take the decision, but they insisted it be scrutinised by an NHS REC instead.

I have had other instances where I have experienced R&D staff as being downright obstructive, but some have been wonderful – see 'Sunny's' story below.

Since the HRA have taken over the processing of research ethics and governance in 2016, R&D departments have had less of a role in the research approvals process. Before then, they had responsibility for **scrutinising all research projects in their Trusts for compliance with the regulations**. (That assumes that they were aware of the regulations and could interpret them correctly.) However, since then they have had their involvement limited to a) confirming the Trust's capacity to host the research; and b) to setting up the panels which will confer the Trust's willingness to sponsor research which their staff are involved in.

Example 2: 'Sunny's' Story

'Sunny' was a student on the MSc in Trauma & Orthopaedics who I supervised. He was in prospect of winning the prize for being the first MSc T&O student to do a dissertation using **qualitative** methods. It was an interesting approach. He wanted to find out what patients undergoing a total knee replacement understood about, and expected from, their operation, and how what they expected pre-operatively, related to their feelings, post operatively. This could have made a nice cohort study, but he did not have time to do that. (The period to stabilisation post-op was two years.) So, instead, he decided to interview two groups of patients – (i) a group of patients about to undergo surgery, and (ii) a group of patients two years after their surgery. His project was approved by our dissertation panel. Then he obtained sponsorship from his NHS Trust, and applied through IRAS for HRA ethics review. This was in the early days of the HRA, when they were still getting their systems into place and ironing out the bugs in their systems. As a result, it took about four months before his study was approved by the HRA ethics committee. Wonderful news! But then the approved documents were sent back to the HRA for them to confirm approval for the project to proceed, and to the NHS Trust for them to confirm capacity to deliver. He had to chase up the HRA and after about six weeks, the reply came back that he **could not proceed with his study** – what he proposed compromised patients' data protection rights! The Trust Legal team got involved, but the HRA were right. It seems that the Trust had permission (under the Data Protection Act) to approach any of their patients to invite them to participate in research. However, the group of patients in question were followed up as patients for a year and then discharged – then they were no longer patients. So, to invite 'former patients', two years after their operation and a year after their discharge, meant that they did not meet the criteria of 'patients' as defined by the DPA. Because Sunny had spent so long getting final confirmation, he could not conduct the study as proposed, and he did not have enough time to go through the whole process again. He eventually did a **systematic review**, passed, and graduated. He and I are now discussing the feasibility of doing the study – but with only one group of patients and following them up in a cohort study!

How to Apply for HRA REC Approvals: IRAS – The Integrated Research Application Service

The HRA have a network of RECs spread throughout the country. It used to be standard practice for researchers to apply for REC approval from their local REC. So, for example, when I conducted a needs assessment for domiciliary palliative care services in an area in the South of England, which entailed interviews with staff from hospices, hospitals, general practitioners, community nurses, patients who were receiving palliative care, and their relatives/carers, I applied to the local REC. My application was considered, and I was awarded their approval within a month. But that was before a medical school was established locally. Consider how many applications there would be now, and how long the wait would be to get a slot for your project at an REC meeting . . . Yes, it would be a long time. This was particularly the case in London where there are still many medical schools and hospitals. So, the DOH incorporated all the local RECs into a single network and set up a single application portal – the **IRAS.**

Through IRAS you have access to all/any REC in the country. IRAS has a set of standard application forms (to suit all types of project) which allows you to enter the information required just once. Then, when you press the 'SUBMIT' button, your application is checked for completeness and it is directed to the REC with the next available slot. Then your REC meeting may be in 10 days' time. That is what happened when Aalya and I submitted our application (for a study of doctors' and patients' understandings of the seriousness of malignant melanoma), we were given an REC slot (somewhere in Scotland) within two weeks. Not bad – eh? You can usually choose to attend the meeting, or, as we did (because of the distance) agree to be at the end of the phone for the time the meeting was scheduled, in order to be able to provide any answers to questions directly. I was quizzed for about 40 minutes over points where the Committee wanted assurance. But that saved them having to send the application back to me with a list of questions for me to answer, and then send back to them, So, they were able to give their approval *immediately*.

Proportionate review – a scaled-down scrutiny with fewer requirements than the full form – is available for those studies which are considered of 'low risk', for example some qualitative interview studies.

In principle it is a good system, and often, in practice it is too. The one criticism that many people I have spoken to about it have is that the form is not very user-friendly. You have to be prepared to repeat some information and to make sure that you really do understand what information is required in each box! Critics of the IRAS system say the form is too unwieldy, it takes too long with too much attention to minute detail to complete, and that there are insufficient opportunities for proportionate review – they complain that the application for an interview study with a small number of patients is dealt with in almost as much rigour as a major drug trial.

The role of students' supervisors is often taken too lightly in my view. I know lots of university staff who agree to supervise students' research projects in the anticipation that they have little or no responsibilities other than marking the dissertation and putting their name on a publication. So, to awaken them to the realities of the research world, I advise all students to ask their supervisors if they are aware of the part of the IRAS form which supervisors have to sign (where applicable). Here is what it used to look like:

**Supervisors' Declaration On The IRAS Form
(as signed by John on Kavi's application)**

D3. Declaration for student projects by academic supervisor(s)

1. I have read and approved both the research proposal and this application. I am satisfied that the scientific content of the research is satisfactory for an educational qualification at this level.

2. I undertake to fulfil the responsibilities of the supervisor for this study as set out in the UK Policy Framework for Health and Social Care Research.

3. I take responsibility for ensuring that this study is conducted in accordance with the ethical principles underlying the Declaration of Helsinki and good practice guidelines on the proper conduct of research, in conjunction with clinical supervisors as appropriate.

4. I take responsibility for ensuring that the applicant is up to date and complies with the requirements of the law and relevant guidelines relating to security and confidentiality of patient and other personal data, in conjunction with clinical supervisors as appropriate.

In my view, all supervisors should sign this when agreeing to supervise any student doing a research project. You could test your supervisor by asking:

1. 'Are you familiar with the UK Policy Framework for Health and Social Care Research?'
2. 'Are you familiar with the Declaration of Helsinki and good practice guidelines on the proper conduct of research?'
3. 'Have you had GPDR Training?'
4. 'Do you have a current GCP Certificate?'

I advise my students to log on to IRAS and open an account. It is free, and safe! You cannot submit anything until you have the magic numbers – the numbers of the insurance policies which your institution provides! (As I explained above.) So, go on the website, open an account, and explore the site. You can do the e-learning which is freely available to all. Try opening a new project file and complete it – you will be guided through it and signposted to the different sections. You can save it and return to it as often as you want. It is worth the experience because then, hopefully you will not be afraid of the form and the process when you come to do it for real!

Good Clinical Practice (GCP)

Anyone who does research within the NHS or has to submit an HRA REC application, must have a valid **GCP certificate**. There is free training provided for NHS and other staff. I recommend to all my students to do the course and complete the assessment. The online version should take you about two to four hours – depending on the modules you include, and how familiar you are already with the material. The **National Institute for Health Research (NIHR)** provides both live and online training in GCP.

GCP is the 'international ethical, scientific and practical standard to which all clinical research is conducted' (NIHR). **NIHR** point out that:

It is important that everyone involved in research is trained or appropriately experienced to perform the specific tasks they are being asked to undertake. GCP training is a requirement set out in the UK Policy Framework for Health and Social Care Research developed by the Health Research Authority for researchers conducting clinical trials of investigational medicinal products (CTIMPs).

They point out that some people might benefit more from other training.

Different types of research may require different training, and some researchers are already well trained and competent in their area of expertise. Some researchers doing other types of clinical trials may also benefit from undertaking GCP training but other training may be more relevant.

And, for those who want it, GCP training is available from lots of sources – some private – as well as *free* from NIHR (**www.nihr.ac.uk/health-and-care-professionals/ learning-and-support/good-clinical-practice.htm**; National Institute for Health Research 2020).

The GCP courses cover:

1. ethical conduct;
2. protocols;
3. benefit–risk assessment;
4. review by IEC/IRC;
5. informed consent
6. continuing review/ongoing benefit–risk assessment;
7. records and reporting of incidents;
8. confidentiality/privacy.

The GCP training is geared to ensuring that all people involved in research in Health and Social Care are equipped to meet the requirements of the **Declaration of Helsinki** (World Medical Association 2013). I have done the training several times and have a few certificates to prove it. I have found the online training to be very good. The versions I did were clear and informative.

Do It!

If you have to fill out an IRAS form for HRA REC approval, you will be asked to provide details of the GCP certification for *each of the researchers* in the study.

GDPR

The **European Union (EU) GDPR** is the directive which governs how we deal with people's – including research participants' – **personal data.** 'Personal data' means 'any information relating to an identified or identifiable natural person ("data subject"); an identifiable natural person is one who can be identified, directly or indirectly, in particular by reference to an identifier such as a name, an identification number, location data, and online identifier or to one or more factors specific to the physical, physiological, genetic, mental, economic, cultural or social identity of that natural person' (GDPR 2018).

All research projects must be **GDPR-compliant,** and all researchers should have completed a minimum of a basic course to familiarise them with the GDPR requirements. Most large organisations, like universities and NHS Trusts, provide free training for their staff. Check with your organisation to see if you can access it. There are large penalties for breaches of data protection – as well as reputational damage.

Essentially, we should not gather any more personal data than we need. It should be gathered for a legitimate purpose. It should be accurate. We have a responsibility to allow anyone to have access to their data which we store, so that a) they know what he have; and b) they are assured it is accurate. All personal data should be stored in a secure way, and only transmitted to appropriate others via secure means. When it is no longer needed, it should be disposed of in a secure manner. Any breaches of data security must be reported to appropriate persons immediately. So, think twice before putting any personal data on a memory stick and carrying it around with you – unless it has a high level of encryption to protect the contents. Likewise, do not store personal data on a pc or laptop, unless it is password protected or properly encrypted. And please, never send anyone's personal data to anyone overseas without getting the permission of the person concerned! Ask in your organisation (e.g. university) who is responsible for data protection compliance and reporting of breaches.

One of the best ways of dealing with this is to keep personal data only on a central research computer and to have all data – which is transported, sent between places or people, or analysed – **anonymised.** This means that it is impossible for any third party to be able to tell whose information it is. In research, it is standard practice to avoid collecting any more personal information (often referred to as **demographic information**) than is absolutely necessary. We also tend to use **study serial numbers (SSN)** – a way of giving each individual in the study a serial number – in place of names. Lists of names and who has which SSN must be kept securely in locked locations and/or password-protected computers.

If in doubt, ask someone responsible for help or advice.

Research Conducted Overseas

For all projects conducted overseas, you are likely to need twin scrutiny of your project. You will probably require some form of institutional or REC approval in this country. Then you are likely to require **Local REC** approval within the country where the study fieldwork will take place. In this instance it is normally the student's responsibility to identify the correct channels and – with the supervisor's agreement – go through them to obtain the necessary consents. Be prepared in such cases not to be too surprised if the documentation differs from the sort of documentation you might expect in the UK. In some poorer countries, REC approvals are not as important as food or drug supplies.

> When Princewill got his approval from our medical school REC that approval was subject to his getting local approval in Nigeria. He sought advice from people he knew in Nigeria and got approval from a **local government office**. When another of my students carried out a study of barriers to care for people with HIV/AIDS in Western Nigeria, he got our medical school REC approval and then he got ethics clearance from **the hospital** where he did his fieldwork in Nigeria. Two of my supervisees (from Zambia) planned brilliant studies. One was interested in the knowledge, attitudes, and practices (KAP) of traditional healers in Zambia with regard to the treatment of people with malaria. The other was interested in the KAP of traditional healers in Zambia with regard to the treatment of people with HIV/AIDS. Both got REC approval from our medical school, then, when they went to Zambia, found that **the university REC** (their local REC) could not process their applications because the staff were on strike! After more than six months, when the strike was over, they went to submit their applications for REC approval and were told it would cost them the equivalent of about £550 each, for the REC to process their applications. They could not afford such sums (they were already paying international students fees for their MSc course) and had to change their projects to do systematic reviews instead. That was such a shame!

Research Passports/Honorary Contracts

Research passports were introduced as a means of enabling researchers to have a single means of identification which gave them access to all NHS Trusts – rather than having to obtain honorary contracts with each Trust. In fact, this has not worked well, and you will usually have to approach each NHS Trust where you hope to do your research and ask them for an **Honorary Appointment.** R&D Departments are the gatekeepers for this and can make it as easy or as difficult as they wish. If you think about it, from a health and safety and from a security point of view, you can't allow just anyone to wander into wards and clinics asking to see patients or staff – you need an **ID badge.** If you slip on a wet floor and injure yourself, you need to be covered for damages by the Trust. The answer – getting an honorary appointment from the Trust. Don't be surprised if this is a thorough business. We all have to go through it – including a **CRB check.** Safety and security – let this be your new mantra!

Example 3: Kavi's Story

Kavi's research involved him interviewing cancer patients. He applied for and obtained dissertation panel approval. He agreed access to patients and cooperation from a local consultant. He applied for and was awarded university sponsorship. He applied for and was awarded full approval from an NHS REC. He applied for and was awarded – after a long delay – approval from his local R&D department. He applied for and was awarded a research passport from the local Trust. He thought he was ready to go ahead. What do you think?

Of course he wasn't. His local R&D department insisted that three of his other collaborators – his supervisor (me), a professor from another university, and his co-supervisor from another university – all have research passports too, even though none of them would ever set foot in the NHS site for this project!

Once this was completed, he began his interviews. He completed the study and we are in the process of preparing it for publication.

Student Safety

In addition to concerns for patients' safety, RECs are increasingly aware of issues around researchers' safety. Physical safety in laboratories is covered by the Health and Safety regulations. I cover some of the issues about safety in laboratories in Appendix C. It is both yours and the lab manager's responsibilities to ensure safety and safe behaviour in labs. So do acquaint yourself with the local protocols for lab safety.

In observational research, we have to be aware of any physical risks which researchers might face. For example, before we allow any of our students to go overseas to take part in research, we have to conduct a risk assessment which takes into account the prevalence of any contagious or communicable diseases and ensure that everyone who goes has the necessary jabs or medicines (especially anti-malarials) before we approve their taking part in the project. We also have to assure ourselves of the safety and security of any country where the fieldwork for the research is being conducted. The first question to ask is, 'Is it a war zone?' Here the UK Foreign Commonwealth & Development Office (FCDO) website can provide very useful guidance and advice about safety and health issues in different countries. You can visit the website for free and up-to-date information at: **www.gov.uk/foreign-travel-advice**.

On a research trip to Pakistan in 1984, I came back (to Hong Kong) with hepatitis A. Whilst in Pakistan, I was very careful to only eat only cooked meals (I avoided salads), and drank only bottled or canned drinks (other than tea and coffee). Several of the people I was visiting, laughed, gently, at me and said, 'I can see you are being very careful!' I still got ill.

I had to go to Peshawar in the North West Frontier or Pakistan. I asked my hosts about the chances of visiting the Khyber Pass (I was interested in the history of the area). 'You mustn't go there!' I was told, 'People will think you are CIA and kidnap you!' Pity! – but I did not go. Later, I was interviewing a couple of British missionaries about the work that they were doing. During the interview I noticed that they had both sunk down in their chairs so that they were almost supine. It was then that I noticed the sound of what I had though was firecrackers (common in Hong Kong at weddings). 'Those aren't firecrackers, are they?' I asked. 'No, that's gunfire.' They explained 'When tribesmen and their families flee here from the war across the border in Afghanistan, they don't surrender their weapons. They are as well armed as the border guards. And they bring all their weapons and their tribal rivalries with them. So, of an evening, when spirits are high, they open the tent flap and loose off a few rounds from their AK 47s in the general direction of their enemies, and of course no one knows where these will end up in a mile or so. We had one come through the wall of the flat and ping around a bit before the bullet landed on the floor, spent!' I sank lower in my chair and we carried on the interview from a supine position! But I did not really think that was a really risky situation.

The most threatened I felt in that trip was during an interview I conducted with an English woman who was running a small school for deaf children. During the interview, she constantly and deliberately made a point of ensuring that her veil covered her face. As I glanced at my driver and my guide who were watching from the doorway, I realised that they were keeping an eye on her, and she seemed to feel most uncomfortable – as did I thereafter. I felt it was a very threatening situation for both of us. I felt that this interview had been engineered to test us both. So, I ended the interview as soon as possible, thanked her and left. I had not thought of this as a risky trip until I was writing this chapter . . .

When doing research in other countries it is *essential* to brief yourself fully on the health and the political situation there – and to get to know the local customs and rules of behaviour of that country. One of our students did a project which involved her interviewing the wives of men who had HIV/Aids in Zimbabwe. Can you imagine the sorts of problems which she might have faced in doing that? In the end, we agreed to her project, but she had to arrange to have a male **'chaperone'** drive her to the address where each interview was to take place; he had to wait there until the interview was over; then he had to drive her back home.

One of my co-supervisees – 'Leah' – had passed through all the necessary approvals and was conducting her individual, face-to-face interviews. One day she reported that she had completed an interview in a participant's home. She was pleased because the interview had gone very well and he was very helpful. Then, at the end of the interview, when she was preparing to leave, he produced a bottle of vodka and invited her to join him for a drink. This may have been a genuine and generous offer, but alarm bells went off in her head. She quickly excused herself and left. As soon as she shared this experience with us, we realised that we had omitted to agree a safety procedure for occasions when she might be interviewing a participant alone, in their own home. Therefore, the following 'lone worker' procedures were put in place for the future.

1. She would inform one of her supervisors when she was going to do each interview.
2. Immediately before going to the interview, she would phone or text her supervisor to let them know.
3. As soon as the interview was over, she would phone the supervisor to let them know she had finished and that she was OK.
4. If she had not phoned within an hour, the supervisor would phone her and say 'are you OK?' If she answered 'Yes . . .' The supervisor would phone the police. If she answered 'No – everything is going well' the supervisor would know she was safe and would not alert the Police. **'Yes'** was the **trigger word** for 'I need help!'

Similar procedures have been used by other students. One student who was interviewing youth gang members established a similar protocol to that outlined above with 'Leah'. Many Health and Local Authority staff are well-versed in using similar **lone worker procedures** to minimise the risks of working alone in the community.

As supervisors we have to bear our students' safety in mind – whether it is in relation to safe laboratory procedures, or to the risks of attack in the community. One area less well publicised is the need for concern over students' emotional well-being. For example, if our students are doing projects which expose them to highly emotionally charged topics, such as cancer, death, and dying, child heath, etc., we need to ensure that in addition to being able to signpost their participants to appropriate support agencies, we should enquire about their well-being and, where necessary, signpost *them* to appropriate support agencies.

Can you imagine the sorts of risks which could be potentially faced by researchers doing participant observation? Chris Coulter, writing in 2005, gives a graphic account of the proceedings and her emotional reactions to a Girl's Initiation Ceremony in Northern Sierra Leone. Here is an extract from her account:

January 9th, 2004.

Tears are running down my face. There is a full moon, and I am sitting quite close to the fire, but it is late, and I don't think anyone has noticed. For an instant, I become overwhelmed with feelings as the significance of the ritual hit me – to become a woman you have to undergo female circumcision.

I am a woman and also a mother of two daughters, and I can't even conceive of putting my daughters through the physical mutilation of a genital circumcision. I am looking at some of the dances performed by the 58 neophyte girls soon to be initiated and circumcised in the village of Kamadugu Sokorala in northern Sierra Leone. However, I am also an anthropologist, and as I am looking around me at the faces of mothers and fathers, aunts and uncles, I can see nothing but joy, happiness, and pride. These mothers do not hesitate for a second in putting their daughters through this, what I see as an ordeal. No, they are proud and enthusiastic. The girls also seem happy; they are the center of attention; they seem proud to share something with the older women, some secret separating them from their younger sisters.

(Coulter 2005)

You get a strong sense of the moral dilemmas faced by this very emotionally and culturally sensitive researcher. The question which is not addressed in this paper, is what support she needed and what she had access to before, during, and after her study.

The **Social Research Association** (SRA) published its **Ethical Guidelines** in 2003. *These recognise the potential for physical and mental harm that may be involved particularly in Social Research. The SRA provides useful guides and training for those involved in social research. The Ethical Guidelines can be purchased as a hard copy (Price £10.00) or downloaded free. Printed copies of this guide can be obtained from: admin@the-sra.org.uk. A free version can be downloaded from the web site:* **www.the-sra.org.uk**.

Social researchers have a moral obligation to attempt to minimise the risk of physical and/or mental harm to themselves and to their colleagues from the conduct of research. Research managers may, in addition, have a legal obligation in terms of health and safety regulations to ensure that risk to field researchers is minimised . . .

The qualitative study of dangerous or threatening groups may place the researcher in some situations of particular personal risk, but all research entailing direct contact with the public presents a risk potential. Researchers should maintain awareness of such risk to themselves and their colleagues and make every effort to diminish the dangers.

(SRA 2003)

Bloor et al. (2010) in their paper on 'Unprepared for the Worst: Risks of Harm for Qualitative Researchers' discuss the sorts of damage, and provide examples, of both physical and emotional harm which can arise from some types of social research.

. . . emotional upset can occur through contact with research participants going through painful or traumatic events (for example, the upset experienced by Coulter 2005 when she witnessed female circumcision rites in Sierra Leone), or even through learning of painful events witnessed by others (for example, the 'pain by proxy' experienced by Moran-Ellis [1997] interviewing professionals involved in child protection). Emotional upset can also occur through the isolation – social and/or geographical – of fieldwork (e.g. Palriwala, 2007), through the emergent resistance or antagonism of some research participants or gatekeepers (e.g. Schramm 2005) or both through a combination of both isolation and antagonism (e.g. Sampson and Thomas, 2003). Additionally, emotional upset can itself trigger a range of physical and psychiatric symptoms – gastro-intestinal problems, insomnia and nightmares, headaches, exhaustion and depression (cf. the review by Dickson-Swift et al. 2006).

(Bloor et al. 2010)

In their review, Bloor et al. note that there seems to be a lot of concern from institutions and ethics committees, about *participants' safety,* and about the physical safety of researchers, but very little attention being paid to emotional traumas inherent for researchers in some types of research. In their enquiry into issues of *researcher safety,* they reported:

> *One person contrasted university practice unfavourably with the 'regular and excellent supervision' she had previously experienced as a probation officer, where risk management was 'part of the professional culture of the organisation'. Another person contrasted the 'antiquated' response of his university to his own distressing fieldwork experiences with the active management of risk experienced by friends of his in journalism. He concluded that he found it 'ironic' that much of the specialist expertise in country analysis and security training that is offered to business, governments and agencies comes from the university sector.*
>
> *(Bloor et al. 2010)*

I must say, that in all the years I have been involved in research into cancer and death and dying, no university person (other than friends like Mick) has ever asked me about my feelings and whether the research had an impact upon me. And quite often it did. Once I interviewed this lovely man about his wife's death at home. It was a very traumatic even and it went on for a long time. The interview lasted about four hours. I kept checking that he was OK to keep going, and he confirmed that he was. At the end of it, I was emotionally spent. I had to drive home a long way and the interview went through my mind over and over. Several times, I have been in tears with the person I was interviewing. Sometimes you cannot help it – when they start, it triggers the same reaction in me! But never – never – have I been asked about it by my bosses, or offered any de-briefing or support in my organisation.

There are some kinds of work I could not and would not do. I could not research subjects like child abuse. I have dealt with consequences of it enough in my psychotherapy practice. As a result of that training, I have a network of people who I can, and sometimes do, approach for support or advice about difficult issues in my therapy and my research work. As a result, I think I am good at providing support for my supervisees and being able to signpost them to supports where necessary. I am particularly concerned that we do support our junior researchers in particular and agree with the conclusions that Mick and his colleagues make.

> *For example, grantholders have had to develop an expertise in the completion of applications for ethical approval, which has given them a practised grasp of the sort of ethical issues that exercise ethics committees. By incorporating a question on researcher safety into ethics committee application forms, one is encouraging grantholders to develop an expertise in addressing this issue.*
>
> *(Bloor et al. 2010)*

Competence

I am glad to see that the issue of **researcher competence** is being increasingly emphasised in recent years. I have always stressed the importance of this to my students – competence in the ability to conduct your study is an ethical requirement.

Interviewing skills and **focus group skills** are other areas where in the health-care field, people assume a greater expertise than they actually have. Just because they talk to patients or clients every day, they assume expertise. (I used to come up against this all the time when James Thompson and I were working on the development of communications skills training in medicine.) I have listened to recordings and read transcripts of interviews with student researchers who have not attended any interview-skills training – even when I was offering them (free of charge) to all our students – which have been so appalling.

Julie Mooney-Somers and Anna Olsen in 2017 wrote an article which highlighted the fact that, without understanding the technicalities of qualitative research, it is difficult to describe or address the ethical issues involved in qualitative research. And that, although the Australian National Statement on the Ethical Conduct of Research Involving Humans requires researchers to demonstrate that they have the appropriate experience, qualifications, and competence for the research they propose, it is the ethics committees who have to judge researchers' competence. Hence, their article provided researchers and members of ethics committees with guidance on how to assess qualitative research competence. They point out that 'We've come a long way since qualitative methods had to be self-taught or when the attitude of "how hard can it be to do a few interviews" was acceptable.' They highlight the wider availability of training available these days. (Check it out if you are interested.) Publications showing your ability are one form of evidence. Certificates of attendance at specific training courses are another. (I always give participants at my research skills workshops a Certificate of Attendance and encourage them to add it as an appendix to any REC application.) Mooney-Somers and Olsen (2017) state:

> 'we believe that in recommending that researchers make explicit their expertise, and that ethical review committees formally consider the competence of researchers, the merit and integrity of proposals are more likely to be appropriately understood. These efforts should raise the status of qualitative research in demonstrating it is not an endeavour that can be lightly undertaken by novices. Instead, it encompasses a diverse range of approaches that require training, expertise and reflection if they are to be used ethically.
>
> *(Mooney-Somers and Olsen 2017)*

To my mind, RECs should ensure that their membership includes people of sufficient proven expertise or competence (even though some may have to be co-opted on to the REC for specific meetings) to provide a fair and professional review of **all** the proposals which they consider.

Publications

It is an ethical imperative that you publish – or otherwise disseminate – the results of your research. *We must not waste our participants' time!* Think about giving presentations at professional conferences. Talk to others about your work. Let it be known about.

It is becoming more common to inform your research participants about the results of your research. One way of informing research participants about the results of your research is to offer then an **executive summary** of the results. This should be written in an easy-to-read format (without academic jargon!) and in a brief form. As Oliver (2010) says, 'Consideration should be given to ensuring that they have access to the research results in an understandable format' (Oliver 2010, p. 17).

To Sum Up

In this chapter, I have tried to lead you through the minefield of the processes you need to go through and the different sets of issues which you need to be aware of when conducting research responsibly. Because of the complexity of the subject, it would take a separate chapter to cover the regulations in each country; therefore, I have provided a detailed account of the UK regulations and procedures – as exemplars of good practice. Hopefully, you will be able to extrapolate from this to any other country that you work in. These procedures may seem very restrictive, but I hope that you will agree that, having read the last chapter, there is a need for open and close scrutiny of all research to protect both those who are being researched and those who are conducting the research. I have pointed out the difference between 'research, 'audit', and 'service evaluations' and pointed out that not everything called 'research' is subject to formal HRA approval. However, if you are a student and are planning to do a research study, then you do need to check with your institution, what approvals you will need before you can properly begin to do your study. I have tried to show something of the complexity of the processes here. Likewise, students' supervisors need to be aware of their responsibilities in ensuring that the basic ethical principles, which guide modern healthcare research, are being followed properly. Normally students cannot expect to be the CI/PI for a research project – that is the supervisor's responsibility – the buck stops there! So, both students and supervisors need to be aware of the regulations governing the conduct of research, and for both your sakes, need to follow the regulations.

I know that there is a lot of material there, and it is a very dry subject, but it is a necessary and an important one. Do persevere and you will get it right.

Research is the art of the possible!

References

Bloor M, Fincham B, and Sampson H. (2010). Unprepared for the worst: risks of harm for qualitative researchers. *Methodological Innovations Online* 5(1), 45–55.

Coulter C. (2005). Reflections from the field: a girl's initiation ceremony in northern Sierra Leone. *Anthropology Quarterly* 78(2), 431–444.

Health Research Authority (2020). UK Policy Framework for Health and Social Care Research. Available at www.hra.nhs.uk/planning-and-improving-research/policies-standards-legislation/uk-policy-framework-health-social-care-research (accessed 18 September 2020).

Mooney-Somers J and Olsen A. (2017). Ethical review and qualitative research competence: guidance for reviewers and applicants. *Research Ethics* 13(3–4), 128–138.

National Institute for Health Research (2020). *Good Clinical Practice (GCP)*. Available at: www.nihr.ac.uk/health-and-care-professionals/learning-and-support/good-clinical-practice. htm (accessed 18 September 2020).

Oliver P. (2010). *The Student's Guide To Research Ethics*. Open University Press: Maidenhead.

Palriwala R. (2007). Fieldwork in a post-colonial anthropology: Experience and the comparative. *Social Anthropology* 13(2), 151–170.

World Medical Association (2013). WMA Declaration of Helsinki – Ethical Principles for Medical Research Involving Human Subjects. Available at: www.wma.net/policies-post/wma-declaration-of-helsinki-ethical-principles-for-medical-research-involving-human-subjects/ (accessed 16 September 2020).

Further Resources

For a full guide to all HRA citations and further information, visit the HRA website at: **https://www.hra.nhs.uk/**

For all NIHR sources, visit the NIHR website at: **https://www.nihr.ac.uk/**

For further information about the EU GDPR regulations and compliance, visit the GDPR websites at: **https://gdpr.eu/** and **https://gdpr-info.eu/**

For all WMA sources, visit the WMA website at: **https://www.wma.net/**

APPENDIX A

Research Skills

Obtaining Informed Consent

Introduction

Obtaining informed consent (OIC) is an essential requirement for any research project involving human participants. But more than that, if you do it well, it will set the mood for the whole of your participants' experience of the project. There are two main aspects of OIC that I shall cover: (i) *giving information orally* about the research and what is wanted from the potential participant; and (ii) *giving written information* about the research and what is wanted from the potential participant.

I first obtained informed consent for interviews I was conducting for a PhD student whilst I was at Aberdeen in 1968. I have done it thousands of times over the years since then and I hope I do it fairly well. I have been running workshops on Obtaining Informed Consent for all of our MSc students since 2009 and they have been well evaluated. So, I feel qualified to share my thoughts and experiences about this process with you.

Giving Information about the Research and What Is Wanted from the Potential Participant in Obtaining Informed Consent

If possible, it is worthwhile alerting potential participants in advance that they may be approached and invited to take part in a research study. This allows them to prepare themselves and to rehearse saying 'No'. I say this because in my experience of recruiting hospital patients for research projects, I have found that most tend to be only too willing to help and take part. This is probably part of their gratitude for the treatment they have received whilst in hospital, and you get comments like 'Oh, I'm very pleased to be able to do whatever it takes to help you, especially after what all the lovely staff here have done for me.' This feeling of obligation or indebtedness is very common in hospital and clinic patients, who, I believe, often find it difficult to refuse – even though inwardly they might like to. Therefore, one of the first things which I say when I am obtaining IC is: **'You don't have to take part if you don't want to.'**

Demystifying Research for Medical & Healthcare Students: An Essential Guide, First Edition. John L. Anderson.
© 2022 John Wiley & Sons Ltd. Published 2022 by John Wiley & Sons Ltd.
Companion website: www.wiley.com/go/Anderson/DemystifyingResearch

Giving Oral Information

So, I might approach a patient who is waiting in an out-patient clinic and the conversation might be something like this:

JA: Hello. Mr Smith?

MR S: Oh, hello.

JA: My name is John Anderson (JA extends his hand and shakes hands with Mr Smith). I hope that the clinic nurses have warned you that I might speak to you to invite you to take part in a research project which I am doing, but I will say this, *you don't have to if you don't want to.*

MR S: Oh, hello. They did mention it. Yes, I'd like to help. If there's anything I can do . . . I'm only too happy to help.

JA: You're only too happy to help? Well I'm very pleased to hear that, but I do mean it when I say that *you don't have to if you don't want to.* Before you decide, let me explain the project to you. Is that OK?

MR S: Yes, that will be fine.

JA: May I sit down here?

MR S: Yes, please do.

JA: Well. I am a researcher from the Brighton & Sussex Medical School and I am involved with some colleagues here in doing a project about *patients' expectations of total knee replacement operations,* and I would like to interview you to find out what your thoughts about this are. My colleagues are orthopaedic surgeons – I gather that you will be seeing one soon?

MR S: Is it Dr Ramaghastalan?

JA: Yes, Mr Ramaghastalan, that's right. Well, I am doing this study with him and two other surgeons. What I understand they are finding is that they *don't feel that they are 'getting it right'* when they explain these operations to patients, because some of their patients complain that they did not expect what happened. So we are doing this study to find out what patients are told – and what they understand will happen – before they have the operations; then we are following patients up some time after their operations to find out how they are progressing and to check if things have turned out the way they (the patients) expected. Then we may develop a training workshop out of our results to help improve the way they communicate with their patients. Does that make sense to you?

MR S: Yes it does. It's about time someone sorted them out!

JA: Good. I can see that you might be able to tell me a lot?

MR S: Yes, I can tell you lots of things from my experience . . .

JA: That's good, and I'd like to hear more about your experiences. Shall I tell you what we would want of you if you do take part? And, again, I'd like to emphasise, that *you don't have to if you don't want to. . .*

MR S: (Laughs) Sure, go ahead.

JA: OK. So, what I'd like to do today is to record the consultation you have with the surgeon – Mr R. – I'll see you as you go into his consulting room, and I'll pop this recorder in there . . .

MR S: Is it on? Is it recording us?

JA: No, don't worry, it's not switched on just yet! Look – the red light isn't on. I'll start the recorder just before the start of your consultation and leave it in there, and I'll collect it later. Then – if you are happy to proceed – I shall meet you back here after the consultation, and I'll take you to a private room where we won't be disturbed and I'd like to interview you to find out about what was said in the consultation, what you understand about it, what you understand about the operation, and what you feel about it. I'll audio-record the interview if that is OK with you. Does that make sense to you?

MR S: Yes that does make sense and I'm happy to do it.

JA: Good. The interview should last about 30–40 minutes, but if you want to, *you can stop at any time you want.* So, if you are too tired, or if you get fed up with the sound of my voice, or for any other reason, we can stop – and that will be OK. Then at the end of the interview, I shall give you this brief questionnaire about your quality of life to take home with you to complete and send back to me. I'll give you a stamped addressed envelope to return it in. How are you doing? Do you understand all this so far?

MR S: Yes, I do, that's very clear, thank you.

JA: Great! . . . But I'm afraid that's not the last you'll see of me – that is if you are still happy to take part!

MR S: (Nods)

JA: Because I would like to see you again when you first come back for your *one-year check-up* and then again at your *two-year follow-up,* when I'll interview you again to see how you have been getting on and to see that your feelings are about the operation and the treatment you have had. And I shall give you a questionnaire to complete each time I see you. But . . .

MR S: (Laughs) But *I don't have to if I don't want to!?*

JA: Yes. Exactly so. *You don't have to do it if you don't want to!* Now, I've been talking for long enough. *Is there anything you'd like to ask me at this point?*

MR S: No that's all clear.

JA: No? OK. Let me say a bit more about the study. As you can tell, we are interested in how well the surgeons do their job of preparing you for the operation . . .

MR S: Well, I can't say about this lot here, but I've met others who couldn't prepare a boiled egg let alone tell you about an operation!

JA: (Laughs) Yes, Doctor-patient communication is an interest of mine, I have been involved in it as a researcher and a teacher for about 45 years now . . .

MR S: You don't look that old!

JA: What's that? . . . I don't look that old? How lovely you are to say that, but I am! Now, I should tell you that the study is *funded* by a small grant from the *XXXX Hospitals NHS Trust.* The research has been *approved* by the *Health Research Authority XXXX Research Ethics Committee.* I don't expect that there are any *risks* involved from your taking part, but if you get *upset* with anything we talk about, I can refer you to someone you can talk to about it. Is that OK?

MR S: Yes.

JA: There are three things I'd like to emphasise:

1. This research is entirely *voluntary.* That's right, *you don't have to do it if you don't want to!*
2. Everything you say to me will be completely *confidential* – I won't tell anyone else apart from my research colleagues anything that you say to me. I'll keep it strictly confidential. And you will be *anonymous* – there won't be any names on my questionnaires, the recordings or the questionnaires you complete. Instead, I shall put a *Study Serial Number* on those. I am the only person who will know who has said what, and I won't share that with anyone else.

3. The third thing is, and this is very important, *whether or not you take part will not affect the treatment you get in any way.*

Is that clear?

MR S: As a bell!

JA: Is there anything you would like to ask at this point? (Pause)

MR S: No, that's all fine.

JA: No? OK. Please feel free to phone up at any time to ask any questions that come to you later. Now, I'm going to ask you, *would you be willing to take part?*

MR S: Yes, as I said, I am only too happy to help out in any way I can.

JA: You would, well that's great, I am very pleased, and I'd like to say *thank you!*

MR S: You're most welcome.

JA: (Nods) So, let me remind you of what that will entail:

- I shall record your consultation.
- Then we'll meet back here.
- I'll take you to a private room for the interview – it should last 30–40 minutes.
- Then I'll give you a questionnaire to complete when you get home.
- Then, I'll see you again in one years' time.
- And again in two years' time – to interview you and get you to complete a questionnaire each time.

How does that sound?

MR S: Yes, you definitely earn your pay! That's fine by me.

JA: OK?

MR S: Yes.

JA: Great. Remember, that *you can stop or withdraw from the study at any time and you don't have to say why . . .*

MR S: I know – *thank you.*

JA: Now the last thing I have to do, and this is for your protection and to show you that I've done my job properly. Here is an *information sheet* about the study – you can take it away with you. This has my name in there and the names of my research colleagues – you can contact any of us to ask for more information and there is a name and number there of the *Director of the R&D Department* in the hospital, who you can contact if you have any complaints about the study.

MR S: This is all very thorough, I must say. I'm happy with everything.

JA: No, I mean it, *if you are not happy with anything about the study, please contact the Director of the R&D Department* and let her know. Lastly, I have a **consent form** which I need you to read and sign before we can go any further with the study.

MR S: A consent form?

JA: Yes, a consent form. It says 'Patients Expectations About Total Knee Replacement' – that's the title of the study.

1. I have been given a copy of the Participants' Information Sheet about the study. I understand what it says and I have had the opportunity to ask any questions I wanted and I have had these answered to my satisfaction. *If you are happy with that, please just put your initials in the box at the side there.*

MR S: I see.

JA: OK.

> **2.** I understand that my participation in this study is completely voluntary and I can withdraw from it at any time, without my statutory rights being affected in any way. *If you are happy with that, please just put your initials in the box at the side there.*

MR S: OK.

JA: Another box to fill:

> **3.** I understand that I may be contacted for further participation in the study approximately one year and two years later, and I give my consent to being contacted for this.

MR S: That's OK. So you will get in touch with me when it's time for my next follow up?

JA: Yes, the hospital will get in touch to let you know when your follow-up visits are and I shall get in touch with you then to arrange to meet.

MR S: That's good. I wouldn't like to be left guessing!

JA: No, that shouldn't happen. Now almost the last one . . .

> **4.** I understand that my consultation with the surgeon today will be audio-recorded for the purpose of this research. *If you are happy with that, please just put your initials in the box at the side there.*

MR S: Yes.

JA: That's good. And this is the last one . . .

> **5.** I agree to take part in this study. *If you are happy with that, please just put your initials in the box at the side there.*

MR S: It's a *yes* to all of them!

JA: Good. Then I shall sign it here to say that I have explained the study to you, so *I sign here, and I print my name here – JOHN ANDERSON – and I put the date here.* Then if you can do the same – *sign here, print your name here, and put the date here.*

MR S: My name . . . J.o.h.n. S.m.i.t.h. (Prints name) and sign . . . here?

JA: (Nods) Yes just there (pointing).

MR S: Uhuh. (Signs and dates the form).

JA: Thank you. Now we both complete *another copy* of the consent form – one is for you to keep and take away with you, so you know who you have seen today and one is for me to keep for my records.

BOTH COMPLETE THE SECOND COPY

JA: OK, *we are all done.* (JA stands) Thank you very much Mr Smith.

MR S: Yes? Well that was pretty painless,

JA: (JA extends his hand and shakes hands with Mr Smith), I'll see you back here after you have seen the surgeon. Bye for now.

MR S: Bye, see you soon.

(JA LEAVES.)

. . . And that's the sort of thing which I used to do for a living – and which I still do, from time to time.

NB – I do not pretend that this is perfect. One of the main things I tried to do was to emphasise, that, no matter how grateful, how **indebted** patients feel, and no matter how much they want to help, I want them to be sure that they *don't have to do it if they don't want to!* I realise that in some instances, in some situations, things might be different, and it is more difficult to recruit participants, but we should not put undue coercion on people to take part. We must, above all, be scrupulously honest with those people who might help us by agreeing to take part in our studies. *Take your time and explain things properly.*

Talking about **coercion,** one of my students 'Tina Favier' did a study to investigate mothers' feeding habits of their children. She got two schools – one in a relatively well-to-do part of the town and another from a relatively deprived part of the town – to announce her research and invite mothers to volunteer to take part in focus group discussions on the topic of child feeding. She offered, as an **incentive** a £25.00 shopping voucher to everyone who took part. (Her study was supported by the Local Authority where she worked.) Tina's study was quite innovative. She also invited anyone who was willing to let her accompany them on a shopping trip, so that she could see at first hand what their food shopping preferences were and to ask them about their choices of foods and the reasons why – a form of **quasi-participant observation.** Nice study! (**Aside:** I remember the trouble I had to go to get the REC to approve this study. They obviously did not understand – or approve of – this kind of approach. So, I had to do a lot of extra digging in the literature to find examples of this sort of approach being used in similar studies!) So, she had two focus groups, one of mothers from a relatively *well-to-do* part of the town and another from a relatively *deprived* part of the town. At the end of the focus group discussions, she asked them all to say *why* they had volunteered for the study. She was surprised to hear several of the mums in the group from the relatively deprived part of the town saying that the money had been a strong incentive. One of them pointed out that, because she was on benefits, £25.00 was about *half of her weekly shopping budget!* Sometimes, we academics forget how well-off we are compared to some of the people who we depend upon to help us by taking part in our research! Well done 'Tina'!

Giving people gifts or payment for taking part in research is OK. It is a fairly common practice in research to make payments for participants, particularly in experimental studies. In fact, a postal survey of GPs, which had one of the highest response rates, offered as a prize a brace of pheasants and a bottle of malt whiskey! (That researcher knew his target population!) We just have to make sure that the gift or financial inducement we offer is not 'An offer they couldn't refuse'!

Giving Written Information

Now let's consider the printed **PIS** – the **Participant Information Sheet** – which we give to the participant to explain all about the study and which also contains important contact information such as:

- The researcher's/interviewer's details.
- The chief investigator/principal investigator's (your supervisor's) details.
- The director of R&D's details.
- Contact names, phone numbers, and addresses of possible sources of support in case of any participant experiencing emotional distress.

You can download examples of PIS and Consent Forms from many sources, including the HRA. The sorts of information contained in PIS at most medical school falls into these headings:

- Study title.
- Invitation to participate.
- Purpose of the study.
- Why I have been invited to participate.
- Do I have to take part?
- What taking part will involve.
- What are the possible disadvantages and risks of taking part?
- What are the possible benefits of taking part?
- Will my information in this study be kept confidential?
- What will I do if I agree to take part?
- What will happen if I don't want to carry on with the study?
- What will happen to the results of the research study?
- Who is organising and funding the research?
- Payment for taking part/expenses.
- Who has approved this study?
- Contact for further information.
- Contact person for complaints.
- Contacts for support.
- Insurance.
- Thank you.
- Date – information sheets should be dated. The title, version number and date it was written, should be shown in the footer of the document.

Yes, it does sound like a lot. And yes, it may be overkill; but rather be comprehensive, than miss something out! But knowing what to include is only a part of the equation. If people can't read it or if they can't understand it, *we are in trouble!*

The Next Issue Is: Can Everyone Read it and Understand it?

We can test the **readability** of anything we write. Dr Rudolf Flesch who was an enthusiastic writing teacher and someone who promoted writing in plain English, created the **Flesch Reading Ease Test** (Flesch 1948). Later, working with Peter Kincaid, for the American Navy, they developed the **Flesch–Kincaid Grade Level Test.** The F–K formula became a military standard for assessing the reading difficulty of Army manuals. You can download free reading ease calculators from the internet. And I shall take you through them now. Microsoft Word can also calculate the Reading Ease of a document for you. (More on that later.)

The Flesch Reading-Ease Score is measured using the following formula:

$$206.835 - 1.015 \left(\frac{\text{total words}}{\text{total sentences}} \right) - 84.6 \left(\frac{\text{total syllables}}{\text{total words}} \right)$$

Memorise it! Got it? Good!

Reading-ease scores vary between 0 and 100. The lower the score, the more difficult it is to read. So, higher scores reflect writing that is easier to read. The following Table A.1 shows how readability relates to different types of written material and educational grades.

I remember in the 1970s reading an article in an orthopaedic journal. It reported on the development of an 'easy to read' information leaflet for patients (over the years I have lost my copy of the article and its source – sorry). I was amazed at it. Not because it was easy to read, but because it was so spectacularly difficult to read. It scored in the very difficult band of Reading-Ease. I reckoned that the poor bloke who wrote it wanted to impress his consultant boss – and the editor of the journal in which it was published!

So, Reading-Ease goes from 0 to 30 for *Very Difficult* pieces of writing – usually accessed by postgraduates in the high-end scientific journals. *Difficult* includes RE scores of 30–50, is readily understood by undergraduates, and is found in most academic journals. *Fairly Difficult* includes RE scores of 50–60, is accessible to grade 10–12 students and is found in 'quality' publications. *Standard* RE scores of 60–70 are understandable by students in grades 8–9 and are found in *Digest* level publications. RE scores of 70–80 are *Fairly Easy*; scores of 80–90 are *Easy* and scores of 90–100 are *Very Easy*.

Hey, wait a minute, did I just say *Digest*? Does that ring a bell? Yes, it does – the **Reader's Digest**. It always had interesting stuff in it and it was always *easy to read*. I have always admired it as a very slickly presented, but professional publication. It has a readability score of about 65, according the *Wikipedia* entry for 'Flesch–Kincaid readability tests' (the same entry cites a score of 57.9 for the novel *Moby Dick,* while 'one particularly long sentence about sharks in chapter 64 has a readability score of −146.77.' The same entry, tells us that 'The cat sat on the mat' scores 116, the US Department of Defence 'uses the reading ease test as the standard test of readability for its documents and forms, and Florida requires that insurance policies have a Flesch reading ease score of 45 or greater' (Wikipedia 2020).

Let's see how you might grade newspapers in this way. Use Table A.2 to fill in the Gaps, and work out which newspapers fit in where.

Illiteracy is more widespread that you might think. The **National Literacy Trust** (NLT) estimates that 16% of adults in the UK are 'functionally illiterate' (NLT 2020). Remember that when you plan a study of people in the UK. Ask yourself 'Who might I be excluding if I pitch the reading-ease level of my information sheets too hard?' Keep it simple! As a rule of thumb, ***use short words and short sentences! And avoid jargon***.

You used to be able to set Microsoft Word to calculate the readability statistics of a document or a part of a document. Fortunately, the version I am using on my laptop

TABLE A.1   Flesch reading-ease scores.

Reading Ease	Difficulty	Educational Level	Typical Magazine Style
0–30	Very difficult	Postgraduate	Scientific
30–50	Difficult	Undergraduate	Academic
50–60	Fairly difficult	Grade 10–12	Quality
60–70	Standard	Grade 8–9	Digest
70–80	Fairly easy	Grade 7	Slick fiction
80–90	Easy	Grade 6	Pulp fiction
90–100	Very easy	Grade 5	Comic

seems to check and comment on the 'accessibility' of my document for me. Let me guide you to set up word to give you readability statistics.

1. Click on 'File' – top left of the screen.
2. Select 'Options' – bottom left of the screen.
3. Click on 'Proofing' – the third option down from the top left of the box.
4. The dialogue box that opens has a section about half-way down which says 'When correcting spelling and grammar in Word'. The fifth option down the list is 'Show readability statistics' Tick that box.
5. Click on 'OK' and exit.
6. Now Word is set to show readability statistics.
7. In my previous version, by highlighting a block of text I could check the statistics for that block. I clicked on 'Review', then did a spell check of the text. When that was finished, I clicked 'OK' and the readability stats came up with the Flesch scores. I loved that – it was easy and controllable.

In the workshops I do on Obtaining Informed Consent, I ask my students to send in a piece of text of up to 500 words on how they might describe 'confidentiality' in a PIS. Then I supply them with the results. It is a nice bit of fun, but it gets the point across – we tend to over-estimate our abilities to communicate easily and effectively.

Let me share with you one of my students' work. 'Valerie' is a lovely person. I co-supervised her MSc Cardiology dissertation of communicating with patients about erectile dysfunction – a warning sign for heart failure. She scored 44.5 on her first attempt – which was in the 'difficult' zone. She was upset at this and was determined to get it better. So she did it again and got 78.6 – in the 'fairly easy' zone. Better! But that was not good enough for our 'Valerie'. She did two more attempts until she hit the jackpot and got a score of 100 – 'Very easy'! Well done 'Valerie'!

Here are her first, second, and fourth versions.

1. 'Confidentiality – this means keeping information about you as safe as possible. We will be collecting data about you. The paper records will be kept in a locked filing cabinet. Computer records will be encrypted and password protected. You will, wherever possible, be identified by a code number, not your real name. Your information will be shared across the people running this trial however this would normally not be

TABLE A.2 Reading Ease scores in newspapers and magazines.

Reading Ease	Difficulty	Typical newspapers	Typical Magazine Style
0–30	Very difficult		Scientific
30–50	Difficult		Academic
50–60	Fairly difficult		Quality
60–70	Standard		Digest
70–80	Fairly easy		Slick fiction
80–90	Easy		Pulp fiction
90–100	Very easy		Comic

connected to your name. The people running this trial include not only your doctors but also other specialists. You will not be identified, or identifiable in any publication or presentation arising from this trial.' (**Flesch Reading Ease Score = 44.5**)

2. 'All the data about you will be kept confidential. Only the trial staff will have access to it. It will be stored safely in a locked cabinet. We shall not use your name and it will not be possible to identify you in any reports we write.' (**Flesch Reading Ease Score = 78.6**)

3. **There is no. 3.**

4. 'You and I will talk. I shall write it down. I will not tell them it was you. I will keep it a secret. Hush. I will write about what you say. I will not tell them it was you. If you don't want to help, you can go. I won't say anything.' (Reading Ease = 100)

You see, it can be done. Have a go yourself. Thank you for that 'Valerie'!

To Sum Up

In this appendix I have discussed various issues around obtaining informed consent. I began by considering how we might give information about our study to potential participants **orally.** I used an example of the sorts of things I would say – to give you something to think about. (NB: my use of **repetition** was informed by a study which I did in Hong Kong of patients' recall of information, in which we found that information which was repeated, was *three times more likely to be correctly recalled* than information which was not.) Then I discussed briefly giving payments or inducements to research participants – and concluded that we need to strike a balance between a fair reward for their time and effort and offering unduly high levels of inducements which people might find impossible to resist.

Then I discussed presenting information in **written** form – such as in a **Participant Information Sheet** (PIS). I talked about the **Flesch Formula for Reading-Ease** and suggested that we might use that to check the readability of our documents.

I want to say that one of the most important things to be able to do in research is to describe your study to a potential participant. Most people who I have observed try it out for the first time, have a lot of difficulty in doing this. So, my conclusion and my advice to you is: *practise* this before you do it for real. Get a colleague or a friend to help you by pretending to be a potential participant and make sure they give you *honest feedback. Repeat* your practice until you are good at it. Then *repeat* it even more times until you are perfect! *Good luck!*

References

Favier T. (201X). Mothers' beliefs about Child Feeding. University of Brighton MSc Dissertation.

Flesch R. (1948). A new readability yardstick. *Journal of Applied Psychology* 32(3), 221–233. doi:10.1037/h0057532

National Literacy Trust (2020). Adult literacy. Available at: https://literacytrust.org.uk/parents-and-families/adult-literacy (accessed 22 September 2020).

Wikipedia (2020). Flesch–Kincaid readability tests. Available at: https://en.wikipedia.org/wiki/Flesch–Kincaid:readability_tests (accessed 22 September 2020).

APPENDIX B

Research Skills

Searching the Literature

Introduction

One of the most essential skills for all researchers is to be able to search the literature to find articles published on the topic you want to research. My best advice here is to consult your **local librarian** and ask for their help – they are usually most helpful and can save you lots of time and energy.

They are likely to help you to identify the most appropriate **publications databases**. These tend to be discipline specific and include publications from journals relating to Medicine, Nursing, Physiotherapy, Psychology, Sociology, etc. Some of the most commonly used ones include:

Health:

- PUBMED
- CINAHL
- Ccochrane
- Embase
- British Nursing Index.

Social Sciences:

- PsychINFO
- ASSIA
- ERIC.

General Science:

- ISI Web of Science

Demystifying Research for Medical & Healthcare Students: An Essential Guide, First Edition. John L. Anderson.
© 2022 John Wiley & Sons Ltd. Published 2022 by John Wiley & Sons Ltd.
Companion website: www.wiley.com/go/Anderson/DemystifyingResearch

Conducting a Literature Search

The development of such online resources has revolutionised the process of literature searching. When I did literature searching as a student and in my earlier research studies, I had to go along to libraries such as the Royal Society of Medicine library, The British Museum library, and others, to *physically* search through all of the journals relevant to my searches, by hand. It took ages. Now, a few clicks of the mouse is all it takes to bring all of those resources to your laptop screen.

But first you have to decide upon your search criteria – the search terms you will use to find articles that might be of interest. Search engines allow you to search their databases using different 'fields' – categories of information about the published articles held in that database. These can include:

- Author
- Date
- Journal
- Language
- Title
- Title word
- Text word
- MeSH terms – **Me**dical **S**ubject **H**eadings – used in PUBMED and CINAHL to reflect subject content
- Etc.

So, the first thing you have do is to develop your search questions. One of the most common way of doing this is to use the '**PICO**' formula. This stands for Population, Intervention, Comparison, and Outcomes. As you can see, this is immediately biased towards searching for research articles on randomised control trials. However, it is still a useful starting point for most studies. This is shown in **Table B.1**.

Using this guide can help you to decide what elements to put into a search engine such as those described above for different specialties. You can create a search string by using several terms by adding 'AND' or 'OR' or 'NOT'. These links are called '**Boolean Operators**' – it's a library term. If you search for 'doctors' AND 'nurses' you will get all the results that include **both** doctors and nurses – but not articles with only doctors or only nurses. If you search for 'doctors' OR 'nurses' you will get all articles which have either doctors or nurses. If you search for 'doctors' NOT 'nurses' you will get all articles with doctors, but ones which also include nurses will be excluded from your search results. NB – the databases do this for you.

Another useful shorthand is to use the '**wildcard' character** – usually an asterisk '*' or a dollar sign '$'. These work like this:

Med* will include medicine/medical/medico- etc.
Nurs* will include nursing/nurses/nursery etc.
Phys$ will include physio/physiotherapy/physiological/physical etc.

TABLE B.1   Using the PICO formula for defining search criteria.

PICO	Meaning	Examples
P	Population, Participants, Patients, People, Problem	Who are you interested in studying – what sort of people/patients/participants? With what sorts of characteristics, etc. In what settings, etc. Try to focus it down as closely as you can to be relevant to the study you are doing.
I	Interventions	Clinical – what treatments, or tests will be included? For what diagnoses or illnesses.
C	Comparisons, Controls	What control or comparison groups will you look for (if any)?
O	Outcomes	Include clinical outcomes – e.g. mortality; reduction of symptoms, etc.
		Think about patient-defined outcomes such as quality of life; function; acceptability of treatment, etc.

They will include any words with the letters before the wildcard in them as being parts of your search. So, the thing to remember when you use 'wildcards' is to think carefully about how you use them – otherwise you may get thousands of unexpected or irrelevant articles! But it certainly saves time through not having to specify a long string of 'OR' links in your search.

Try them out.

NB: Databases change their inclusions from time to time. This can be confusing because a journal which was included in 2020 might not be included in 2021. It is always worth using **more than one search engine**. This increases your likelihood of getting a comprehensive search. For example, when Seb and I first searched the literature to find out what had been published on *dyslexia* in *medical students/medical education* (Shaw, Malik & Anderson, 2017) we turned to our old favourite – **PUBMED.** So, we did our searches using the search terms 'dyslexia' and 'medical*' – nothing! There must be something. . . So, I did a **Google** search – three results!

These were:

- Ricketts, C., Brice, J. and Coombes, L. (2010). 'Are multiple choice tests fair to medical students with specific learning disabilities?' *Adv Health Sci Educ Theory Pract.* 15: 265–75.
- Gibson, S. and Leinster, S. (2011). 'How do students with dyslexia perform in extended matching questions, short answer questions and observed structured clinical examinations?' *Adv Health Sci Educ Theory Pract.* 16: 395–404.
- Mckendree, J. and Snowling, M. J. (2011). 'Examination results of medical students with dyslexia.' *Med Educ.* 45: 176–82.

But these were all in non-PUBMED indexed journals. Yes – *Medical Education* was not included within PUBMed at that time. These would have been picked up if we had searched an **Educational database** – such as ERIC – we should have identified them straightaway.

Librarians usually warn you against using Google. I use it, and I suspect you are used to using it. So it can be an easy starting point for your first search.

My advice is to ALWAYS **use more than one database.** Find out from your librarian what the main databases for your subject are and search within these.

Once you have identified your literature, the next step is to **search the references** in the published papers that you have identified. This is a simple check to make sure that you have not missed anything of interest. Every now and then, you might find a crucial paper that you have overlooked in your other searches.

The Grey Literature

What do we mean by this? 'Grey Literature' refers to written work which has not been published in academic journals. It includes things like: MSc dissertations and PhD theses; conference papers; unpublished papers; research in progress; reports; government documents; and so on. Much of the grey literature is difficult to find. People who are well-established in their field tend to know a lot about what is going on; for example, by attending conferences, reading the newspapers, networking, etc. For example, I was aware of the work which my colleague, Harry Witchel had been involved in because I had heard him talking about it and I Googled it. (See Chapter 3 on Real Life Experiments.) You probably won't pick up much from the grey literature but, occasionally, you find a nugget of pure gold! It is an essential source for those of you who go on to conduct a systematic review. My librarian colleague, Annemarie Frank, signposted me to 'the most comprehensive list of grey literature databases produced by Public Health England on the King's College website attached' **https://libguides.kcl. ac.uk/systematicreview/greylit**. Have a look at it.

De-duplication

Once you have accessed full copies of all of your studies, the next step is to check for duplicates – many might be the same as ones you have found in other databases. You can discard the duplicates. That will reduce the numbers. The next thing to look out for is the same study being published with a slightly different title and emphasis in different journals. These are a nuisance, because they are more difficult to spot as the authors may be switched around. Discard duplicates.

Keep Records of all Your Searches and the Results

Make sure you keep a record of each of your searches. Note the date and time, the search engine/database you used, and the search terms you used. Next, do the search and note the number of 'hits' or results you get. These will usually be listed in date order – most recent first. That is the easy part! Now the hard work begins. You have to go through each one of the articles that are identified to sort out those which might be relevant from those which are obviously not relevant. So, you might get, say, 7345 results. Don't worry – you can get through those in about three days! Or you might wish to re-define your search to make it more specific. Then you narrow it down to 862 results. That's better. Looking at the **titles** will, in most cases, help you to decide on the really irrelevant ones. For others, you may need to read the **abstract** (usually available freely within the database), and that will tell you if you can exclude that article or not. However, for many, you will need the **full version** of the paper to judge. Many sources allow you to access free copies of their articles. For others, you might be able to access them using your university or college's account – ask your librarian about this. For some you may not be able to access a copy online – in these cases, speak to your librarian about how to get a copy, for example via inter-library loan. etc. Most university and NHS Trust libraries have resources to allow healthcare students to access articles in the journals they need.

   Now – keeping records . . . As you go through the list of articles, **NOTE DOWN** those which look interesting (year, title, author) – and note which you can get immediately and those which you need to ask your librarian for help with. Then note the date you request copies and the date they arrive. By keeping good records, you can easily move on to the next step.

The Prisma Diagram

One of the clearest ways of displaying your search results is in a **Prisma diagram.** An example of this is shown in **Figure B.1**. I have taken it from Aalya Al-Assaf's MSc dissertation work which was a systematic review of the literature on physical activity and ovarian cancer (Al-Assaf, 2014). She used the PICO formula for searching the literature as shown in Table B.2 below.

   She described her search in detail:

An extensive electronic literature search of PubMed, EMBASE, CINAHL, Psych info, AMED, Web of Knowledge, British Nursing Index (BNI), and Cochrane Library was performed. Also, searching for grey literature in NHS evidence, Google search, Brighton and Sussex University Trust Hospital, CINAHL, National Technology Information Service (NTIS), and Cancer Research was conducted. Moreover, references of the identified articles were searched manually to identify any relevant articles. Specialised librarians were consulted to identify the most important databases and to help in creating the suitable combinations of keywords.

A combination of keywords and mesh terms/subject headings were used. Generally, search terms were (Physical activity OR exercise) AND (Ovar* AND (cancer OR neoplasm OR tumour OR malignancy). No time limit for the years of publication was set in the databases in order to identify all the available literature. There was no language restriction to reduce the chance of publication bias as this bias can arise because of limiting the included studies to those only published in one language.

*Additionally, to identify any ongoing trial on the subject of this review, the research registers of ongoing trials (**http://controlled-trials.com**) was also searched. The search was performed in the period between July 2012 to 2/10/2013. Search alarms of the electronic databases were set to update the search weekly to identify any new published study.*

(Al-Assaf, 2014)

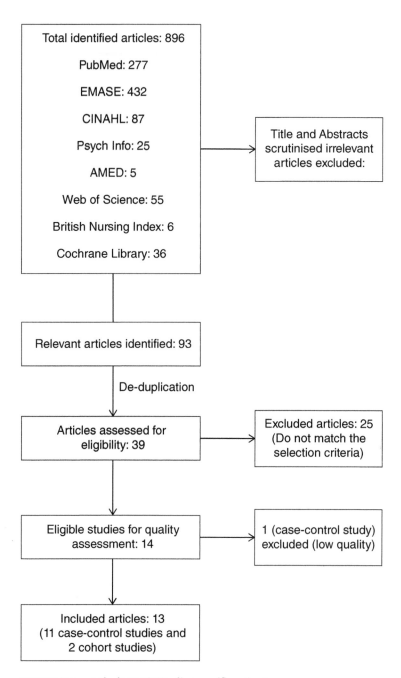

FIGURE B.1   Aalya's PRISMA diagram/flowchart.

Full details of the search strategy were included in an Appendix. This is a really useful thing you can do to save words in a dissertation or thesis where you have a word limit. By including this in an appendix, it is there for the markers to see and yet does not take up valuable words.

TABLE B.2 Dr Assaf's PICO Search Criteria.

PICO criteria:	Specifically:
1 - Population:	women from different age groups, social and cultural background to increase generalisability and size of the sample
2 - Exposure/ Intervention:	physical activity that is defined according to the WHO as 'any movement of the body that is created by skeletal muscles and spends energy'. Details of measures of PA assessment should be mentioned in the study
3 - Outcome:	ovarian cancer risk
4 - Study Design:	RCTs, non-RCTs, cohort studies, and case-control studies that investigate the effect of PA on OC risk

Source: (Al-Assaf, 2014)

Assessing the Quality of Published Work

If you do decide to conduct a systematic review, then you must perform a **quality assessment** of the studies you find in your search. This is not normally done in most publications where you refer to the literature for discussion. But in a systematic review, the data in the publications you find **IS** your data. Therefore, you need to be confident that the data you include is of sufficiently high quality to be included – hence a form of quality assessment is needed. In her work, Aalya chose to use a two-step approach. Because all of the relevant studies she identified were either case-control studies or cohort studies, she used Elwood's schema for the assessment of cohort studies (Elwood, 2007) and Khan's for cohort studies (Khan et al., 2001). Then she repeated the quality assessment using the **Scottish Intercollegiate Guidelines Network (SIGN)** methodology checklists for cohort studies and for case-control studies (SIGN, 2004a, b). Poor quality studies were discarded.

Aalya and I went through this process together – I offer to validate my students' quality assessments when they do systematic reviews. It is always best to get help from your supervisor or a friend or colleague to do this, to confirm that you are not biased in any way.

The most rigorous quality assessment that I have been involved in was as part of a Cochrane Review along with Aalya and other colleagues (Rutjies et al., 2018). In honour of Archie Cochrane, **'Cochrane Centres'** have been established throughout the world. They promote high quality systematic reviews of clinical interventions and assessments and, to this end, they have teams of dedicates librarian staff, statisticians, and clinical experts on hand to support the professional (clinicians and academics who they engage as subject specialists to do the reviews). The Cochrane database is one of the ones which you can search, as Aalya did, for appropriate trials.

Data Extraction

In a systematic review, it is essential to decide upon what data you are looking for in the studies you find – before you begin your search. This can be formed into a **data extraction sheet** which you use to search each of your identified studies for their results. The PICO system can be used to help you determine what to look for in the studies you find. This will provide you with your **results.**

Data Analysis

The next task in a systematic review will be to analyse your results. This can be done in two ways:

1. Using appropriate **statistical tests** – as in a **meta analysis.** In a meta analysis, you can pool all the data that is similar – or comparable – and analyse it. This grouped data usually benefits from having larger numbers than just one study and is more powerful – it has **greater generalisability**. There are statistical tools which you can use to compare the data in different studies and also to analyse the pooled data. But that is another story!

2. Using a **narrative analysis** – where you describe the data (usually when you can't pool it) and draw your conclusions from this analysis.

A narrative analysis can also be used when conducting systematic reviews of **qualitative studies.**

In most studies, our literature review will be summarised in a narrative form, citing statistics from the studies where appropriate.

Wow! There was more there than I had intended, but I thought that this would be useful to those of you who are tempted to do a **systematic review.**

References

Al-Assaf A. (2014). *Physical Activity and Ovarian Cancer: A Systematic Review.* University of Brighton, MSc Dissertation.

Elwood JM. (2007). *Critical Appraisal of Epidemiological Studies and Clinical Trials,* 3rd ed. Oxford University Press: Oxford.

Gibson S and Leinster S. (2011). How do students with dyslexia perform in extended matching questions, short answer questions and observed structured clinical examinations? *Advanced Health Science Education and Theory Practice* 16, 395–404.

Khan KS, ter Riet G, Popay J, et al. (2001). STAGE II – Conducting the review. PHASE 5 – Study quality assessment. In: *Undertaking Systematic Reviews of Research on Effectiveness* (eds. Khan KS, ter Riet G, Popay J. et al.) pp 1–20.

Mckendree J and Snowling MJ. (2011). Examination results of medical students with dyslexia. *Medical Education* 45, 176–182.

Ricketts C, Brice J, and Coombes L. (2010). Are multiple choice tests fair to medical students with specific learning disabilities? *Advanced Health Science Education and Theory Practice* 15, 265–275.

Scottish Intercollegiate Guidelines Network (SIGN) (2004a). Methodology checklist 3: Cohort Studies [online]. March 2004. Available at: www.sign.ac.uk/guidelines/fulltext/50/checklist3. html (accessed 8 November 2012).

Scottish Intercollegiate Guidelines Network (SIGN) (2004b). Notes on the use of methodology checklist 3: Cohort Studies [online]. March 2004. Available at: www.sign.ac.uk/guidelines/full-text/50/notes3.html (accessed 8 November 2012).

Shaw SCK, Malik M, and Anderson JL. (2017). The exam performance of medical students with dyslexia: a review of the literature. *MedEdPublish* https://doi.org/10.15694/mep.2017.000116.

APPENDIX C

Research Skills

Laboratory Safety

Lab Safety Is a Serious Matter

Our concerns are for:

- the researcher
- other people in or near the lab
- the environment
- society in general.

The Researcher's Safety

In the nineteenth century it was common practice for medical researchers to use themselves as 'guinea pigs'. Waldemar Mordecai Haffkine, in Paris, following in the footsteps of Robert Koch (Koch 1882, 1884) Lois Pasteur, and Edward Jenner, created the first vaccines for cholera and plague. To prove his theory that his vaccine would work against cholera, in 1892 he injected himself and then some friends with his vaccine. Although they reported some brief fevers, they did not suffer any ill-effects. He ran into great scepticism from the medical establishment at that time who were committed to the belief that cholera and malaria originated from a 'miasma' which emerged from swampy areas. That same year Max Von Pettenkoffer drank beakers full of cholera bacilli to demonstrate that not all healthy people when exposed to the disease actually succumbed to it. **PLEASE – DON'T TRY THIS AT HOME!**

In 1996, a researcher, Karen Wetterhahn, who was working in a laboratory in Dartmouth College, USA, to study the effects of heavy metals on living organisms, accidentally spilled a drop of **dimethyl mercury** on to her glove. It penetrated the glove, but

Demystifying Research for Medical & Healthcare Students: An Essential Guide, First Edition. John L. Anderson.
© 2022 John Wiley & Sons Ltd. Published 2022 by John Wiley & Sons Ltd.
Companion website: www.wiley.com/go/Anderson/DemystifyingResearch

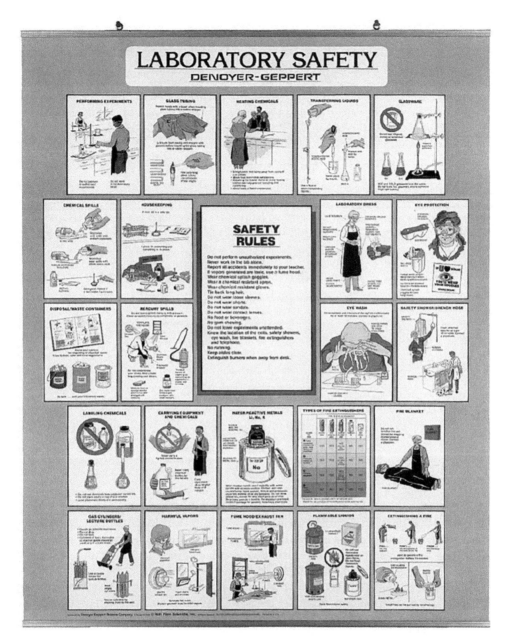

FIGURE C.1   An example of a lab safety poster.

she did not think it was serious. Five months later, she was hospitalised with mercury poisoning – the level was 80 times more than the standard toxicity threshold. She went into a coma and died. John Winn, head of the Dartmouth Chemistry Department, said that 'accepted lab procedures call for the use of gloves in handling dimethyl mercury, but don't necessarily specify what kind . . .'. He and two colleagues warned that latex gloves are 'not suitable for significant, direct contact with aggressive or highly toxic chemicals' and recommended that two pairs of gloves, one of them laminated, be worn.

In addition, says Winn, 'We're trying to urge the chemical community to establish a safer substitute' (Science News Staff, 11 June 1997).

A frightening event in a US lab, which could have harmed naïve researchers in that lab, was reported in *Science* by Jocelyn Kaiser on 8 July 2014.

> *Federal scientists last week discovered a half-dozen forgotten vials of smallpox virus while cleaning out a storage area on the campus of the National Institutes of Health (NIH) in Bethesda, Maryland. Variola, or smallpox, which killed hundreds of millions before it was declared eradicated in 1980 through a worldwide vaccination campaign, is legally stored at only two locations in the United States and Russia.*

> *The six vials of freeze-dried virus, apparently dating from the 1950s, were found by a scientist from the Food and Drug Administration (FDA) on 1 July in a cold storage room that was originally part of an NIH laboratory, but was transferred to FDA in the early 1970s. The FDA laboratory is being moved to the FDA's main campus, according to ABC News, NBC Washington, and a statement today from the Centers for Disease Control and Prevention (CDC). The vials were labeled as containing variola and were packed in a cardboard box along with 10 other vials with unclear labels*

When you are working with dangerous substances, ***clear up properly afterwards***. The lessons are clear to lab bosses and lab workers:

- never let novice researchers work alone;
- always wear proper safety equipment; and
- know what you are working with.

Other People in the Lab

One of the most famous breaches of safety involved the disease **smallpox**. After decades of effort, smallpox had been eradicated in the natural world in 1978. But, in 1978 a medical photographer at Birmingham Medical School (UK) contracted the disease and died. Where she worked was above the smallpox lab at the medical school, and faulty ventilation and shortcomings in technique were blamed.

Ian Sample, the Science Editor at the *Guardian* reported that 'Safety blunders expose lab staff to potentially lethal diseases in the UK' (the *Guardian*, Friday 9 February 2018).

> ***Marburg virus disease*** *is a highly virulent disease that causes haemorrhagic fever, with a fatality ratio of up to 88%. It is in the same family as the virus that causes Ebola virus disease. Two large outbreaks that occurred simultaneously in Marburg and Frankfurt in Germany, and in Belgrade, Serbia, in 1967, led to the initial recognition of the disease. The outbreak was associated with laboratory work using African green monkeys (Cercopithecus aethiops) imported from Uganda. Subsequently, outbreaks and sporadic cases have been reported in Angola, Democratic Republic of the Congo, Kenya, South Africa (in a person with recent travel history to Zimbabwe) and Uganda. In 2008, two independent cases were reported in travellers who visited a cave inhabited by Rousettus bat colonies in Uganda.*

(WHO)

The Environment

In 2011, the UK Health and Safety Executive (**HSE**) took action against an animal health laboratory, the Institute for Animal Health in **Pirbright in Surrey** following two incidents. In the first, a flask containing foot and mouth virus cracked and leaked over a sink. The contents went down a secure drain and did not leak into the environment. In the second, an incinerator which was being used to burn infected cow carcases leaked liquid out of the incinerator – but not out of the building. Another near miss which highlights the need for stringent safety precautions – which were in place and saved further contamination! However, the HSE concluded that in both cases, there were serious breaches of health and safety regulations.

> *The Pirbright site was at the centre of an outbreak of foot-and-mouth disease in August 2007 which led to the slaughter of over 2,100 animals in Surry and Berkshire. Surrey County Council said there was a lack of evidence to pinpoint the exact source of the outbreak. . . (which was) . . . probably due to live virus used in the development of a vaccine leaking from faulty pipework and spreading from the site.*
>
> *(Pallab Ghosh 2011)*

Society in General

Another example of **smallpox** re-emerging was reported in 2002 by Debora Mackenzie in the *New Scientist*. She reported:

> *In 1971, the Soviets were testing smallpox aerosols at their main bioweapons testing range, Vozrozhdeniye Island in the Aral Sea, according to the report by Jonathan Tucker and colleagues at the Monterey Institute for International Studies in Washington. It will be published later this month.*
>
> *A fisheries research vessel passed closer to the island than regulations allowed during the test, and a young female biologist working on deck was infected. She came down with smallpox later in the port town of Aralsk. A total of twelve people there became ill, the town was quarantined and 50,000 people were re-vaccinated.*
>
> *The three who died, a woman and two small children, had never been vaccinated.*
>
> *(Debora Mackenzie 2002)*

This issue was also raised recently during the **Coronavirus pandemic**, when questions were raised about security and safety in research labs – as the following extract from Mark Field's piece in highlights in the *Bulletin of the Atomic Scientists*, 30 March 2020. He cites Professor Richard Ebright of Rutgers University's Waksman Institute of Microbiology, a biosecurity expert who has been speaking out on lab safety since the early 2000s and who concludes that the conspiracy theory linking the COVID-19 outbreak to bioweapons research is untrue. However, he reports that it possible the pandemic arose from an accidental release from a laboratory, such as one of the two in Wuhan which were known to have been studying bat coronaviruses.

Except for SARS-CoV and MERS-CoV, two deadly viruses that have caused outbreaks in the past, coronaviruses have been studied at laboratories that are labelled as operating at a moderate biosafety level known as BSL-2, Ebright says. And, he says, bat coronaviruses have been studied at such labs in and around Wuhan, China, where the new coronavirus first emerged. 'As a result', Ebright says, 'bat coronaviruses at Wuhan [Center for Disease Control] and Wuhan Institute of Virology routinely were collected and studied at BSL-2, which provides only minimal protections against infection of lab workers.'

Higher safety-level labs would be appropriate for a virus with the characteristics of the new coronavirus causing the current pandemic. 'Virus collection, culture, isolation, or animal infection at BSL-2 with a virus having the transmission characteristics of the outbreak virus would pose substantial risk of infection of a lab worker, and from the lab worker, the public', Ebright says.

The Nature Medicine authors 'leave us where we were before: with a basis to rule out [a coronavirus that is] a lab construct, but no basis to rule out a lab accident'.

(Field, 2020. See also Field, 2021)

So, the message is clear – **be safe in labs** and ensure that you follow all safety procedures and protocols, no matter how tedious or unnecessary they might seem. Report all breaches of safety! *Save lives* – including your own!

References

Field M. (2020). Experts know the new coronavirus is not a bioweapon. They disagree on whether it could have leaked from a research lab. Bulletin of the Atomic Scientists, 30 March 2020.

Field M. (2021). The Origins of COVID-19: Evidence Piles up, but the jury's still out. Bulletin of the Atomic Scientists, October 11, 2021.

Ghosh P. (2011). 'Safety incidents' at animal lab. BBC News, 26 May 2011. Available at: www.bbc.co.uk/news/science-environment-13566593 (accessed 21 April 2020).

Kaiser J. (2014). Six vials of smallpox found in US lab. Science, 8 July 2014. Available at: www.sciencemag.org/news/2014/07/six-vials-smallpox-discovered-us-lab ().

Koch R. (1882). Die Aetiologie der Tuberculose [The Etiology of Tuberculosis]. *Berliner Klinische Wochenschrift [Berlin Clinical Weekly]* 19, 221–230.

Koch R. (1884). Sechster ericht der Leiters der deutschen wissenschaftlichen Commission zur Erforschung der Cholera [Sixth Report of the Head of the German Scientific Commission for Research on Cholera]. *Deutsche medizinische Wochenscrift [German Medical Weekly]* 10(12), 191–192.

Mackenzie D. (2002). Soviet smallpox outbreak confirmed. New Scientist, 17 June 2002. Available at: www.newscientist.com/article/dn2415-soviet-smallpox-outbreak-confirmed (accessed 21 April 2020).

Sample I. (2018). Safety blunders expose lab staff to potentially lethal diseases in UK. The Guardian, 9 February 2018.

Science News Staff (1997). Mercury poisoning kills lab chemist. Science. Available at: www.sciencemag.org/news/1997/06/mercury-poisoning-kills-lab-chemist (accessed 18 April 2020).

APPENDIX D

Research Skills

Interviewing

Introduction

Interviewing is one of the commonest ways to collect data. Even in a clinical trial, you may have to speak to your participants to get information from them, e.g. about side-effects, about their clinical history, and so on. We all do 'interviewing' of some sort in our everyday lives. In our conversations with people, we question them about things and they question us. But there is a difference between these interactions and a **professional** interview. In our everyday conversations, it doesn't usually matter if we make mistakes or don't do it right. But there are lots of local customs which govern our ways of interacting.

a. We tend to take these for granted – we engage in them, usually out of our awareness.

b. These conversational conventions are often carried on in the workplace.

c. In our professional work, it is not always possible for us to be aware of when our 'lay' conventions are leading our 'professional' interactions.

What I have observed, over and over again, are doctors, nurses, social workers, and other healthcare professionals (HCPs) who believe they are good at communicating with patients and clients – because they get on well socially with their peers – but who are actually *not very good at it*. What is often passed off as **professional patois** (the jargon or informal speech used by a particular social group) is sometimes downright rudeness. In my four years of psychotherapy training, no one ever taught me communications skills explicitly. And that disappointed me because of my awareness of the importance of these issues from the years I spent (with others) researching and developing communications skills training in medicine. Now, what can we do about it? Well, there are certain rules of thumb which can guide us to be better professional communicators. But the first challenge for us is to be aware that there are differences about how we communicate in a *professional situation* as opposed to a *general social situation*. So, as researchers we have to be professional in the way we give information (exposition skills) and gather information (interview skills) with our research participants. In interviewing one of the key components is the ability to *listen*.

Interviews are **formal** occasions where we collect information from other people. There are three main types of interviews.

Demystifying Research for Medical & Healthcare Students: An Essential Guide, First Edition. John L. Anderson.
© 2022 John Wiley & Sons Ltd. Published 2022 by John Wiley & Sons Ltd.
Companion website: www.wiley.com/go/Anderson/DemystifyingResearch

Unstructured Interviews

Unstructured interviews: These, as the name suggests, have no formal structure at all. These are most commonly found in **qualitative research;** for example, in grounded theory or in phenomenological approaches. In these the interviewer allows the participant to tell her/his own story in her/his own words, in the order that it comes to her/him. So, after explaining the purpose of the interview, the interviewer might then say, 'Tell me about your experiences with. . .' and let the respondent tell her/his story, only occasionally intervening with supplementary questions to clarify or expand on the information given.

Loosely-structured interviews: There are mainly used in qualitative research of all kinds. Here the interviewer may develop a set of topics which have to be addressed during the interview and will use a **'topic guide'** as an aide-memoire to facilitate the interview. NB: the topic guide is *not* a list of questions – if it is, then the interviewer will tend to stick slavishly to the wording in the questions. It is a reminder of the topic areas to be explored using appropriate questions to suit the tone of the interview and the part of the interview that you are in – it will *not* give you set questions to ask.

Semi-structured interviews: These are interviews which have a set of questions to be asked and a suggested order for them to be asked in, but the interviewer can be allowed her/his own discretion to change the wording or the ordering of questions – as appropriate to the interviewee (often found in quantitative studies).

Structured – or highly-structured interviews: We discussed these briefly in Chapter 8 on 'Survey Methods'. These are usually conducted by interviewers using a highly structured **questionnaire**. The theory, remember, is that by asking all the *same questions,* in the *same order* – and crucially with the *same wording* – then you know that each participant has been presented with the same set of **stimuli** to which you want them to respond. Then you can be assured that the answers are all responses to the same set of stimuli. (You can think of this as the **stimulus–response model.**) You don't really need any training in interview skills to be able to do these, a robot can do them just as well. And of course we have the equivalent of robots in our. . .? That's right. . . in our questionnaires!

But, highly structured interviews apart, you do need to be competent at some interview skills. For highly structured interviews, you need to be trained so that you know the interview as well as you know the back of your hand! *In all interviews, you have to be able to listen!*

You can think of an interview as having four main stages or phases.

Phase 1: Introduction

In a research interview this is a crucial part of the process. It is where you explain what you want from the research participant. If (as in the example I gave in Appendix A) you have only just obtained informed consent from your participant, then you should have covered some of this recently, but it is still important, at this point, to recap some of what you have said about the purpose of the interview and what you want to get out of it. **Remember:** you are now working with someone who has agreed to take part in your study – they want to help you. So, *help them by being clear about the information you want to get from them.* Below, I have outlined how the interview that I got consent for might start.

(JA and Mr. Smith have seated themselves in the interview room.)

JA: Hello again, Mr. Smith, it's good to see you again

MrS: It's good to see you too.

JA: OK are you happy to continue?

MrS: Yes, I'm fine, thank you.

JA: Are you sure?

MrS: Yes.

JA: Good. But remember you can stop at any time if you want to. Just say the word – I won't be offended . . . Are you comfortable in this room?

MrS: Yes this is quite cosy.

JA: It is, isn't it. I've put a 'Do Not Disturb' sign on the door to stop anyone interrupting us.

MrS: That's good.

JA: Now, let's begin. I mentioned the purpose of the research to you didn't I?

MrS: Yes you did – it's to find out about what I expect to happen after my total knee replacement.

JA: That's exactly it! And I should also say that you can say whatever you want to say – there are no 'right' or 'wrong' answers to any of my questions. Is that OK?

MrS: Yes, got it.

JA: And I want to emphasise again that I shall not let anyone else know what you have said. Although Mr Ramaghastalan is a member of the research team, I am the only person who will know who has said what. . . what *you* have said.

MrS: Really? How come?

JA: Well, what I do is I give everyone a study serial number and that is all that any of the other researchers see. I keep the names secret, so that they can't tell who said what when they read the transcript of the interviews. How does that sound?

MrS: Yes, that's very clever.

JA: I don't know about that, but it does work. OK, I mentioned to you that I wanted to record the interview, are you happy for me to do that?

MrS: Yes, you go right ahead.

JA: OK, let me switch the recorder on. Yes, it's on – look, you can see the red light, so it's working OK.

MrS: (Chuckles) Yes, I can see it. I'm glad it's working OK.

JA: Yes. As I explained to you when I saw you just before you went in to see Mr Ramaghastalan, I would like to ask you about what you have been told about the operation; about what you understand about what you have been told – and what you don't understand; what you expect as outcomes from the operation – by that I mean how do you think or hope it will benefit you; and I'd like to ask you about how you feel about the information you have been given about the operation. How does that sound to you?

MrS: Yes, you seem to be covering everything there.

> JA: I hope so. Now, I'd like to begin by getting some more information about you. Just so you are aware, I haven't seen your notes or been told anything about you, other than that you are coming in for this operation that I am interested in. So, I'll get some background information from you and then I'll get on to the main topics of the interview, and then, at the end, I'll check that I've got the main points and I'll ask you if there anything you would like to add, and then. . . we can finish.
>
> MRS: That all sounds fine to me. I'll look forward to the finishing bit!
>
> JA: Quite! Now, to begin with some background details. . . How old are you?
>
> MRS: I am 63.
>
> . . .

So, in this vignette, what you can see me doing is:

a. Checking that he is happy to continue.

b. Checking he is happy for the interview to be audio-recorded.

c. Checking he feels comfortable for the interview to be in that place.

d. Being open about switching the recorder on – and showing it to him.

e. Reminding him about what we will be discussing.

f. Checking that that is OK with him.

g. Outlining the structure of the interview.

h. Checking that that is OK with him.

i. Beginning to ask for background details.

I also used what I call the **Three Ps.** These are:

- **Purpose:** I made sure he was aware of the purpose of the interview.
- **Permissions:** I pointed out to him that 'you can say whatever you want to say – there are no "right" or "wrong" answers to any of my questions'.
- **Protections:** I assured him that his answers to my questions were 'secure' by saying 'I want to emphasise again that I shall not let anyone else know what you have said. Although Mr Ramaghastalan is a member of the research team, I am the only person who will know who has said what. . . you have said' and I mentioned the anonymous interview transcripts.

Just to mention some technical details – what I did was to use **explicit categorisation (EC)** to signpost to him what was coming in the interview. Using EC, you say what you are going to say, then you say it, then you say that you have said it. In an interview situation, you say what questions you are going to ask, you ask them, and then you say that you have asked them. It is also referred to as **signposting, chunking,** and **checking.** Essentially, it facilitates the process so that your interviewee (or your audience) knows what is coming up and can mentally prepare to answer the questions (or process the information you give). It is *very effective* – try it!

Notice that I have signposted a phase in the interview in which I shall ask questions about his background details – his age, his work, his marital status, and so on. These data may come in useful later on in the interview – e.g. I might ask a question like, 'How do you think the operation will affect your work?'– and I now know what work he does. Or I might ask a question like, 'Who can you turn to for help and support after the operation?' – and I know if he has a wife who he might be expected to turn to for that. So, this phase can act as a **preparatory phase** in that way.

The second function that this background information phase might have is one of settling down. The beginning of an interview is one where most people are slightly anxious – about what questions to ask and about what answers to give. Researchers often get nervous at this point and rush into it – thus making silly mistakes. For you as an interviewer, it is a time to *slow right down,* to think about the words which will come out of your mouth before you put your foot in there! We all tend to rush at the beginning, so make sure you take. . . your. . . time. . .! And what better phase of the interview to put your foot right in it than asking questions about the interviewee's background? These are usually relatively neutral questions which you don't have to worry too much about. Mind you, another law for interviews is that 'There is no such thing as a neutral topic!' I have begun interviews with this phase and occasionally I have asked someone what their marital status is (e.g. 'Are you married or single, or. . .') and have met 'That's just it – my wife died last week and my life has just fallen apart since then, and . . .' **HELP!** What to do? Enter psychotherapist mode, 'Oh, I am sorry to hear that. I truly am? Do you want to talk about it?' Oh no! I've just opened a Pandora's Box! Rule 5 about interviews – **NEVER** ask a question if you don't think you can deal with the answer. But, having said that, it will probably happen to us all at some time.

OK, so I have covered the explanations, structuring, signposting, and the background information. I would now like to cover the following points as well:

1. facilitation
2. silence
3. probing in depth
4. clarification
5. re-focusing
6. dealing with tears and other issues
7. endings
8. managing recordings
9. transcriptions.

Facilitation

Facilitation refers to the means by which we encourage the interviewee to tell her/his story in their own words and in the order they would wish to give it. So, you might begin with a question like: 'Tell me what you expect from the operation?' *Then you wait*. You give the interviewee time to think about their answer and to reply with it. One of the commonest mistakes in interviewing, is haste or impatience. Golden Rule 2 of interviews is *to be patient*. Don't rush in with another question, then another, then another, then another. I remember a student who asked me for advice on analysing her interview data. When I read the transcripts of her interviews, I was surprised that they were full of multiple questions – she did not wait for her interviewees to answer her initial question and rattled off a series of others! But that is typical of a novice interviewer without any training.

We can facilitate responses by:

- Being attentive.
- Looking (NOT staring!) at the respondent.
- Nodding.
- Smiling (appropriately!)
- Saying things like 'Yes', 'Uh huh', to acknowledge that you are listening.
- Saying things like 'Go on. . .' 'Tell me more. . .', to encourage more information.

All of these are used with the intention of encouraging the interviewee to talk. NB – the word 'Yes' can be used in three ways: (i) as an answer to a question; (ii) to confirm that you have heard what the other person is saying; and (iii) to shut someone up – e.g. 'YES!' (I've heard enough!).

Silence

As you can see from the above, some interviewers – particularly novice interviewers – are very threatened by silences. Don't be. Sometimes, people need time to think about what they want to say. Sometimes people are upset and they have to pause before they can go on. Use silences to encourage interviewees to go on and say more. Silences can be uncomfortable for both interviewees and interviewers. So you will both feel the pressure to say something to fill the silence. Some police interrogators use this as a standard technique to put pressure on someone they are questioning. Practise it with a friend – BUT be careful to remain an interviewer rather than an interrogator!

Probing in Depth

At times in an interview, you may have to probe to get more information, especially if the interviewee seems reticent about giving a full answer to your question. The message you want to get across is 'It's OK, I don't want to force you, but I'd like to hear more about. . .' This is where you have to be sensitive to your interviewee and not put too much pressure on her/him to provide more information. You can use phrases like, 'Tell me more about. . .' or 'You mentioned. . .', and so on.

Clarification

As with probing, you have to exercise your own discretion and tact in how far to push your interviewee. Again – be straightforward and polite. Make it clear what you want.

For example, 'When you said "you were confused" what exactly did you mean by that?' When clarifying inconsistencies, again be clear and straightforward, 'I'm sorry, can I clarify. . . Earlier you said that X happened, but just now you said that Y happened. Have I misunderstood you, or missed something? Which was it?' Above all, be polite.

Re-Focusing

At times our interviewees may stray from the point or go on. . . and on. . . and on about something. This is where you have to gently but firmly bring them back to the point.

I remember on one occasion, in the early days when we were testing our History-Taking Training for Medical Students, one student volunteer, let's call him 'Martin', was given the task of getting a medical history from a patient in 15 minutes. Unfortunately for 'Martin', this patient had a long and convoluted story! 'Martin' began by asking, 'Can you tell me when your problem fist started?' The Patient replied, 'Do you mean at the very start of my problem?' 'Martin' said 'Yes – please.' And off the patient went. After 12 minutes, of hearing about his army service and the pains he first experienced during the desert warfare in 1942, and how, despite attempts to treat them, they had kept on coming back and being treated. . . 'Martin' eventually asked the patient, 'And when was this?' To which the patient replied, 'That would have been in, let me see. . . 1947'! – a long way from 1972!

Lesson learned – say, 'That's is very interesting, but can I bring you back to the present. . .'

And that is all you need to do – be polite, but don't be embarrassed or beat about the bush. Be open with your interviewee and let them know that you want them to focus on the issue you are interested in. Remember, YOU have set the agenda and the interviewee will take their lead from you. So, if you allow someone to be joking and flippant, they are likely to continue to be joking and flippant. Keep them to the point.

Dealing with Sensitive Topics

You are now asking 'What does Anderson mean by a "sensitive topic"?' *Any* topic can be a sensitive topic. I have found that the most sensitive topic I have asked people about is 'How much do you earn?' Now, that's a sensitive topic. But I have dealt comfortably with topics such as cancer, death, and dying, and so on. They are often labelled as 'sensitive topics'. There is a snobbery in research circles – 'Oh, I deal in sensitive topics, and I train other people how to handle them!' *Every topic is a potential sensitive one. What you need is training in how to deal sensitively with any topic.*

Be **humane.** Try to be sensitive to how your interviewee is being. Do they look uncomfortable? Are there tears in their eyes? Does their voice tremble? Try to be **empathic** (show the ability to be aware of and understanding of other people's feelings).

Dealing with Tears

I have lost track of the number of times someone I have been interviewing has broken into tears during the interview. And I have lost count of the number of times I have joined them – or held it together for the interview and been in tears later. Crying is a natural response to a painful experience – whether that pain is physical or psychological. It is almost universal at times of grief and loss. Therefore, if one of your interviewees starts to cry during an interview – **do not panic!** Pause and observe. Try to gauge how upset the interviewee is. Do not interrupt with some automatic attempt to comfort: *'Oh, there, there, don't you cry now. Everything will be alright soon.'* Never make promises you can't keep or give assurances which aren't true – no matter how good your intentions are. We interviewers can't make someone's cancer disappear. We can't make the world a safer or a better place. We can't do away with poverty, human suffering, war, and false politicians – more is the pity. But we can be strong and say things like, 'I am truly sorry to hear that'. 'Do you need to take a minute to yourself?' 'Would you like a tissue?' or 'Would you like us to stop there?' The answer to this last one is usually (but not always) 'No'. A better question to ask is 'Are you OK to continue?' Show that you are sensitive, that you *do* care, but that you are not panicking.

Endings

Do end the interview! I have had some which could have gone on and on and on. When you have asked all the questions you want to ask, say something like:

JA: Well, that's all I want to ask. Let's see, we have covered your background information; then we discussed what you had been told about the operation and the likely benefits of it; you told me that you had understood all the information Mr R had given you, and you seemed quite happy with it; you mentioned that you had spoken to a chap who had had the same operation, but he had had some problems afterwards – but that hadn't put you off; we discussed the benefits that you expected from the operation – full mobility after 1–2 years; and the side effects – occasional pain and/or stiffness; and overall, you had been given all the information you wanted and you were 'reasonably happy' – your words – with how well you had been prepared for the operation overall.

MRS: Yes, that about sums it up.

JA: Is there anything that you think I could have asked about that I left out??

MRS: No. You've been very thorough.

JA: Phew! Is there anything you would like to add?

MRS: No.

JA: Or anything else you would like to ask me?

MRS: Yes, there is one thing, I forgot to ask earlier, what will you do with the results of your study, when you have spoken to everybody else?

JA: Yes, I shall be speaking to about fifty people like yourself who are going to have total knee replacements. Then when I have finished doing the interviews, I shall have the recording transcribed (typed out) and start to analyse the information we get. Then we plan to publish the results in a professional journal (that's a posh way of saying an orthopaedics magazine) and perhaps give presentations at conferences. I hope, if it is possible, to go on to use what we have learned in this study, to develop a training programme for junior surgeons to help them improve how they work with their patients. And then, I'll take a break!

(Both laugh)

MRS: You've got your work cut out for you – I don't envy you that!

JA: Indeed! Now, I don't want to delay you any more than I have to, but there is one last question I want to ask you – how have you found this interview?

MRS: You know, I have quite enjoyed it! I was a bit nervous at the beginning. . .

JA: I noticed.

MRS: . . . but you put me at my ease and. . . It's strange. . . You helped me to think about the operation more clearly than I had been, and I'm very grateful to you for that!

JA: That is interesting. Thank you for that. Now, my last words to you just now are to say, **THANK YOU VERY MUCH** for taking part. Here is the questionnaire I mentioned earlier – in this envelope – for you to complete at home and send back to me. I shall be in touch before you come back for your follow-up, to arrange to meet you again.

Is there anything else you want to say?

MRS: No, just that you. . . it has been very nice to meet you.

JA: And lovely to meet you Mr Smith. Let me switch the recorder off and. . .

Here you see I did the final part of my **explicit categorisation**, or the 'signposting, chunking, and checking' – the **checking** part, where I did a very brief recap of the interview. I made sure that I gave Mr Smith ample opportunities to add anything else that he might have wanted to. I gave him his 'homework'; and reminded him of the next part of the study when we would meet again. And I did something which I always do, I asked him how he had found the interview – and wasn't that interesting? It was gratifying to hear that he had actually felt that he benefitted from the interview! You know, so many RECs say to me: but can you ask those questions of those patients at that point in time? I believe it helps make your interviewees aware that you are concerned about what they think and feel. Then I very deliberately and openly said 'Let me switch the recorder off'. Then we left the room, I walked him back to the exit, we shook hands. and he went home.

Managing Recordings

Now you have a recording in your recorder! I like recorders which are as simple as possible – not too many buttons or options to confuse me. Digital recorders tend to have five 'folders' (sub-divisions in their electronic memory) into which you can store your interviews. I like to store each interview in a different folder. (On one good day, I did five interviews.) Storing them in separate folders helps you to remember which one is which.

The first thing to do is to check the recording. Is it there? Hopefully, it is. Once I did a telephone interview which lasted about one and a half hours. I had done lots in the past using a telephone microphone which has a rubber sucker which you attach to back of the earpiece on your phone. Up until then, I had been using corded telephones – you know the ones which are plugged directly into the socket – and that arrangement had worked very well. However, on this one time, I was doing the interview from home and I used my cordless phone. When I listened to the recording all I had was a continuous loud buzzing. Lesson learnt – always test your equipment before you use it. (I remember Princewill saying, after my work with him that he spent hours at home practising until he could use his recorder with his eyes shut!)

Next, transfer your recording on to your (password-protected, secure) computer. Give it the appropriate study serial number – SSN – e.g. A001, etc. and **date it!** That helps to prevent mix-ups. Then you listen to it to check that you have copied it properly. Make sure that your recording does not contain any personal details by which the interviewee can be identified. (Remember your GDPR!) Now make a back-up copy somewhere else – on an encrypted USB stick for example. Then check that that is OK. Then breathe a sigh of relief! Also remember to keep a note of which interviewee has which SSN. *Only after you have done this, delete the file from the recorder.* Do not carry a recorder full of interviews around with you. You will probably be in breach of your research proposal and approvals as well as GDPR!

Always keep your recordings until you publish your work. Any REC will ask how long you will keep your data. Many people, in the false belief that they are being very ultra-correct, say something stupid like 'Recordings will be destroyed/erased once they have been transcribed'. I would prefer that to read 'Recordings will be destroyed/erased once they have been transcribed and checked'. I prefer to keep recordings until the research is published – just in case there are any queries about the authenticity of quotes from publishers. In one study, the transcriber had made an typing error which completely changed the meaning of a section of the interview we had quoted – and this hadn't been picked up until it was being prepared for publication. Imagine it. What could we have done if that recording had been erased before we could check it?

Transcribing Interviews

Interviews should be transcribed **verbatim** – word for word – being exactly the same words as used in the interviews. That means you transcribe them without any editing, additions, subtractions, or amendments. I recommend to my students that they do it themselves – it helps get them closer to the material (part of the process of 'immersion' that I shall talk about in Appendix F on Analysing qualitative data). Some people prefer to use a transcription service. These are usually very good and professional, and they *do* save you a lot of time. But they cost money, so be prepared to pay upwards of £1.00 for every minute of recorded speech to be transcribed – that is £60.00 per hour, or more.

A word of caution about using your secretary to do the transcription. Secretaries can type very fast, but, if they are anything like my sister Doris (who is a medical secretary), they are used to 'tidying-up' the dictations that their bosses give them. It is their job to tidy up both the grammar and the spelling. So 'I'll' is typed 'I shall'; 'Yeah' is typed as 'Yes' and so on. Verbatim transcription requires things to be typed as they are said. With pauses and laughter, etc. noted. So you will have to train, or rather re-train, your secretary to do it properly. The other thing that transcribers can do well is to type within a grid which numbers the lines within the text – very useful when analysing or citing your data.

One last thing about transcription services – they are only human, so they can make mistakes! As I mentioned above, in one study I had used a very good transcription service but they had missed a word out, so when I went to quote this crucial bit, the transcription, as it was, gave exactly the opposite meaning to the text than the real one. I had to go back to the original recording to correct it. ***Always check your transcripts for accuracy*** – even when you do them yourself!

The One-Question Interview

This is perhaps the equivalent to the 'Holy Grail' of qualitative research interviews. In theory, if you have briefed your participant fully and clearly, so that they understand what the purpose of your research is, and what you want from them, then after your introduction, you should be able (in theory, at least) to just sit back and say something like: 'OK now please tell me about. . .' Then you can sit back and listen, only interrupting where necessary to clarify what has been said. This is essentially the approach which Cheryl Beck used in her Descriptive Phenomenological study of women with post-partum depression in Chapter 13).

> *Please describe a situation in which you experienced postpartum depression. Share all the thoughts, perceptions and feelings you can recall until you have no more to say about the situation.*
>
> *(Beck 1992)*

Multiple and Leading Questions

Don't ask multiple questions! Don't ask leading questions!

I have noticed it is very common for all sorts of clinicians to ask multiple and leading questions. **Multiple questions** are where you ask one question, then – before the patient/client can reply – you ask another – and then maybe another. For example:

DR: What do you yourself. . . eh. . . Think about this? Has anybody made any suggestions, or are you worried in any way about it? (From 'Just Sign This Form')

NRS: Hello Mrs. Jones, Are you in any pain? Any headache? Or any other pain? Do you need any pain medication?

The problems with multiple questions are: (i) when the person does answer, you can't usually tell which question they are answering; and (ii) by asking too many questions all at once, you do not give them time to tell their story.

Leading questions are, as the name suggests, questions which tend to lead the person being questioned to one answer rather than another. Those of you who are fans of courtroom dramas will have heard the judge occasionally give a lawyer a telling off, saying something like, 'Disregard that last question. Counsel is leading the witness!' It is something you shouldn't do. The danger is that you get false information, **biased** information, when in research we aim to get the truth. So, avoid questions which tend to favour one response rather than any other.

Interviewing People you Know

Sometimes we are put in an invidious situation, someone we know is a participant in our research. Strictly speaking we should not interview that person. However, depending on the nature of the research, we might use an approach which defines the boundaries between us as 'Interviewer' and 'Interviewee', rather than friends.

Let me tell you about an experience which helped me clarify this.

In 1975 I was considering buying a house for the first time. One of my karate students (JH) was a financial advisor, so I asked him if I could get some advice about mortgages etc., from him. He suggested I should phone his office and make an appointment to see him there. So I went to see him in his office. I was impressed. It was a very big, nice office. He greeted me from behind his big desk.

JH: 'Now John', he began, 'before we go any further, I want you to know that in here, I'm not your friend'.

JA: 'But that's the whole reason I came to see you. I thought that you'd be able to get me a good deal. . . I want to be your friend'.

JH: 'John', he said mellifluously, 'I get everyone the best deal I can. It's what I do. That's my job, and I am good at it'. (He was good at his job, and the investment he advised me to make eventually paid out handsome dividends! I looked at his car in the car park – an Aston Martin DB5 – yes, he must be good at his job! Thank you JH!)

Can you see the point I am trying to make? When we are a nurse, for example, and we are doing research and one of the people we have in our study is a patient whom you know well, you will find yourself in two conflicting roles – nurse vs researcher. So at times like these you have to establish clear boundaries – e.g. 'Why hello, Mrs McLean, I didn't expect to see you here. So, let's begin by getting things straight. Today, I'm not your nurse. I am seeing you as a researcher, so it would be unethical for me to discuss your care or treatment today. Do you understand that?'

Interviewing colleagues is more difficult. What if, during your interview, you find out something which changes your opinion of that individual? Would you be able to prevent yourself from acting differently towards her/him when s/he was 'your colleague' again as opposed to a 'participant' in your study? You can see how fraught with danger doing insider-research (interviewing people within your own organisation) is. Avoid it wherever possible, and – *bosses should never conduct research on people who work for them! Never!*

King et al. (2019) have this to say about 'interviewer role conflicts':

Probably the most common example of this is where the researcher is also a practicing health or social care professional and is interviewing members of the service user group they work with in their professional life . . . If you are in such a position, the key requirement is to be clear from the start where the boundary lies between your researcher and professional roles. In general, our advice would be to tell participants explicitly that you are not in a position to deal personally with any health or social care problems they may talk about in their interviews as you are there only in the capacity of a researcher.

(King et al. 2019, pp. 87–88)

I have tried to give you some insights from practical experience into different aspect of interviewing – as well as some of the issues you may encounter in doing interviews. This is largely geared towards qualitative interviews, but is also relevant to quantitative interviews too. I hope this is of some use to help you inform your own practice.

References

Beck CT. (1992). The lived experience of postpartum depression: a phenomenological study. *Nursing Research* 41(3), 166–170.

King N, Horrocks C, and Brooks J. (2019). *Interviews in Qualitative Research*. Sage: London.

APPENDIX E

Research Skills

Focus Groups

Introduction

Focus groups are most often used in ethnographic approaches. I have said a lot about them in my earlier Chapter 11 on ethnographic approaches, so I shall be briefer here and concentrate on aspects of focus group work that are not often covered elsewhere, whilst emphasising important points I made before. The same general rules that apply in individual interviews also apply to focus groups – some with minor alterations.

Numbers

The ideal number for a focus group discussion is **6 to 10 people**. Any more and it becomes a crowd which does not allow all participants much of an opportunity to contribute. Less than six and it becomes too intimate for a *useful group* discussion.

Participants

It is best, in my view, to have a relatively **homogeneous** group. So, you have to consider and come to your own decisions about the following issues. Are there advantages to having a mixed sex group rather than a single sex group? Will your group discussion run better with a mix of kinds of participants such as healthcare professionals (HCPs) – where you have to question the effects of mixing professions versus the effects of keeping to one group at a time. As a general rule of thumb, I tend not to mix doctors with other HCPs because of issues of status and power.

Demystifying Research for Medical & Healthcare Students: An Essential Guide, First Edition. John L. Anderson.
© 2022 John Wiley & Sons Ltd. Published 2022 by John Wiley & Sons Ltd.
Companion website: www.wiley.com/go/Anderson/DemystifyingResearch

The Setting

Always ensure that you have a **private room** in which you can hold the discussion without fear of interruption. Bear in mind that group discussions can become quite animated and may cause disruption to those in nearby rooms. Rachel (who you met in the Chapter 14 on Grounded Theory) told me about a very uncomfortable experience she had in one focus group discussion she was running. She had obtained access to a consultant oncologist's patients to enrol some of them into a series of focus group discussions she was running. In one group, part of the way through the discussion, the door to the room suddenly burst open and the consultant popped in and said, 'Hello ladies. Everything going okay?' Rachel had to hastily take him outside and remind him that although they were his patients, *in that room* they were her research participants! You can imagine the effect on the group – the interruption killed the discussion. And Rachel had put up a 'Do Not Disturb' notice on the door.

I prefer to sit around a table if possible. I realise that some focus group facilitators prefer to sit in a circle of comfy chairs, but that smacks of **'excess informality'** to me. Remember that you are there for a research purpose – not for a social get together. Having a table, also provides participants with somewhere to put any papers or drinks (bottled water only, please! The chinking of teacups really stands out in a recording!). It is also the best place to put your recorder or microphone – remember to do a dry run to test your recording equipment. Make sure it picks up voices from all parts of the room. You can use a stereo microphone or two recorders with stereo microphones.

Facilitator and Co-facilitator

The facilitator has the responsibility to manage the group. I mean *manage*. In addition to facilitating the discussion, the facilitator has the responsibility for maintaining order in the group. The co-facilitator's role is to help the facilitator in this. If you do a lot of focus-group work, then you may find that you work with the same facilitator/co-facilitator a lot. This is a good thing because it allows you to know one another and to know how each other works. Then you can trust one another and work well as a team. You don't want any surprises when you are in the middle of running the group discussion (as I have had). It is important to be able to trust one another. There is nothing more embarrassing in a focus group (FG) discussion than to witness two facilitators battling for control over the group. So, before you go begin, you and your co-facilitator must agree on who does what. I also like to agree on a means of **signals for communicating** – which I shall present below.

Issues of Social Power

It is important that you are respected as the professional researcher leading the group, otherwise you could end up with chaos. However, you don't want your status to confer an image of power which might **intimidate** group participants or predispose participants to give you answers that they think you would like. Remember what Princewill did. As a doctor running FG discussions with rural women in Nigeria, he was aware of this dilemma, so he did some things to try to narrow the social distance effect between himself and his participants.

- He dressed in his tribal robes to show he was one of them.
- He spoke the local language and dialect.
- He emphasised that it was their beliefs he wanted to hear about and that they, therefore were the 'experts' in the room.
- He was quite deferential towards them, rather than imperious and arrogant like many of the doctors they had probably met before.

It worked. The mothers in his FG discussions entered into the discussions with enthusiasm and openness.

Dominant/Reticent Participants

Sometimes in a focus group, you will find some people who talk too much (**dominants**) and some who talk too little or not at all (**reticents**). When you find that someone is tending to hog the discussion and is not giving others a chance to contribute, your job will be to rein them in in order to give others a chance to say what they want to. So, you may have to say something like, 'OK Philip, we have heard what your views on the matter are. Now it's time to hear what others have to say.' Be calm, be polite, but be assertive. When someone is not saying anything at all, the challenge for you is to bring them into the discussion and you might have to be quite direct about it. So, you might have to say something like. 'What about you Yvonne? What do you think about this?' Don't be afraid to exert your 'authority'. Participants will expect you to manage the group and maintain order. There is a comfort to them in that. Remember you are the group *manager*.

Dealing with Disclosures

This is something which your REC may have asked you to consider and to specify in your application for REC approval. You should be clear in your own mind about when you have to report any inappropriate practices. At the beginning of the group when setting the **ground rules,** you should clarify this point and alert everyone that 'If you disclose anything which causes me concern, or is inappropriate practice, I shall have to report that to the Chief Investigator of the study and s/he will decide whether or not to take it any further.' But this is something which should already be mentioned in your PIS and when you obtain informed consent.

The Structure of a Focus Group Discussion

I tend to structure my group discussions along these lines:

1. **Introduction:** In this you give the participants a reminder of the purpose of the group discussion; you outline the **ground rules** for the group, and possibly, invite them to add anything else which they think is appropriate. You remind them that you will be recording the discussion, check everyone agrees to this, and then – *switch the recorder on.* (You might include any 'housekeeping' information here – e.g. 'If the fire alarm goes off. . .' 'The lavatories are. . .' 'If anyone needs to stop. . .', etc. Emphasise boundary issues, like 'No shouting', 'No physical violence', etc. You might give everyone copies of printed material such as the ground rules and any questions you want them to discuss. (NB: if you are using FGs as a means of asking a lot of people questions at the same time, as a general rule of thumb. Limit your questions to *12 – max.*)

2. **Introductions:** Start with yourself, then go around the table and invite everyone to say their name clearly, e.g. 'My name is. . .' Some researchers invite participants to say what their name is and any one other thing about themselves that they are happy to share with the group. If you do this and it begins 'Hi all, my name's Damien, and I'd an Arsenal fan!' – followed by an uproar. . . think carefully about what you might invite. Make sure that you get them to say a few words before their name – such as 'my name is. . .' so that you (or whoever is transcribing the recordings) can become familiar with the voice and recognise it.

3. **Icebreaker:** At this point you might say something like, 'Now I'd like us to do an "icebreaker." It is a brief exercise to get us all talking and maybe have some fun. So, I'd like you to discuss for a few minutes what are your thoughts about what is the best type of food in the world?' – or something relatively neutral which you decide yourself. Bear in mind that you want to get everyone talking, so it has to be something anyone can join in, and it should be a 'neutral' topic which is unlikely to raise tempers, or other emotions. During the icebreaker, you and the co-facilitator should try to keep out of the discussion. Instead, use this time as an opportunity to *observe your group in action.* Look out for who talks too much and who hardly talks at all.

4. **Re-focus:** 'Well that was fun wasn't it!' (You wish!) 'Now let's get down to the main reason we are here – to discuss. . .'

5. **Explanation:** Remind the group of the main discussion topic and the questions you want them to discuss.

6. **Main discussion:** Remind them of the main topic(s) or question(s), then sit back and let them get on with it. A good group will run itself. It will require very little 'management' and the less you intervene the better. Be prepared to intervene when necessary but avoid making yourself the focal point of the group, when they talk to you rather than each other; and when they look to you to confirm that answers are 'right' or 'wrong'. Interventions, e.g. clarifications or probing, such as 'Marcus, can you tell everyone what exactly you mean by. . .'. Or 'What do you mean by that Clarissa?' are OK. Sit down, sit back and enjoy the process.

7. **Summing-up and additional comments:** A brief recap may help to confirm that you have covered all the points that you wanted to. Ask if anyone has anything important that they want to say.

8. **Ending:** This is where you say anything you want to before the group breaks up. Thank everyone. Deal with any loose ends. Give everyone their expenses claims forms. Tell them that they are the best group that you have worked with. . . today!

9. Now send them home.

Ground Rules

The sorts of ground rules you might have are:

1. Respect each other.
2. Confidentiality – 'what is said in this room stays in this room'.
3. One person talks at a time – no talking over each other.
4. Give people time to talk.
5. Don't hog the discussion.
6. If you need to have a break, use this sign – 'T'.
7. No shouting/abuse/swearing/violence, etc.
8. Any other rules the group wants to introduce.

Communications Between Facilitators (Signals)

I have found that it is essential to agree who does what in focus groups. If you are a lone researcher, you might get a colleague to help you as your co-facilitator. (NB: make sure that you have declared this on any REC application and with any R&D department which you have to deal with. See Chapter 19 on Regulations and Permissions.) It is best to agree in advance a series of non-verbal communications – **hand signals** that you can use to communicate discretely without disturbing the group or the flow of the discussion.

One of my supervisees, 'Audrey' who you met in Chapter 19, did a study of the attitudes of hospital doctors, nurses, and HCAs to influenza vaccinations. She conducted focus groups with nurses and HCAs and interviews with doctors. (Doctors don't usually do focus groups.) She asked me to help her by co-facilitating her first ever focus group. I did that gladly. (That's what supervisors [as CIs] are for.) Fortunately, she had recently attended one of my workshops on focus groups, so I was confident that she knew the ropes. Before the meeting we met and we went over our signals and agreed the signals, etc. About halfway through the discussion, which was going fine, I saw her put both hands up to the sides of her face – the sign for **'HELP! Please take over'**. So, I did for a few minutes then she signalled 'Can I come in?' and I signalled back 'yes, come in and she took over again. In our debriefing she told me that she had 'frozen'. She had panicked (it is likely that my presence, rather than comforting her, made her even more nervous) and froze – hence the 'hands to the face'. Thank goodness we had agreed the signals beforehand!

Here are a few of the ones I use. You can make your own up. But don't let them get over-complicated.

1. **Can I come in/contribute?**

   Left hand palm up on the table towards the facilitator. See **Figure E.1**.

2. **Yes, come in/say something.**

   Move your left hand to touch the right upper arm with your palm. See **Figure E.2**.

3. **No – wait.**

   Left hand palm down on the table. See **Figure E.3**.

4. **Help – Please take over.**

   Both hands palms to the sides of the face. (As in Edward Munch's 'The Scream'.) See **Figure E.4**.

5. **Can you please say something?**

   Left hand to the side of the face. See **Figure E.5**.

6. **Draw attention to a group member.**

   Right hand finger taps gently to the left if that is where the person you want to draw attention to is, or left-hand finger taps gently to the right. See **Figures E.6** and **E.7**.

   Add any you want – *but don't over-complicate it!*
   There – nothing to it! Is there?

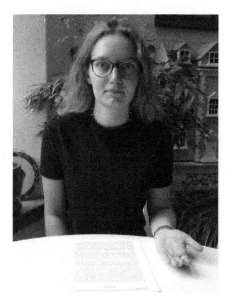

FIGURE E.1   'Can I contribute?'

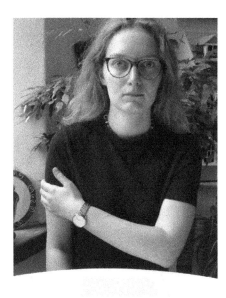

FIGURE E.2 'Yes, you can say something.'

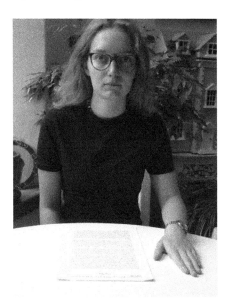

FIGURE E.3 'No – wait.'

In Chapter 11, I covered the use of focus groups in some detail. In this chapter I have focused on the 'How to do it' aspects. I began by presenting different issues that you might have to address when you are planning to use focus group discussions in you research. Then I discussed how you might structure your FGs and suggested ways of doing this. I discussed ground rules and finally showed you some simple signals that I use for communicating between FG facilitators. I covered how to manage your recordings and transcribing in Appendix D on Interviewing.

 I wish you luck and I hope you enjoy running focus groups.

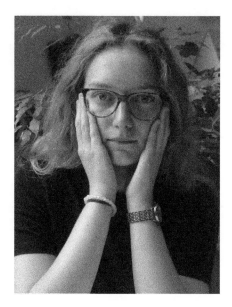

FIGURE E.4 'HELP! Please take over.'

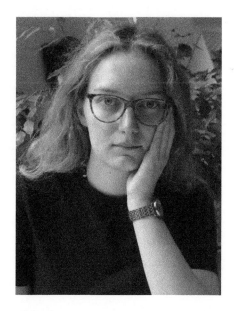

FIGURE E.5 'Please say something.'

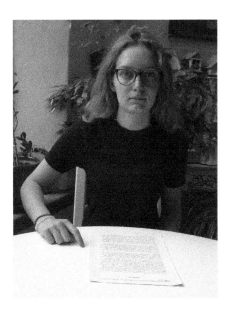

FIGURE E.6 'Look at her/him over there.'

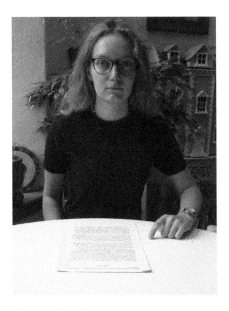

FIGURE E.7 'Look at her/him over there.'

Additional Reading

Barbour and Kitzinger. (1999). *Developing Focus Group Research: Politics, Theory and Practice.* Sage: London.
Bloor M. (2001). *Focus Groups in Social Research.* Sage: London.
Kreuger and Casey. (2000). *Focus Groups: A Practical Guide.* Sage: London.
Stewart DW. (2006). *Focus Groups: Theory & Practice.* Sage: London.

APPENDIX F

Research Skills

Analysing Qualitative Data

Introduction

In this chapter I shall introduce you to, and try to show you how to do, a **General Thematic Analysis (GTA)**, and I will also introduce you to a **Framework Approach** to analysing qualitative data. We have already looked at an example of how data was analysed in **Grounded Theory.** If you get the hang of a GTA, then it is relatively easy to pick up other types of qualitative data analysis. It is usually an inductive process in which the data determines the emerging themes.

General Thematic Analysis (GTA)

There are several steps in a Thematic Analysis:

1. **Immersion or familiarisation:** If you have done your own transcribing, you have already started the process of immersing yourself in the data and becoming familiar with it. Read and re-read your transcripts, listen to your recordings over and over.
2. **Record the emerging themes:** As you immerse yourself in the data, you will probably find that concepts or issues or **themes** jump out of the text at you. Note them down. As you go through the data for the first time, you will become aware of the initial emerging themes. Note them down. Be careful not to note down everything that was said. Ask yourself, 'What can I call this theme?' That may prevent you noting spurious text/conversation as 'themes'.
3. **Record the secondary themes:** As you read it more and more, other themes, which were not obvious the first time around, will become apparent to you. Note them down.
4. **Verify the themes:** This is the process by which you use someone else to 'interrogate' you about your **coding** (the process of turning plain words into categories). I described this in the work I did with Rachael Ballinger in Chapter 14 on Grounded Theory. In fact, as you can see, I favour doing this in a team, as do most others. The

Demystifying Research for Medical & Healthcare Students: An Essential Guide, First Edition. John L. Anderson.
© 2022 John Wiley & Sons Ltd. Published 2022 by John Wiley & Sons Ltd.
Companion website: www.wiley.com/go/Anderson/DemystifyingResearch

dangers of sole researchers doing this are that only their interest or bias is seen. If I were a journal editor, I would reject papers which did not confirm data verification by at least one other person. So, when Seb and I did our work, Seb would tend to do the initial coding and then I would verify with him, questioning and making suggestions where appropriate. Then it becomes a truly **iterative** process.

5. **Organise and categorise the themes:** Look for themes which fit neatly into groups of similar themes. Note those which may be linked in any way to other themes.

6. **Describing and reporting the themes:** This is where you write it up and put your **jargon** into words which can be understood by anyone reading your work – a sort of de-construction of your coding! At the same time, you will organise the themes you have into what we call **theme clusters** – you can give a name to the theme cluster which contains all of the sub-themes within it. (Remember Cheryl Beck's work in Chapter 13 on Phenomenology.) Each of the sub-themes should have their own name and there should be a clear and logical link between them all.

Let's have a go at it. Below is a transcript of a meeting between a doctor and a woman who has come into hospital for an operation on a lump she has found on her breast – **'Just Sign this Form'**. I use this as an example because there is a lot of issues in there. It tends to evoke strong emotional responses. For the purpose of this exercise, I only want you to read the first two pages which I have included here.

So, first of all, begin the process of immersion. Read it and keep a pencil and paper with you for noting anything down. Then re-read it and this time make more notes of what strikes you from the extract – yes, you have moved seamlessly on to the process of noting down the **obvious themes** which strike you as **issues of interest** in your research. Here you are interested in communication between the doctor and the patient. NB – because you are doing this 'blind' without any previous briefing, you are doing an **inductive thematic analysis** – you are not testing a hypothesis or searching for the presence or the absence of specific issues or themes.

PAUSE – DON'T READ ON UNTIL YOU HAVE DONE THIS EXERCISE FOR YOURSELF.
WHEN YOU ARE READY MOVE ON, LET'S COMPARE NOTES.

<u>JUST SIGN THIS FORM</u>

DOCTOR: Hello, Mrs Stevenson.
PATIENT: Hello.
DOCTOR: Hello. I'm Dr Store
PATIENT: Umhu.
DOCTOR: How are you feeling at the moment?
PATIENT: Well ___ not very well ___
DOCTOR: In what way?
PATIENT: It's _____
DOCTOR: You worried about the operation?
PATIENT: Yes.
DOCTOR: Yeah. What do you yourself___eh___think about this? Has anybody made any suggestions, or are you worried in any way about it?

PATIENT: Well, they're all said it's nothing to worry about, but, ehn, I mean they've done thorough examinations on me, and it's___it's kind of nerve-racking, you know?

DOCTOR: Mm. Yeah.

PATIENT: And eh___

DOCTOR: Eh, let me explain the position to you___ Ehm, there are many causes of lumps in the breast. Some of which are not too serious and some of which are a little bit more serious. Ehm, very often we don't know the eh, precise cause of a lump until we actually see the lump at operation. In other words, when we're IN there having a look. Now what the normal procedure is, is that we take you up to the operating theatre, and under anaesthetic, we make a small incision, (cough) – excuse me – and eh, take a little piece of the lump in the breast and send it off to the Pathology to look at under the microscope. Now, if this turns out to be a simple lump, ah, we can just take the lump out and leave it at that. Now if on the other hand the lump turns out to be something more serious like a tumour, eh, then in some cases it may be necessary to remove the whole breast.

Now, in your case, we don't as yet know what this lump is. But it is *possible* that it's in fact a tumour. Now, ___we won't know until ___ as I say, we're actually in there, eh, and we've sent the lump off for what's called a frozen section, eh, in other words look at under the microscope. But, eh, by far the safest thing to do, as you know, in any form of tumour of the breast, or any, tumours in general, but particularly of the breast, ehm, the earlier you remove it ___ ehm ___

PATIENT: What? Your breast or the tumour?

DOCTOR: The tumour *or* the breast. Eh the better the chance of a permanent cure. Now ___ in cases of *tumours* of the breast, the only treatment really is to remove the whole breast. And there's a very good chance in fact an almost certain chance, eh, particularly in your case if this is a tumour, that will <u>cure</u> you. And you can then forget that the rest of your life. Now the point about removing a breast is that ___

PATIENT: So do you think it is a tumour?

DOCTOR: I really don't know, it may be, and it may not be.

PATIENT: Ehm, if it is a tumour, I mean, you're going to do the whole operation there and then?

DOCTOR: <u>Yeah</u>_____Because, that is by far the best way of doing it.

PATIENT: (sighs)___And what about Radium?

DOCTOR: Well radium in this sort of case, ___ehm___is not the best form of treatment. You see there are two sorts of tumours of the breast, (clears throat). There's one sort which is confined to the breast and if it's removed early, if the breast is removed, then that takes away all the tumour and you're cured.

The other sort, which is what happens if you wait for months and months and months, before actually diagnosing it. The tumour has already spread outside the breast, and then, radium can be used for treatment. But in that case, it's only something that will___eh___will work temporarily, eh, but won't actually cure you. And in your case, if it is a tumour, to be certain of an absolute cure, unfortunately, it will be necessary to actually remove the breast. Now, if this is the case___obviously your worried about ehn, not having the breast afterwards, and, and so forth. And you're relatively young aren't you? Twenty-nine, I think it says_____

PATIENT: Oh yes, I'm very young still.

DOCTOR: Ehm_____

PATIENT: Can't you just___ Can't you just___ leave that second stage so that I___ I mean I don't get any decision in it at all then do I?

DOCTOR: Well___ the decision is entirely yours in fact. Eh___ I mean obviously we won't and can't do anything that you don't agree to. But, eh, the advice, my advice, and certainly the advice of all the doctors looking after you would be that if this *does* turn out to be a tumour, to go ahead and remove the breast.

Ah___ Now if this is the case. Eh, firstly, you will be cured, and secondly, eh these days there are very, very good artificial breasts that can be used afterwards. Which people will come and talk to you about and show you examples and you can wear___ which, eh___ you know, apart from obviously yourself people won't know that you're any different. Ehm, just to take an example, eh (clears throat) I've got, ehn, an aunt who had a breast removed, eh, what, it must be about six years ago now, and ehn, she's perfectly all right and perfectly healthy and cured and, eh, just to look at her, with her clothes on at any rate, ehm, you wouldn't notice any difference at all. She looks like she's like a plump woman. I know that ehm*!*

PATIENT: You can say the same about somebody with a wooden leg on with their clothes on, couldn't you!

DOCTOR: Well no that's not true because somebody with a wooden leg limps. Ehm. Are you married?

PATIENT: No.

DOCTOR: You're not? are you___ Any prospect of getting married in the near future? Have you got a regular boyfriend or _____?

PATIENT: Yes, I have.

Okay, let's see what we have. Now, don't be worried if you come up with a different set of codes or issues to me or to others who you are doing this with. You are almost bound to because we all have our own ways of looking at and interpreting things. Here are some of my thoughts below. (See Table F.1.)

1. On reading this transcript again the first thing that occurs to me is that the doctor seems to be quite empathic. So, I have noted **empathy** as a possible theme. And, when asked to point to evidence of that, I point to:

'**DR:** How are you feeling at the moment?'
'**DR:** In what way?'
'**DR:** You worried about the operation?'

TABLE F.1   **Emerging themes from 'Just sign this form'.**

Emergent Themes	
Theme	**Example**
1. Empathy	'How are you feeling at the moment?'
	'You worried about the operation?'
2. False empathy	Interrupting and changing the subject
	'she looks like she's like a plump woman'
3. De-personalisation	'when we're IN there'
	'the breast'
4. Searching	'what about radium?'
	'Can't you just. . . Leave that second stage'
	'you think it's a probability don't you?'
5. Why don't you . . . Yes but. . .	'I don't get any decision . . .'/'Well. . .'
	'no possibility of radium?'/ 'Well in your case it's not the right treatment.'

Emergent Themes	
Theme	**Example**
'Erosion'	A pattern that runs through the interaction in which the Surgeon is constantly wearing away the patient's defences to the point at which she eventually agrees to sign the form.

These three early questions are suggestive to me of an **empathic approach by the doctor.**

What do you think? Can you see it?

2. Then, as we read on through the text of the transcript, I realise that, rather than being truly empathic, he seems to displaying what I would call a 'false empathy'. And I note it down. And, when asked to point to evidence of that, I point to:

PTNT: . . . it's kind of nerve-racking, you know?
DR: Mm. Yeah.
PTNT: And, eh . . .
DR: Eh, let me explain the position to you . . .

Here the doctor, who up to this point in time seems to be being understanding and interested in the patient's point of view, suddenly changes the pattern of his contribution. He starts to interrupt the patient and then changes the subject to proceed with his own agenda of explaining the operation. *The empathy was not genuine.* This lack of empathy is also demonstrated later:

DR: . . . obviously you are worried about ehm, not having the breast afterwards, and, and so forth . . .

> **DR:**   . . . And secondly, eh, these days there are very, very good artificial breasts . . . She looks like she's like a plump woman . . .

> What do you think? Can you see it?

3. The next theme that I noted was the fact that he was talking to the patient as though she was a 'thing' rather than a real person. I called this **de-personalisation**. This is demonstrated by his constant reference to her breast as 'the breast' and by:

> **DR:**   . . . when we're IN there having a look . . .
> Can you find any other examples of this?
> What do you think? Can you see it?

4. The next thing I noted was that the patient was constantly seeking alternatives. I called this **searching.** Here are examples:

> **PTNT:**   . . . And what about radium?'
> **PTNT:**   Can't you just . . . Can't you just . . . leave that second stage so that I . . .

> What do you think? Can you see it?

5. As I read through it, I noticed a pattern that I had not noticed previously. In Transactional Analysis, it is referred to as a **Game** – a series of interactions which have hidden agendas, and which end up with both parties experiencing familiar payoffs. So, I called this 'Why don't you . . . Yes, but . . .' (Berne 1964) The patient repeatedly asks for alternatives to having her breast removed, but the doctor keeps giving, what on the face of it are, good reasons for not choosing any of the alternatives. For example:

> **PTNT:**   . . . And what about radium?
> **DR:**   Well, radium in this sort of case . . . Ehm . . . Is not the best sort of treatment . . .
> **PTNT:**   . . . I do not get any decision in it at all then do I?
> **DR:**   Well the decision is entirely yours in fact.
> **PTNT:**   . . . You could say the same about somebody with a wooden leg on with their clothes on could not you!
> **DR:**   Well no that's not true because somebody with a wooden leg limps . . .

> In all of these the **payoffs** are: for the doctor – 'I'm right!' and for the patient: 'Oh silly me!'

> What do you think? Can you see it?

6. As you read through, I got the sense that the doctor is wearing the patient's defences down. He keeps putting up arguments in favour of what he wants, which she – as a lay person – *cannot* challenge. Any options she makes, are discounted as not being possible, or not the best treatment for her. I called this a process of **erosion,** which is a sort of meta-theme running through the whole interaction and which encompasses several other sub-themes. In fact, it may be interpreted as his main 'strategy' or the pattern he adopts to obtain his goal – getting the consent form signed, *which she eventually does.* In the full study (as opposed to just this one extract), we might look out for this as a pattern among all of the doctors in the study, otherwise, it would be a sole example.

What do you think? Can you see it?

There. That wasn't too painful was it? Please, now take a moment to note down your own feelings about this example.

When you have done this, then ask yourself, 'Could I remain impersonal and unbiased in analysing this consultation?' Most people have, in my experience, been strongly influenced by this at an emotional level and could not be totally dispassionate about it. *But,* they could still analyse it and justify the themes that they identified in the consultation – or in this case, part of the consultation.

Framework Analysis

A **Framework Analysis** is slightly more rigorous and, therefore, more work than a GTA. You can either begin with a list of 'themes' or 'issues' which you are looking for – this is a **deductive approach** – or you can allow your themes and issues to emerge from the data in a more 'organic' way – this is an **inductive approach.** Let's look at the steps involved in this approach.

1. **Identifying the themes** – first, you can create your framework by listing all of the key themes and issues – this can provide the **framework** for the analysis.

2. **Indexing** – next, check *each case* to see if these themes are present – and make a note (**index**) of them where they are – e.g. 'false empathy (FE)' – p1/p2.

3. **Charting** – re-organise the data within your thematic framework and form **charts** – these group all common themes together into **theme clusters**.

4. **Mapping** – using charts to make a **map** of the themes and the theme clusters to show the range and the inter-connections between them – and give names to them.

5. **Interpretation** – define the inter-connections between themes and **theme clusters**.

This is an extremely rigorous method of coding and organising your data. It sounds complicated, but if you take your time and try it out, then it is relatively easy. You can think of your framework as a) one which originates **in the existing theory** which you use for defining your framework (a deductive approach); or b) your framework emerges **from your data** in the shape of the list of themes you have identified (an inductive approach). You make a list of them all and then you go through every case to check for all/any of the themes on your list – your framework – and you index them as you go. Try it with the example above.

In projects where you have followed a topic guide for your interviews or focus groups, then the topic guide might form an initial guide also for the development of your framework – I suggest to my students that they get a sheet of A3 paper (twice the size of A4). Draw columns down the paper and label them with the topic areas or theme clusters, as appropriate. See Table F.2.

Then you can use this to list the different themes that emerge under each of the topic headings – or in the framework (Table F.3). As you do this, index it by saying where it is in your data. So, if an example of 'empathy' was found in Case 1, and it was at line 58 of the transcript, give the reference point as 1/58. If there is another example

TABLE F.2 Blank grid.

Topic 1	Topic 2	Topic 3	Topic 4	Topic 5	Notes:

TABLE F.3 Filling in the grid.

Topic 1	Topic 2	Topic 3	Topic 4	Topic 5	Notes:
Empathy (1/58) (1/143) (2/32)	De-personalisation (1/19–29)(3/2)				

of it in Case 1, and it was at line 143 note it as 1/143. If there was an example in Case 2 which was at line 32, note it as 2/32. . . and so on. If your transcripts are not line-numbered, don't worry, use the page numbers instead – e.g. 2/1 for Case 1, Page 1, but write in the margin of the appropriate page of the transcript annotation to signpost where it is – e.g. 'E' (for Empathy). Use a highlighter to mark the text if you wish – anything so that you can easily find that example again.

Use the 'Notes' column to write down any ideas or questions that come to you. You can also use it for any 'Aha' moments (**lightbulb moments**) you have! In this way you can record your emerging themes and index them at the same time.

Colaizzi's Approach

Colaizzi developed a seven-step approach for a phenomenological analysis (1978). Edward and Welch (2011) added an extra stem which you may or may not find useful.

Colaizzi's Seven Step Method with the Inclusion of an Additional Step

1. *Transcribing all the subjects' descriptions. In this section of the analysis process, participant narratives are transcribed from the audio-taped interviews held with each individual. According to Colaizzi's (1978a) process, the narratives do not need to be transcribed verbatim, as long as the essence of what the participant was communicating is caught in the transcription. Individual transcriptions of interview are then validated by the respective participant.*
2. *Extracting significant statements [statements that directly relate to the phenomenon under investigation]. Any statements in the participants' narratives that relate directly to the phenomenon under investigation are considered significant. Significant statements are extracted from each of the narratives and numbered. The significant statements are numerically entered into a list (i.e. 1, 2, 3, 4 . . .) that is, an assemblage of all significant statements.*
3. *Creating formulated meanings. In this stage of analysis, Colaizzi (1978a) recommends that the researcher attempts to formulate more general*

restatements or meanings for each significant statement extracted from the participant's narratives.

4. Aggregating formulated meanings into theme clusters. Colaizzi (1978a) suggests that the researcher assign or organise formulated meanings into groups of similar type. In other words, the formulated meanings are grouped into theme clusters. That is, some statements may relate to, for example, faith while other statements relate to self-awareness and so on.

5. Developing an exhaustive description [that is, a comprehensive description of the experience as articulated by participants]. An exhaustive description is developed through a synthesis of all theme clusters and associated formulated meanings explicated by the researcher (Colaizzi 1978a).

6. **Additional step** – Researcher interpretative analysis of symbolic representations – from the articulation of the symbolic representation (which occurred during participant interview).

7. Identifying the fundamental structure of the phenomenon. The fundamental structure refers to 'the essence of the experiential phenomenon as it is revealed by explication' through a rigorous analysis of the exhaustive description of the phenomenon.

8. Returning to participants for validation. A follow-up appointment is made between the researcher and each participant for the purpose of validating the essence of the phenomenon with participants. Any alterations are made according to participant feedback to ensure their intended meaning is conveyed in the fundamental structure of the phenomenon. Integration of additional information provided by participants for inclusion into the final description of the phenomenon occurs at this point. (Edward and Welch 2011)

Verification

As I said, it is absolutely necessary for you to get help from someone else to do this. Hopefully, if you are part of a team, then other members will roll up their sleeves and get stuck in and help you. Here are two examples of **verification** and how it is presented in the publication of the works.

Each discussion, lasting 1 hour, was audio-taped and transcribed. The transcripts were assessed for emerging themes by separate researchers (AE, EM and RP), which were then agreed by discussion. All data were then classified independently by three researchers (AE, EM, and RP) according to these themes and agreement over classification again achieved by discussion.

(Edwards et al. 1998)

Data analysis: SS transcribed the audio-recordings verbatim. This facilitated his immersion in the data. He then conducted a general thematic analysis. Due to SS' own dyslexic difficulties, a template analysis was used to facilitate the initial, open coding of the transcripts. This enabled him to maintain a sense of structure, and to visualise his themes – bypassing his inherent weaknesses with *the written form. SS then conducted axial coding. JA verified this analysis in an iterative process, where differences were resolved by discussion and re-analysis. Both authors agreed on the final theme clusters, and a clear meta-theme was extracted.*

(Shaw and Anderson 2018)

'Quantifying' Qualitative Data

Generally speaking, we *don't* do this. However, I was so impressed by the work that one of my supervisees did that I couldn't resist showing you how she presented some of her data. She did a study of how clinicians made decisions about the prescription of antibiotics for people with diabetic leg ulcers. She presented a list of all of her themes in a table, but also visually and numerically showed how often these themes emerged from the interviews with her 18 respondents (**Figure F.1**) This shows very clearly which themes were very commonly experienced and which were relatively rare. In this way she got around the often-experienced dilemma of when to include a theme (e.g. if very few people report it) or not. Have a look and see for yourself. Might it be a useful way for you to present any of your data?

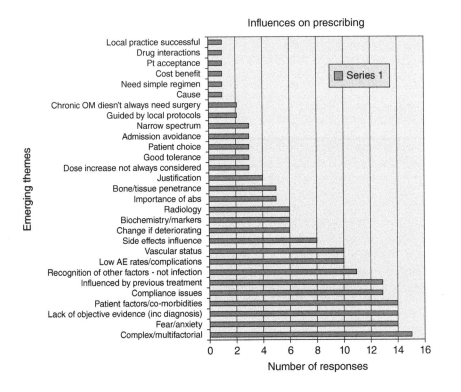

FIGURE F.1 Debbie Sharman's presentation of her data.

I have introduced you to two models of qualitative data analysis (QDA) in this appendix – a **General Thematic Analysis** and a **Framework Analysis.** There are many more approaches to QDA, but these are two of the most widely used. (I had previously given you a description of how I conducted an analysis of data in a Grounded Theory approach.) I have given you as an example a transcript of a consultation between a doctor and a patient to practice on – and have shown you some of my tentative analysis. I have given you a suggestion for a way of recording and indexing your themes. Finally, I have emphasised the need for **verification** and shown you a couple of examples of how these are described in publications.

Now a word of caution. I can see a trend in QDA for it to become more elaborate and complex. I question the utility of this – sorry – but I do not think that this is a good thing and I suspect that the temptation is to try to copy Quantitative Data Analysis by having similarly complicated processes. Keep it simple. It works. So, 'if it ain't broke, don't try to fix it!' is my advice.

References

Berne E. (1964). Games People Play – The Basic Hand Book of Transactional Analysis. Ballantine Books: New York.

Colaizzi P. (1978a). Psychological research as the phenomenologist's view it. In Existential-Phenomenological Alternatives for Psychology (Vale R and King M, eds.), pp. 48–71. Oxford University Press: New York.

Edward K-L and Welch T. (2011). The extension of Colaizzi's method of phenomenological enquiry. *Contemporary Nurse* 39(2), 163–171.

Edwards A, Matthews E, Pill R, et al. (1998). Communication about risk: diversity among primary care professionals. *Family Practice* 15(4), 296–300.

Shaw SCK and Anderson JL. (2018). The experiences of medical students with dyslexia: an interpretive phenomenological study. *Dyslexia* 24(3), 1–14.

APPENDIX G

Research Skills

Writing Research Reports

Overview

I do not pretend to be able to tell you the best way to write research reports – I do not want to be prescriptive. What I aim to do is to give you some things to think about when you are writing – with a view to getting your message across as clearly as possible and to publish your work successfully. My problem with the guidelines which you will often find when you are considering which journal to publish your work in, is that these often assume a 'scientific stance' which utterly depersonalises the work and makes it unreadable! The following quote from my icon, Archie Cochrane when writing his book *Effectiveness and Efficiency: Random Reflections on Health Services*, embodies what I mean.

> In publishing such papers I have inevitably adopted that standard MRC
> (Medical Research Council) style of writing which passes for scientific English.
> There is a lot to be said for it. It is accurate, meticulous, and almost bias-proof.
> Personal prejudice is concealed. The only drawback from my point of view (and
> I suspect that of others) is that I find it almost unreadable. Unfortunately I have
> become so used to writing that way that I found expressing my own opinion,
> without detailed discussion of possible biases, nearly impossible. As a result
> on many occasions the book came to a halt. I was horrified, being relatively
> unknown, that readers might imagine that I was an experienced respectable
> physician whose opinions everyone accepts on sight. I finally decided that the
> simplest solution was to admit my biases in advance to warn my readers.
>
> *(Cochrane, 1972)*

Notice that in this text, Archie did not use the terms 'the author' but chose to be more human and accessible by using 'I', 'my', etc. I have taken a leaf out of his book in my approach throughout this book. I encourage my students when they are writing their dissertations to do the same – to *own* their text. But I also suggest to them, as I suggest to you, that *when you prepare an article for publishing in a scientific/professional journal, you should follow the guidelines provided by that journal.*

When I went to work with Ann Cartwright in 1970, in addition to the 'research kit' which I mentioned in Chapter 8, I was given a copy of Sir Ernest Gowers' book *The Complete Plain Words* (1954) and told to use it as a guide to writing in plain English. I recommend that and Trish Greenhalgh's book *How to Read a Paper: The Basics of Evidence-based Medicine and Healthcare* (2019) to our students. But, in doing so, I always have Archie's words when he talks about the formulaic MRC style of writing in mind – 'I find it almost unreadable'. The problem with being 'formulaic' – rigidly adhering to strict guidelines – is that this tends to erase all of 'you' and your personality from the text. Thus, I encourage my students to give accounts in the first-person (using 'I', 'me', 'my', etc.) where they can. The main things to bear in mind when you are writing is to ask yourself 'Am I getting across the message I want to get across?', 'Is it understandable?', and 'Will it bore people to death?'

Seb (who you have met earlier) took my advice to heart when he began his auto-ethnography (Shaw, Anderson, & Grant, 2016) and when we submitted it to a leading journal in medical education, one reviewer noted:

> *This paper is beautifully written, it is a compelling story, and it takes on a topic of growing interest around the world . . . They [Seb and John] acknowledge that the findings might not be generalizable and indicate that their aim is to inspire research in the area. While I am supportive of this goal, it is not clear to me that a research journal is the appropriate venue for it . . .*
>
> *(Shaw et al. 2018)*

We were pleased – until we went on to read the editor's decision, that the reviewers were equivocal about it and he had decided not to publish it! With Alec Grant in our team, we submitted it to *The Qualitative Report* and they accepted it immediately. In fact, one of the things I like about *The Qualitative Report* is that the editors encourage authors to be personal – to say how the research developed, how they contributed to it, and how it impacted upon them.

In the account I mentioned earlier of Sir Charles Fletchers report of the first clinical use of penicillin (Fletcher, 1984), Sir Charles gives a very personal account of that work and of his involvement in it and freely uses 'I', 'my', etc. This helps us as readers to picture him on his bicycle getting the urine from the patient to the lab so that the penicillin could be extracted from it – it engages us! I remember one senior clinical manager in the NHS giving an account of a Health Minister's visit to the hospital he worked in as a consultant. He was the last of a host of clinical leads who was to give a presentation to the visitor. All of the others over-ran their time, so that when it came to his turn, he was told that he only had five minutes, not twenty to give his presentation. So, he said to the visitor, I could bore you with lots of statistics (as the previous consultants had done), but we don't have time to do that, so I'm going to tell you a story. And he gave a brief account of a patient of his and the issues that he was faced with. The visitor kept asking him to say more, and after forty-five minutes they were still deep in conversation, with the visitor listening keenly to his every word. (He commented that he had inadvertently made it very personal by telling his story about one real person who was admitted to the hospital needing care. This made it interesting and impactful! Remember the words ascribed to Joe Stalin – 'A million deaths is a statistic. One death is a tragedy!') He was later offered a job as a government advisor. And, in answer to your question –'Was it Archie?' – no it was not. But it was a like-minded individual who also cared about the people who were patients under his care – more than about the statistics of people in general.

You should know me well enough now that you have got this far through my book, to know that I admit that each has its place. But I despise the pseudo-science of technological jargon which, to my mind is mainly designed to keep information from falling into the wrong hands – the ordinary man or woman who form the basis for the statistics, So, to my mind, it seems that the sorts of reports which make the most impact are those that resonate with the listeners or the readers. Now, I concede that there are some kinds of study which automatically lend themselves to a more 'formal' presentation than others, but that does not mean that they should lose all of the humanity behind the science – we can be **overly impersonal**.

What do you Want to Say?

Before you begin to write, think about the main messages that you want to get across. I guess that most of you will begin to think in terms of saying what you did and why. I'd suggest that you begin by considering the *end-point* – what is the *message* (the conclusions) that you want other people to take from your research? What *lessons* can others learn from your study? That is something which you may be shy about – especially if you are a novice researcher. Hence, remember Mick Bloor's words – 'Research is the art of the possible'. You will have done your best, within the time you had to do the research, the resources you had, the supports you had and the response rate and results that you had. (I have faith in you.) So, **be proud of your achievements** and present them as the best that could be done in those circumstances. When I supervised one of Seb's projects, he only managed to get three students to participate in his study. Shock, horror – what to do? After the initial panic, we decided that the best way to present the results was in the form of three individual case studies and then draw out common themes by linking them to the theoretical perspective that we were following – that was Martin Seligman's theory of Learned Helplessness (Abramson, Gaber & Seligman, 1980). This worked well for us and was very well received when we presented a paper on it at a Medical Education conference. 'But can you get such a paper published?' I can hear you asking. Then we had an e-mail congratulating us on its acceptance for publication (Shaw & Anderson, 2021). So, you see, that even a very small-scale study can have an impact when it is analysed and presented in the right way. Take heart!

Two of the main things to bear in mind are:

a. What are your tutors'/the journal's rules about the style? Many will insist on it being impersonal – 'The author conducted a double-blind, randomised, control trial . . ..' Others will allow you to use your own style. (I always say that if Archie says it is OK to use 'I' etc., then that's good enough for me!)

b. What sort of structure, or format, do they want you to use? This should be clearly stated in your essay/dissertation/thesis guidelines. Journals usually have notes or guidance for authors which will define the sort of format they prefer.

Whilst I have my own preferences, I'm afraid that I would always make sure that I followed my tutors' guidelines (to get as good a mark as possible) and my journal editor's and reviewers' requirements (to give me a better chance of getting it published).

The sort of format which is quite common is:

1. **Introduction and background to the study.** In this you briefly describe why you wanted to do the study you did. Try to simply outline what the issues were and why you were interested in them. Mention whether or not there has been any recent research on the topic and why it might be necessary to do it your way. Say what your research question is and state any hypotheses (or hunches) you have.

2. **Literature review.** Show that you have done a proper search of the literature, giving names of the databases (search engines) you have used, what search terms you used, and when. Give an account of the results of this search and discuss some of the more relevant studies (if any). By relating other studies – or the lack of them – to your own proposal, you can show the justification for doing your study. If these have led to you re-defining your research question, say how and re-state your revised question.

3. **Methodology and methods.** Clearly state what you did in a simple step-by-step account of the process, from identifying participants, to recruiting them and to doing what the study required you to do with them. Give details of the methods – lab work/interviews/focus groups/PO etc., and name any validated, or approved, tolls such as questionnaires and measures you used. Give reasons for any decisions you had to make. Say how you analysed the data. Mention any research ethics approvals which were required and sought.

4. **Results.** Begin by describing your participants – how many, what sort, etc. Then give details of the results of your data analyses. Note that at this point you usually provide a bare description of the results – without any discussion of them.

5. **Discussion.** This is the section where you discuss your results in more detail – did they surprise you? How did they compare with previous research and other researchers' findings. Be creative in offering explanations for your findings and what the implications (e.g. for practice) are.

6. **Conclusions.** Keep this section brief. Say what the main points for the reader to take away from your report are. Is there a need for further research? What were the limitations and strengths of your study?

7. **Acknowledgements.** This is where you say 'thank you' to everyone who helped by taking part (participants), and who contributed (colleagues).

NB – the above sections 1–6 are often briefly included in an **abstract** which goes at the beginning of the report.

Writing in English as a Second Language

Many of my students have had English as a second language, and many of them have found it difficult to write essays or research reports. My main advice to them is:

1. **Keep it simple.** If English is your second language, then the language of the healthcare professional is your third language, and the language of the healthcare professional researcher is a fourth language – with each of these layers getting

more and more complex. So, don't worry about being as impressive as your tutors, do your best to **make yourself understood.**

2. **Write things as you would say them.** Clarity often comes with being straight forward. Think about it. Do you normally say things like 'this researcher, after long and arduous deliberations, made the decision to write about theories and concepts in a remarkably obtuse manner'. No, I bet you don't. You are more likely to say something like, 'After thinking it through, I decided to write about things as simply as possible' – sort of thing. If you find it hard to get words onto paper, **say them in your mind, or out loud, and write down what you have said.**

3. **Write a draft in your first language and translate that into English.** This does add time, but you get better at it and you become quicker.

4. **Get advice from a friend or tutor.** It is OK to ask people to have a look at what you have written and to say if it makes sense to them and if they can understand it or not. This sort of advice is not about plagiarising (copying without acknowledgement) others' work. You need not be afraid to ask your tutors for this sort of help – it's what we get paid for!

5. **Use short words and short sentences.** When I discussed 'Obtaining Informed Consent', I introduced you to the idea of **'reading-ease'.** The same applies here. As a general rule, if you do not understand what you have written, then others are not likely to either.

6. **Don't be ashamed or embarrassed.** I spent six years living and teaching in Hong Kong, and I know what it is like not to be fluent in the language of the people around me. It happens. We have to learn to live with it and do the best we can.

7. **Use university or college support services.** Most universities and colleges offer help with reading and writing and with talking in English, to overseas students. Make the most of what is on offer.

A 'Writing Blank'

How many times do you experience this? I just did! The best way I have found to deal with it is to write the first word of a new sentence – and just carry on from there. Then you can return to this place – but make sure you remember to do this – and carry on filling in the gaps.

What can I say next? I know . . . That's about all I have to say on this subject. See what I mean?

A lot of my students found the beginning of their report the most difficult. So I wrote a few openers for them – for example:

'My interest in this began when . . .'

'This is a very important topic. It concerns . . .'

'Archie Cochrane once wrote . . .'

And I would leave it up to them to take it from there. The Chinese philosopher, Lao Tzu, is often credited with saying: 'A journey of a thousand miles begins with a single step.'

How true! Maxwell Akin writes:

Nevertheless, though, I sit down and I begin writing. I take that first step, I start writing whatever comes to mind that pertains to the topic I've chosen and the structure that I'm working with, and I find that something happens.

In no time at all, I'm putting material onto the page that I'm proud of, that's fun to write, and that is in alignment with the themes and ideas that I had been nurturing. Rather than being a challenging and tedious process, the writing process is actually quite fun and surprisingly effortless.

It all begins, though, with that first word. There's just one word — one single step — at first, and then that word leads to another word. Soon enough, there's one-sentence. And then, there's a paragraph. Until, of course, there's an entire essay.

None of it happens, without that first word. None of it can take place without that single-step in the right direction.

(Akin, 2015)

Now it's your turn – here you go. **'The . . .'**

Good luck! Remember: 'Research is the art of the possible'.

References

Abramson KY, Gaber J, and Seligman MEP. (1980). Learned helplessness in humans: an attributional analysis. In Human Helplessness: *Theory and Applications* (Gaber J and Seligman MEP, eds.), pp. 3–34. Academic Press: New York.

Akin M. (2015). A journey of a thousand miles. Available at: https://maxwellakin.medium.com/a-journey-of-a-thousand-miles-53140d371fa4 (accessed 5 March 2021).

Cochrane AL. (1972). Effectiveness and efficiency: Random reflections on health services. Nuffield Provincial Hospitals Trust.

Fletcher C. (1984). First clinical use of penicillin. *British Medical Journal* 289: 1721–1723.

Gowers E. (1954). The *Complete Plain Words*. Her Majesty's Stationery Office (HMSO): London.

Greenhalgh T. (2019). *How to Read a Paper: The Basics of Evidence–based Medicine and Healthcare*. Wiley-Blackwell: New York.

Shaw SCK, Anderson JL, and Grant AJ. (2016). Studying medicine with dyslexia: a collaborative autoethnography. *The Qualitative Report* 21(11), 2036–2054.

Shaw SCK and Anderson JL. (2021). Coping with medical school: an interpretive phenomenological study. *The Qualitative Report* 26(6), 1864–80.

POSTSCRIPT

In this book, I have tried to give an outline of the main research approaches used in healthcare research. My aim has been to 'demystify' research so that students and healthcare professionals can be better equipped to understand different research methods – and, I hope, feel better able to do your own research.

I have covered quantitative methods, qualitative methods, and mixed methods. In doing this, I have tried to teach by examples and cases of research studies. I have used some examples from very famous people, from my own students' work and from research I have been involved in myself. In doing this, I have let those researchers' own words speak for themselves and added commentaries where necessary. I hope that this has been useful.

I have also added chapters on research ethics and governance. These are not research methods in their own right, but they underpin all ethical research projects. By giving examples of some horror stories and unfortunate experiences, I hope that you will appreciate the importance of these issues and be guided to conduct ethical research and to avoid the 'dark side'!

In the appendices, I have tried to give more practical advice on different research skills. I hope that these too, will be useful to you. Remember – keep a Research Log!

My teaching is very interactive. I enjoy the participation of my students in the classroom, and I thrive on the feedback I get from them. Teaching online in 2020 and 2021 was a new challenge for me. I still enjoyed teaching, but missed the full dynamics of the interactive nature of the classroom. Writing this book has also been a challenge for me. It is a wee bit scary to write it and to send it out into the public domain – to you and others like you. 'How will it go down?' is my constant worry.

SO, please feel free to send me any feedback and suggestions for future updates. These will be most welcome! Please send any correspondence about the book to j.anderson@bsms.ac.uk; and medicalstudent@wiley.com. I shall try to reply to all communications.

I wish you good fortune in your research. Now, I have only two more things to say to you:

1. '**Don't Panic!**' And,
2. Remember – '**Research is the art of the possible!**'

John L. Anderson

7 February 2022

Demystifying Research for Medical & Healthcare Students: An Essential Guide, First Edition. John L. Anderson.
© 2022 John Wiley & Sons Ltd. Published 2022 by John Wiley & Sons Ltd.
Companion website: www.wiley.com/go/Anderson/DemystifyingResearch

Index

A

acute respiratory infection (ARI), 131
    Focused Ethnographic Study of, 134–141
    Adams, D., 1
Ajuied, A., 96
Al-Assaf, A., 76
Almoners, 82
analytical autoethnography, 147
    approach, 152
analytic induction, 129, 142
analytic reflexivity, 147
Anderson, J.L., 106, 24–25, 71–73, 88–94, 96–97,
        101–105, 130–142, 145–146, 165–171, 179–184,
        194–198, 217–220
anthropologists, 108
anthropology, 7, 108
applied research, 3
Arkenau, H.-T., 43, 46
arthroscopic partial meniscectomy *vs.* Sham
        surgery, 60–62
assisted autoethnography, 145, 155
Attarwala, H., 45
attributional analysis, of learned helplessness, 25
autobiographical accounts, 144
autobiography, 145
autoethnographies, 124, 144
    analytic vs evocative autoethnographies, 147
    case study, 148
    collaborative, 145–146
    echocardiographer, 152–154
    hypothetico-deductive, 155
    hypothetico-inductive, 144, 155
    method, 149–152
    vs. participant observation, 154
    types of, 147
    ulcerative colitis, 148

B

Ballinger, R., 43, 179-184
Barbour, R., 122
Bartlett, J., 86
Beagan, B., 114
Beck Depression Inventory (BDI), 164
Beck, C., 161–165
Becker, H., 114–117, 119, 120–122
bias, 25, 63, 294
BIA 10-2474 trial, 45–46
blaming the victim, 206
blinding, 51–53
    of staff, 58

Bloor, M., 3, 125–130, 253–4
blue skies research, 3
Boolean operators, 270
Boston Area Community Health (BACH)
        Survey, 32
bracketing, 160
breast disease treatments, psycho-social
        aspects of, 71–73
Brink, S., 71
Bristol Online Survey, 96

C

CAM *see* Complementary and Alternative
        Medicines (CAM)
Campbell E, 154
cardiology, 70
cardiovascular disease (CVD), risk factors for, 70
Cartwright, A., 87
case-control studies, 5, 69, 80
    depression and disability in people with
        podoconiosis, 83
    matching cases and controls, 85
    measuring suspect variable, 84
    smoking and lung cancer, 81–83
    uses, 84
case series, 194–199
case studies, 186–194
    approach, 7–8, 195
    clinical, 187
    hypothetico-deductive, 186, 198
checking, interviews, 286
Chen, S.C., 46
Chesser, T., 49, 71, 78
Chief/Principal Investigator (CI/PI), 242–243
cholecystectomy RCT, 57–60
cholera epidemic in London, 28
chunking, interviews, 286
clarification, interviewing, 288–289
class stratified sample, 73
clinical case studies, 187
clinical iatrogenesis, 202
clinical trials, 39
    Phase 0, 40
    Phase I, 39–43, 46
    Phase II, 39, 43–44
    safety in, 44–46
clustering, 90
Cochrane, A., 48, 50, 53, 60
Cochrane Centres, 48, 275
coding, 305

Demystifying Research for Medical & Healthcare Students: An Essential Guide, First Edition. John L. Anderson.
© 2022 John Wiley & Sons Ltd. Published 2022 by John Wiley & Sons Ltd.
Companion website: www.wiley.com/go/Anderson/DemystifyingResearch